feeding littles
& beyond

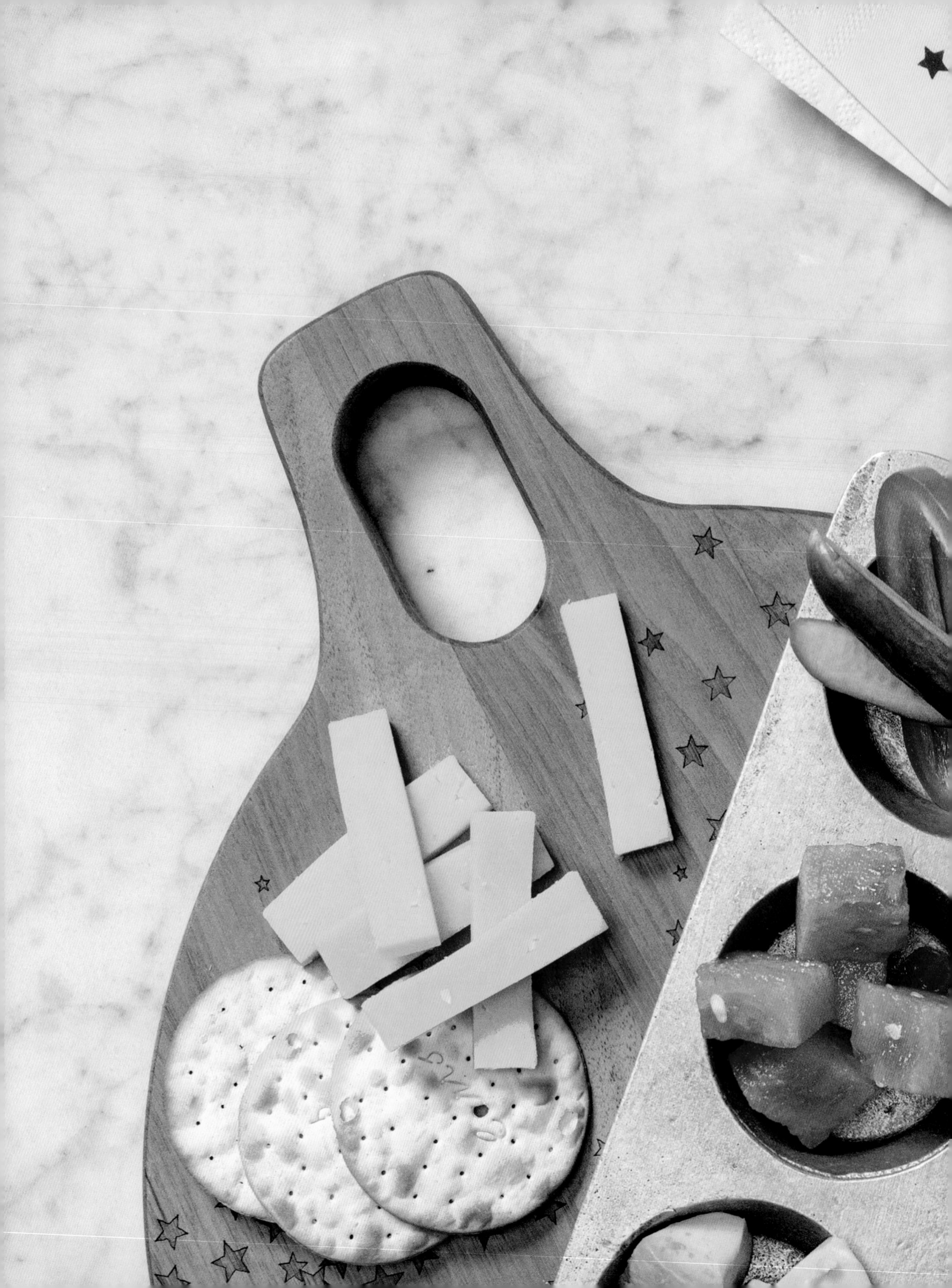

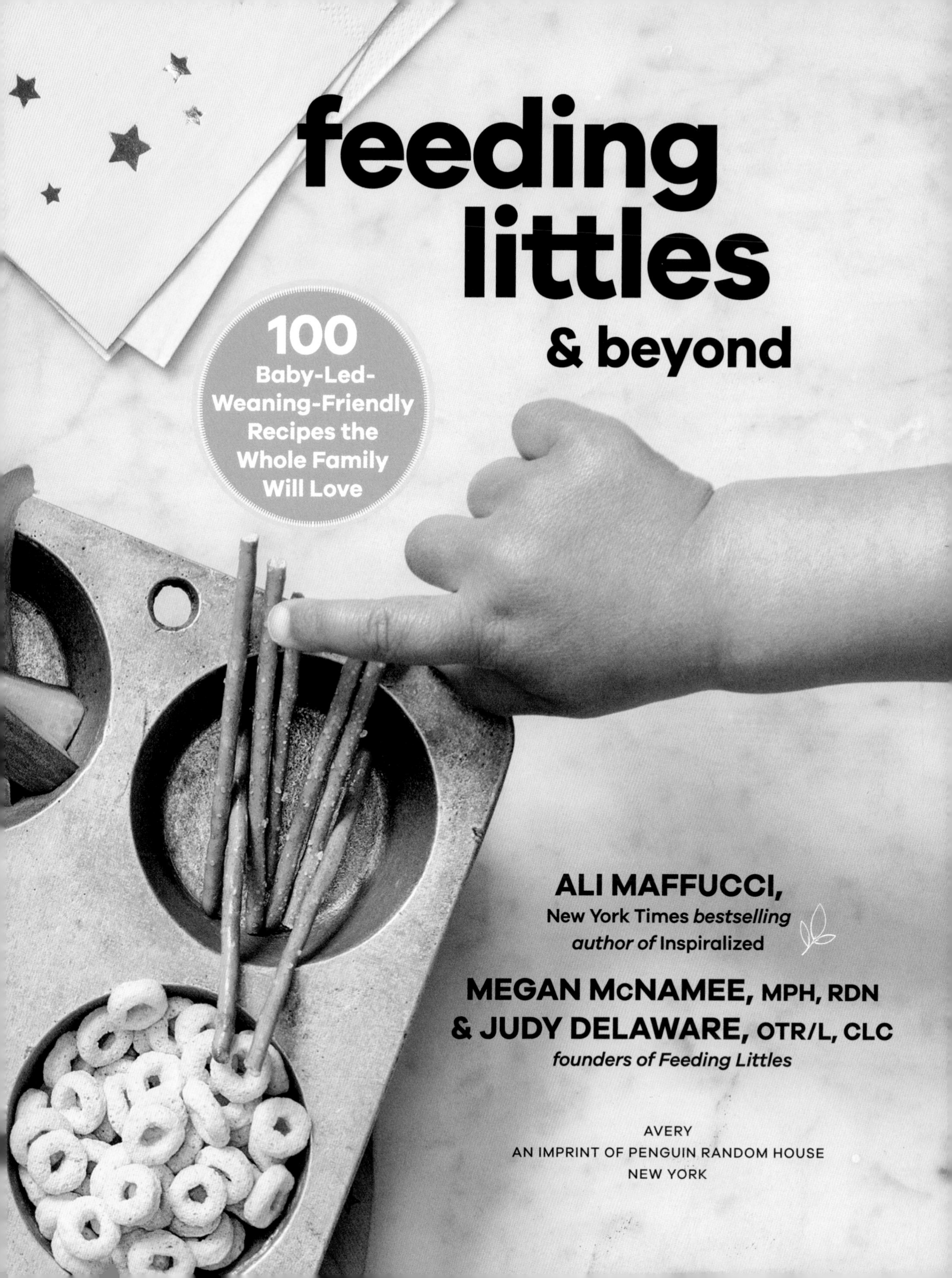

feeding littles & beyond

100 Baby-Led-Weaning-Friendly Recipes the Whole Family Will Love

ALI MAFFUCCI,
New York Times *bestselling author of* Inspiralized

MEGAN McNAMEE, MPH, RDN
& JUDY DELAWARE, OTR/L, CLC
founders of Feeding Littles

AVERY
AN IMPRINT OF PENGUIN RANDOM HOUSE
NEW YORK

AVERY
an imprint of Penguin Random House LLC
penguinrandomhouse.com

Photographs by Evan Sung

Library of Congress Cataloging-in-Publication Data
Names: Maffucci, Ali, author. | McNamee, Megan, author. | Delaware, Judy, author.
Title: Feeding littles & beyond 100 baby-led-weaning-friendly recipes the whole family will love / Ali Maffucci, New York Times bestselling author of Inspiralized, Megan McNamee, MPH, RDN & Judy Delaware, OTR/L, CLC, founders of Feeding Littles.
Other titles: Feeding littles and beyond
Description: New York: Avery, an imprint of Penguin Random House, [2022] | Includes index.
Identifiers: LCCN 2022001080 (print) | LCCN 2022001081 (ebook) | ISBN 9780593419243 (trade paperback) | ISBN 9780593419250 (epub)
Subjects: LCSH: Infants—Weaning. | Infants—Nutrition. | Baby foods. | LCGFT: Cookbooks.
Classification: LCC RJ216 .M2823 2022 (print) | LCC RJ216 (ebook) | DDC 649/.3—dc23/eng/20220121
LC record available at https://lccn.loc.gov/2022001080
LC ebook record available at https://lccn.loc.gov/2022001081

Printed in United States of America
10 9 8 7 6 5 4 3 2

Book design by Lorie Pagnozzi

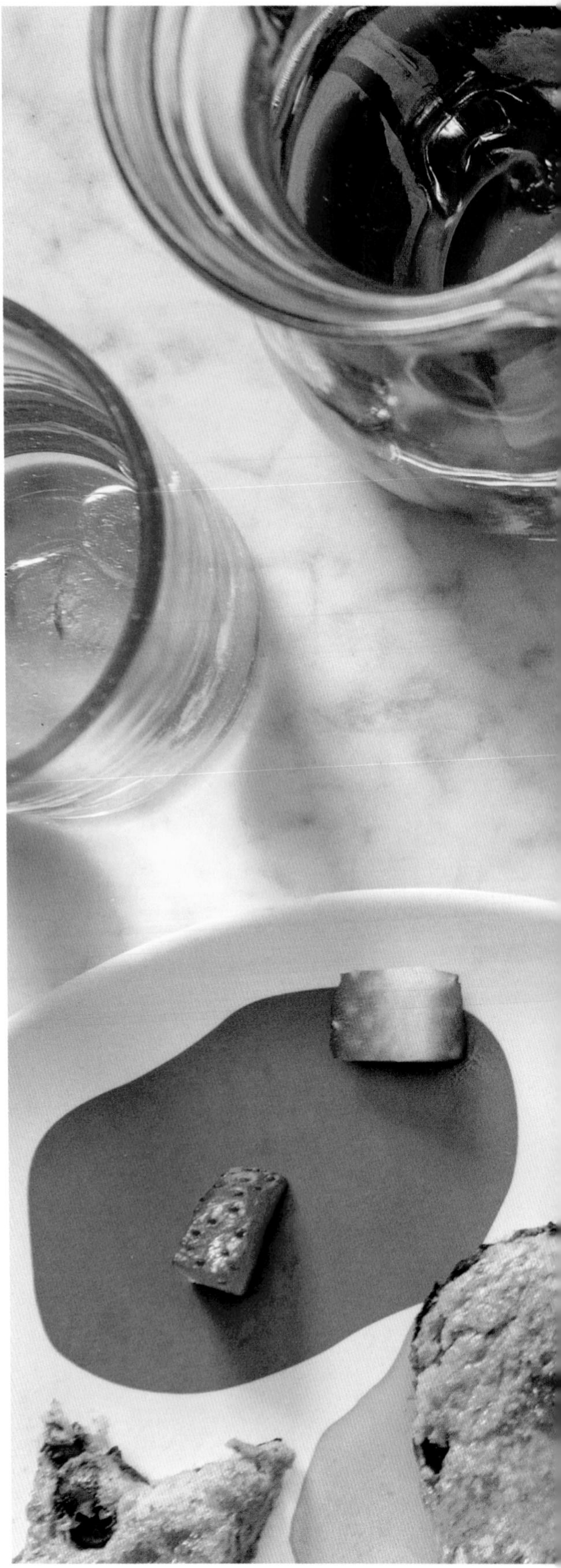

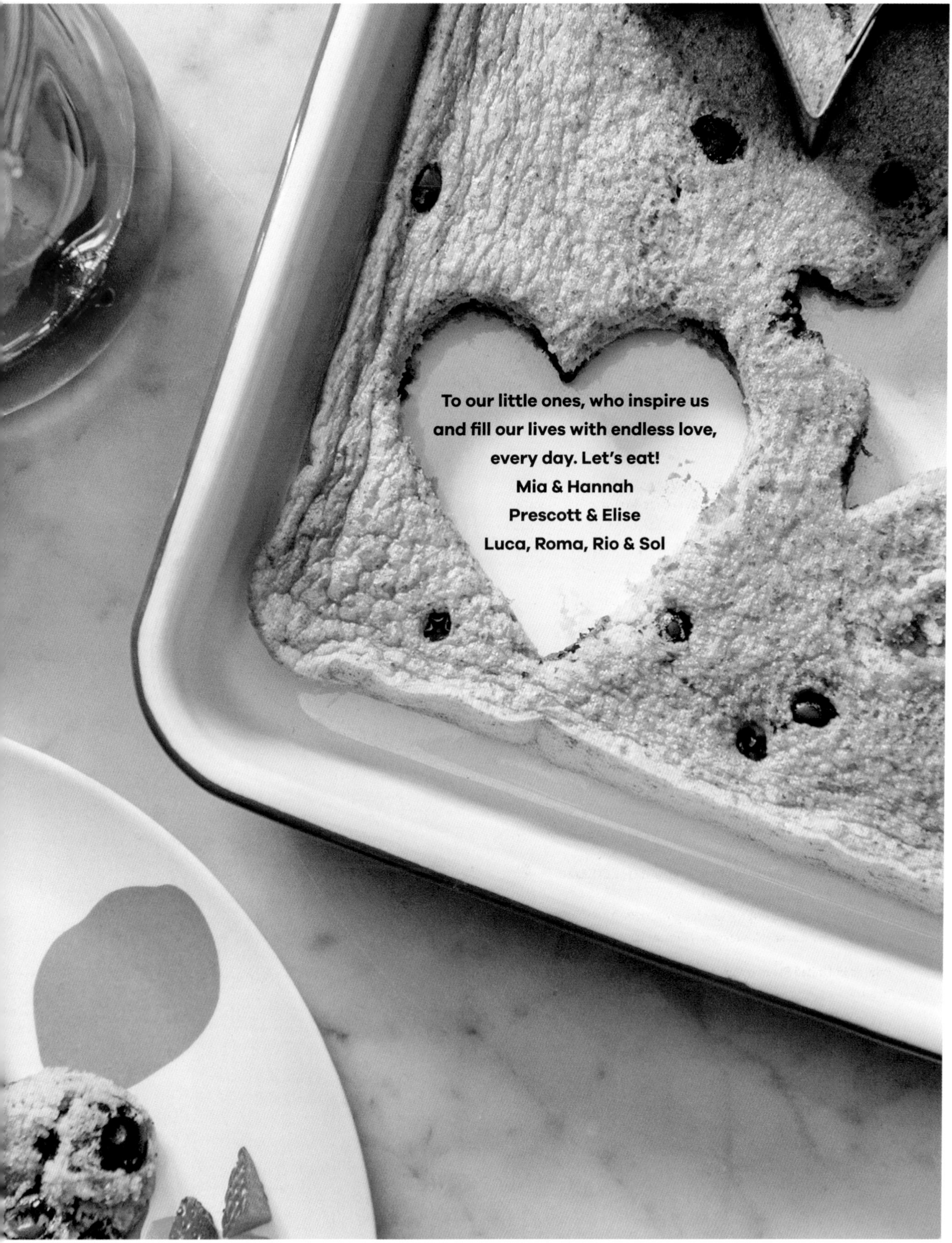

To our little ones, who inspire us
and fill our lives with endless love,
every day. Let's eat!
Mia & Hannah
Prescott & Elise
Luca, Roma, Rio & Sol

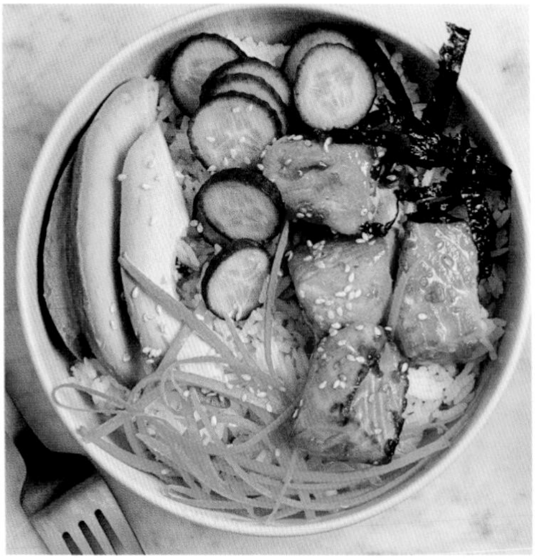
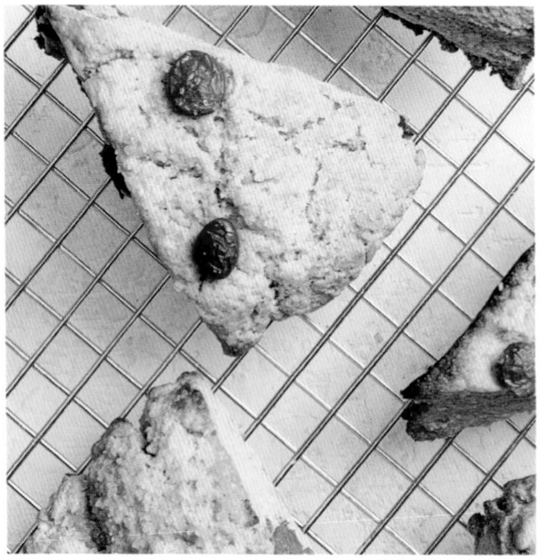
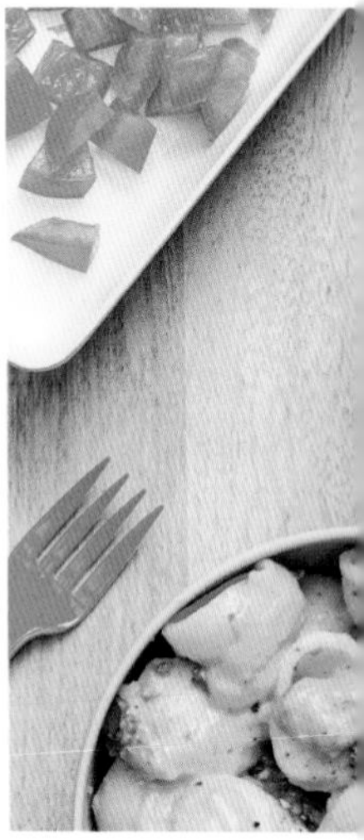
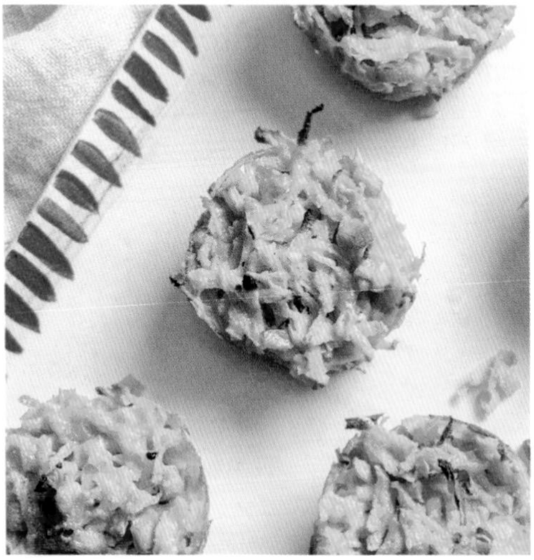

table of contents

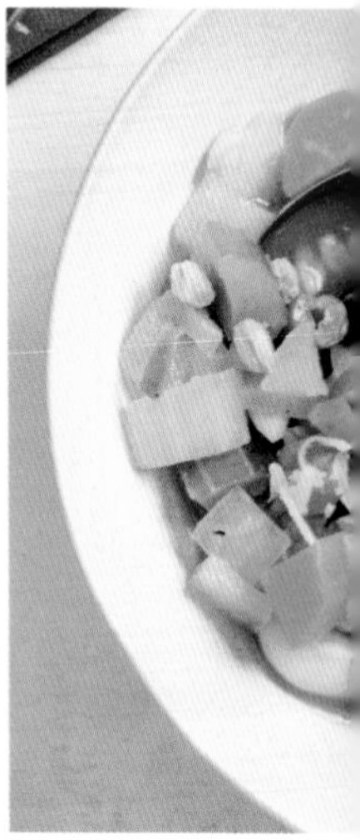
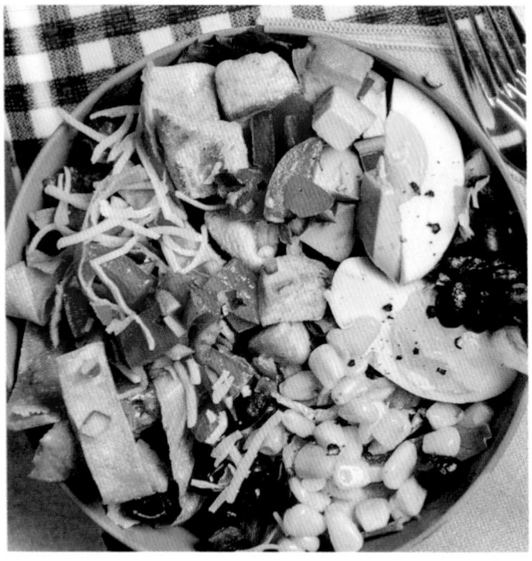
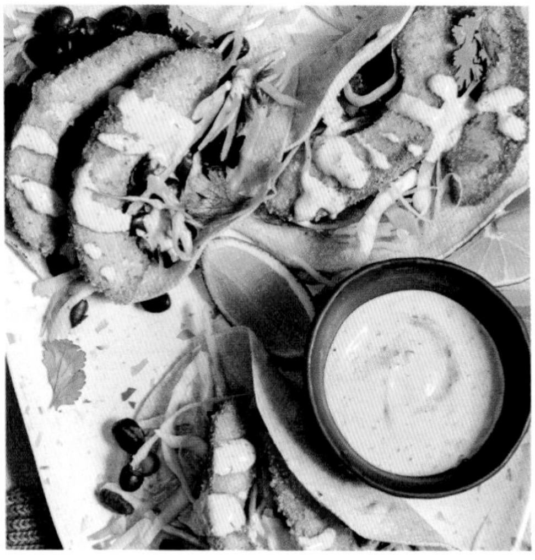
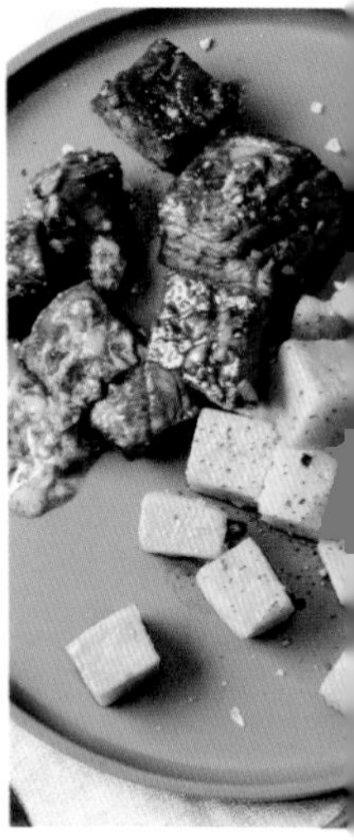

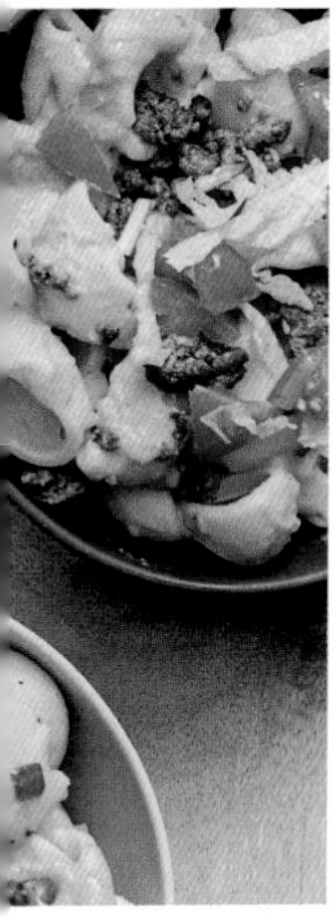
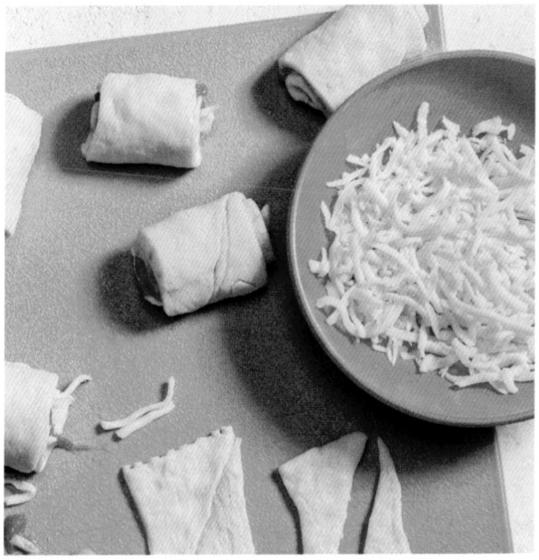
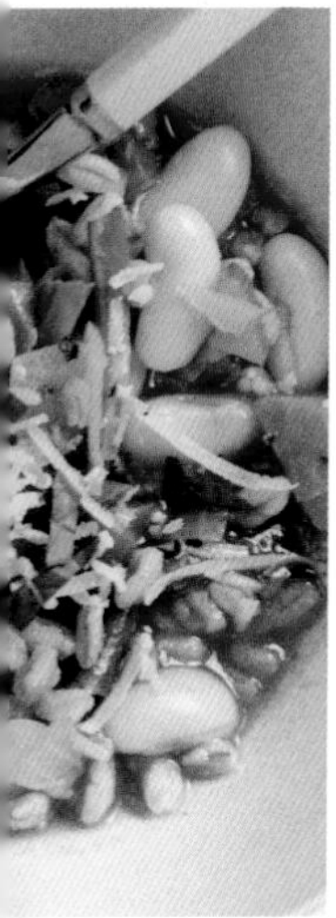
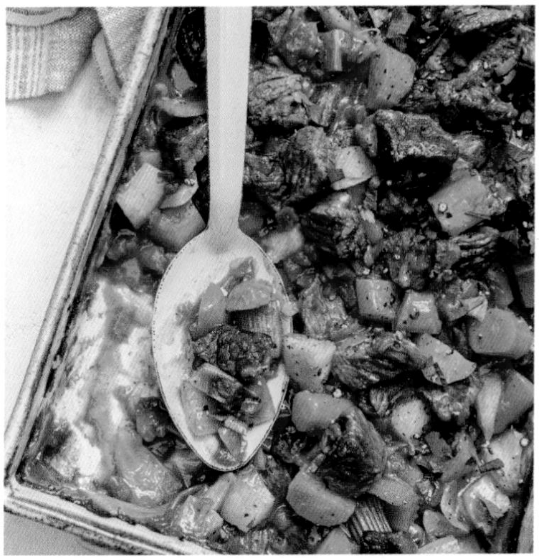
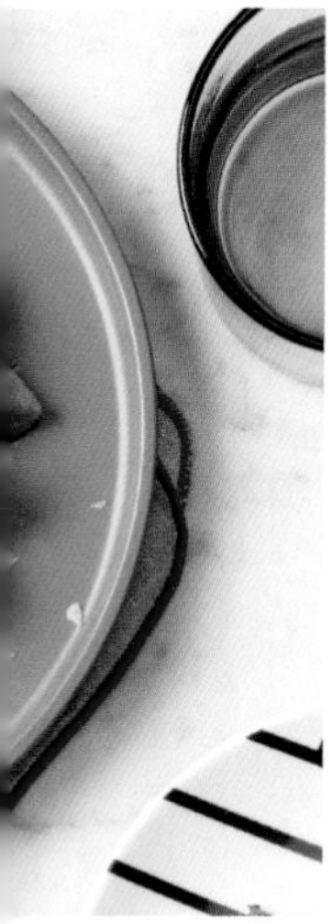
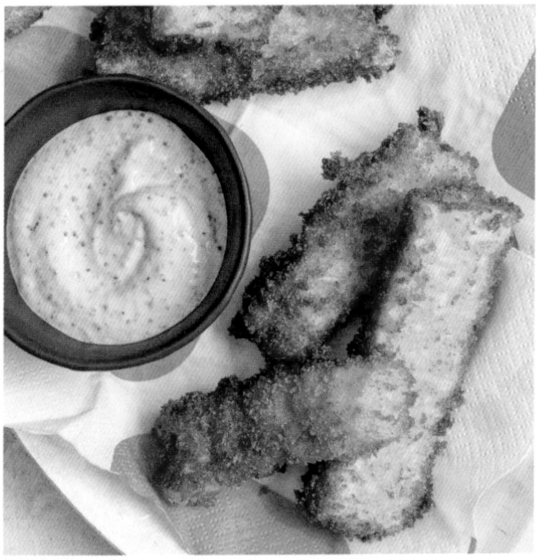

feeding littles
& beyond

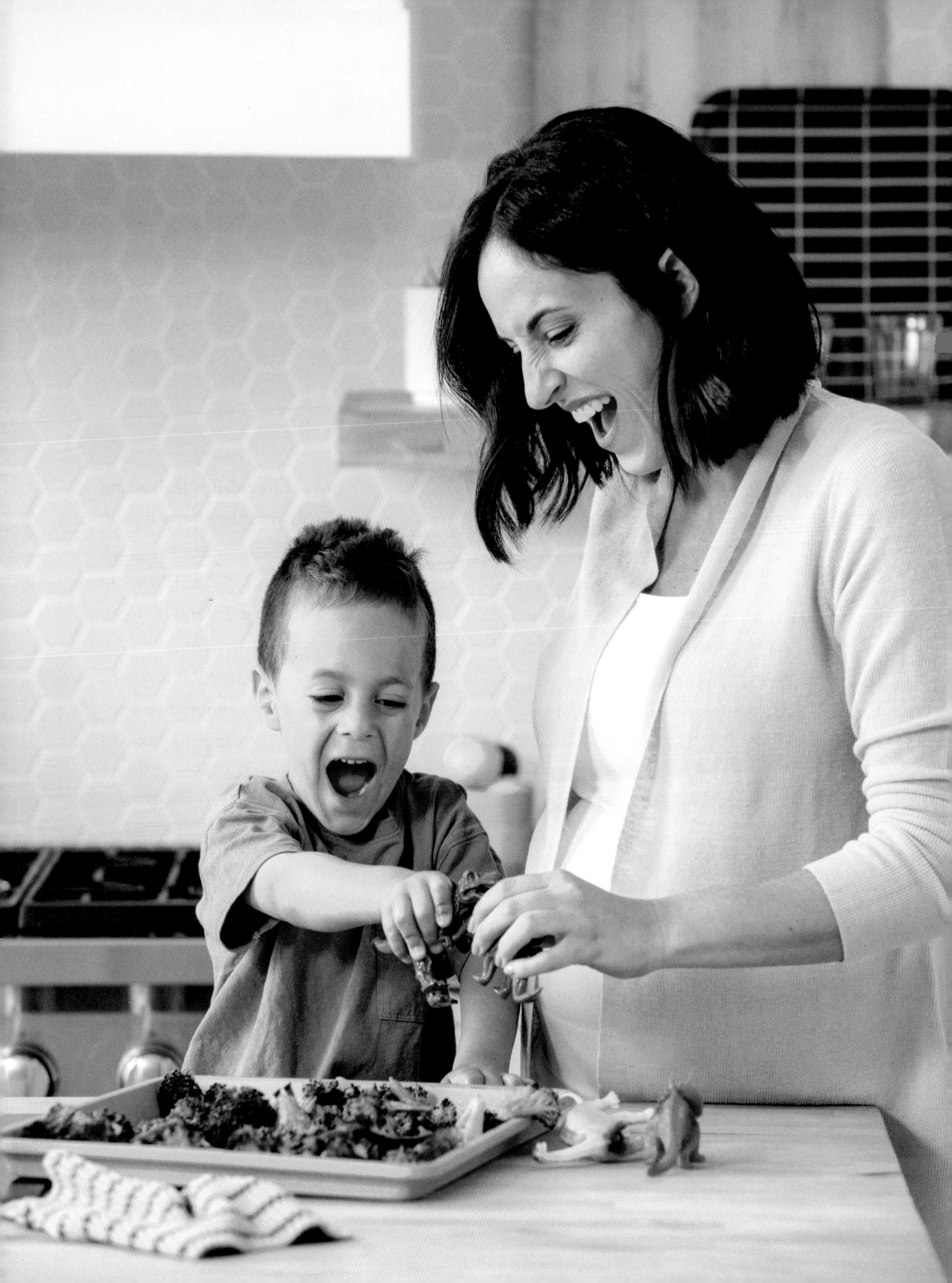

our story: how we came together and why

"Rawr!" my son, Luca, roared as he marched his toy dinosaurs across a broccoli jungle. Looking over the roasted broccoli and plastic dinos scattered on a large sheet pan, I thought to myself, "This is crazy. I'm losing it!" But as we sat there, feeding a stegosaurus a small floret, I watched as Luca, for the first time in his life, brought a piece of broccoli to his mouth, licked it, and ate it. As I stared in disbelief, he started feeding himself and the dinosaurs broccoli, floret by floret, until they had downed a couple of cups. To this day, broccoli is his favorite vegetable.

Why am I sharing this story—and why was my son eating veggies with dinosaurs? It had been a year of countless frustrating and demoralizing mealtimes during which my almost-two-year-old son refused to try any new foods. I needed guidance and reached out to Judy, an occupational therapist who specializes in pediatric feeding therapy and is cofounder of Feeding Littles, an online resource for helping families feed their children. When we chatted, she didn't ask about Luca's picky eating but about his personality, likes, and dislikes. "Well, Judy, he never stops playing. He can't sit still," I told her. Hearing that, she suggested that rather than focusing on mealtime, I bring food into playtime. She gave me the dinosaur idea, and our family's approach to eating changed forever and for the better.

This is just one of the many ways that the dynamic duo at Feeding Littles helped me in my feeding journey with my children, starting when my eldest was just starting solids. I'm humbled, honored, and delighted to be writing this book with them. I cannot wait to see how it positively transforms thousands of struggling parents' journeys. But before I get into what this cookbook is all about and what to expect, I want to share how our partnership came to be and how I learned about the dazzling Megan and Judy of Feeding Littles.

First, I haven't introduced myself yet! Hi, I'm Ali Maffucci, authoring this book alongside Megan and Judy. I'm the founder of Inspiralized, where I was originally dedicated to cooking exclusively with the spiralizer, a kitchen tool that turns vegetables and fruits into noodles. However, after my kids were born, my time became more precious, and I needed to make meals that were appropriate for my kids but could still satisfy me and my husband, and veggie spaghetti wasn't cutting it. Now, you can find me sharing family-friendly recipes for every meal (not just those in noodle form) that use vegetables creatively, in an effort to show people that veggies can be craveable, too.

Back in 2018, after my son Luca's four-month checkup, my pediatrician told me, "You can start feeding him solids." I was over-the-moon excited. As someone who shares their everyday life on social media, I whipped out my phone, opened Instagram, and recorded a video: "Baby food, here we come!"

That's when the messages started pouring in. "Do baby-led weaning; you'll love it." and "You don't have to do purees—there's another way."

And then, "Follow Feeding Littles!"

You may be having a similar reaction to mine: *baby-led-what?!* I had always assumed that toothless babies could only "handle" purees, and I assumed I'd be committing to jarred food, pouch snacks, and flying a spoon of creamed spinach into my baby's mouth, just like on television.

While starting with pureed foods for your baby can be healthy and wonderful if it works for your family, there is indeed another way. Later, Megan and Judy will dive deeper into baby-led weaning or baby-led feeding and the beautiful philosophy around it, but in short it's a way of feeding your baby that skips the spoon-feeding altogether and encourages your kiddos to self-feed finger foods and other safe textures. This way, you don't have to buy or make separate meals for your child, and the whole family can eat together. This method of feeding extends into toddlerhood and sets a foundation for an explorative, positive, and empowering relationship with food and mealtimes.

Sounds ideal, right? That's what I thought, but I was overwhelmed with the how and when. That's where Feeding Littles came in. Their supportive, educational community was exactly what I needed as I embarked on my own journey. Social media tends to create a culture of comparison, and it is so easy for new parents to feel like we're not "doing it right." I could tell immediately that Feeding Littles was a safe place to share my experiences and insecurities, knowing that I would be met with empathy and solid advice. Sign. Me. Up!

I bought their online course, grabbed a glass of wine, and buckled up. You'd think the class was the latest bingeable crime show by the way I was on the edge of my seat. I was captivated. Every principle I learned resonated with me and the way I hoped to raise my littles. The idea of my family gathering around the table to enjoy a meal together was what sealed the deal.

After those first few weeks and months of feeding Luca, I knew Feeding Littles had built

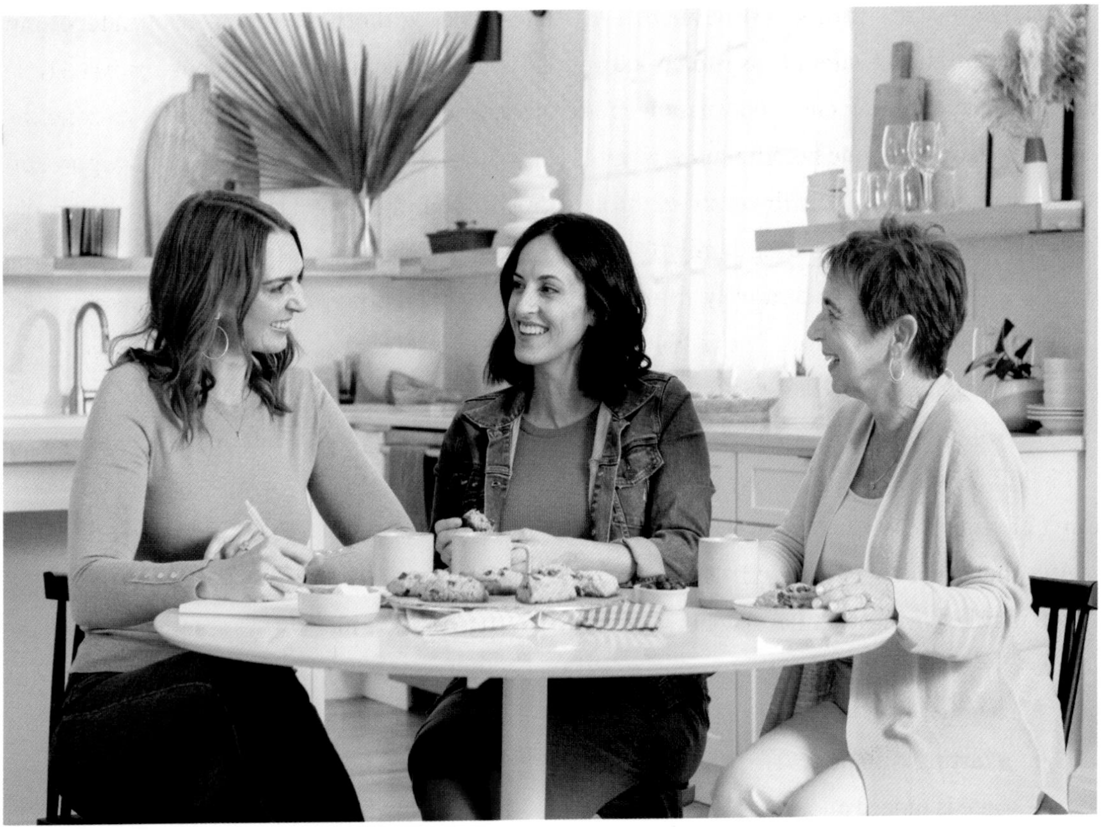

something truly life-changing, and I wanted to meet the masterminds behind it. We connected as anyone in the twenty-first century does: through Instagram. Before you knew it, we collaborated on an e-cookbook called *Inspiralized Littles* (cute, right?).

I wanted everyone to learn about baby-led weaning. However, I didn't have the nutritional knowledge to offer expert advice and could only share my own experience. Of course, when it comes to feeding your babies, you want to make sure you're getting your information from a reliable and professional source, and Megan and Judy are the perfect team: Judy is an occupational therapist who specializes in pediatric feeding development, oral-motor skills, and sensory processing issues as related to feeding, and Megan is a pediatric registered dietitian nutritionist who specializes in maternal and child nutrition and disordered eating prevention.

As for Megan and Judy, they weren't recipe writers. They threw meals together like most families do or had their own favorites and go-tos. They were there to equip parents and childcare providers with the safety and nutritional guidelines necessary to feed their own families safely, with troubleshooting help along the way. But their audience wanted recipes that complemented their feeding philosophy.

That's why we decided to partner on that starter e-book. We were blown away by its reception, so we got the band back together to build something bigger and better: this book.

To this day, choosing baby-led weaning is one of the best parenting decisions I have ever made. After devouring this book, with the qualified and specialized guidance from Megan and Judy and our delicious recipes, I know you'll feel the same way. And hey, if you find yourself feeding broccoli to plastic dinosaurs with your rambunctious toddler, you'll giggle to yourself. We're all in this together, so know that whatever way you choose to feed your family is the right way.

The Story of Feeding Littles

Judy Delaware and Megan McNamee would never have met had it not been for a baby named Jack.

As an occupational therapist specializing in feeding, Judy has worked with thousands of clients in her hometown of Louisville, Colorado. Jack had a severe form of SMA (spinal muscular atrophy), a genetic condition that causes the inability to move, swallow, and eventually breathe. During his short life, Judy went into his family's home and helped him play, develop, and eat in ways that worked for his body. Jack passed away in his mama's arms at just six months of age, but his legacy was just beginning.

Less than two years later, Megan, a dietitian, was teaching baby-led weaning (BLW) to families in Phoenix, Arizona. At the time, BLW was a new concept. Her clients loved letting their babies feed themselves, but they often asked what they should do when their kids became toddlers and began to refuse foods.

As luck would have it, Megan's good friend Sarah—Jack's mom—had just come back from visiting Judy. She excitedly shared how Judy helped Sarah's toddler eat foods she hadn't wanted in months, and that Megan and Judy had to meet. On their first call, they couldn't stop talking. Their philosophies and goals were so closely aligned, and they both brought different areas of expertise. They knew they had to create something together.

The Feeding Littles community grew quickly. It was obvious that parents all over the world wanted positive messages and proactive strategies for handling mealtime, food, body images, and parenting in general. Today, Judy and Megan serve hundreds of thousands of families worldwide every day.

how to use this book

There are many reasons you may have picked up this book. Do any of these sound familiar?

- "My toddler is so picky. There has to be a better way."
- "I'm expecting my first baby, and we want to try baby-led weaning."
- "I'm expecting another baby, and I want to do things differently this time."
- "I'm bored with all the meals I make at home. I need inspiration."
- "I'm so tired of cooking multiple meals at mealtimes to satisfy everyone's preferences. I need a solution."

No matter what your reason, we're glad you're here. While you will find one hundred recipes in this book, this is much more than just a cookbook. If you're feeding your baby solids for the first time and are new to the concept of baby-led weaning, please start with the Basic Guide to Baby-Led Weaning. In this chapter, you'll learn what you need to know to feed your baby safely. Take your time to read through the information, as it's important that you approach feeding your baby with confidence.

After that you can start to safely prepare our recipes for your family. Each one has tip boxes from Megan, Judy, and Ali to equip you with the capabilities to tackle mealtime with support. They include:

- Inspiralized Tips: These are tips from Ali that offer advice on the cooking process, any ingredient swaps that can be made, and general suggestions pertaining to the recipe.
- Feeding Littles Tips: These tips are written by Megan and Judy about feeding techniques for the recipe, as well as nutritional pointers.
- I Can't Even: These tips will be geared toward simplifying the recipe and taking shortcuts to reduce prep or cooking time, on the days when you just "can't even." More on this on page 119.
- Prep Ahead: If a recipe (or certain components or steps) can be prepped ahead, it will be noted here.

We encourage you to read everything in the recipe before you start cooking. There will be safety tips, feeding techniques, and allergen adjustments, and we want you to be prepared before getting in the kitchen.

All of the recipes are written for adult portions. That way, you can decide how many portions to make for your unique family. Generally, we consider one adult portion of a lunch or dinner enough to feed two toddlers. For a baby under one, it would range anywhere from two to four portions, depending on the recipe and how much your baby eats. You know your baby best, so plan accordingly.

And if you're still stumped on how to adequately plate a recipe for your baby, that's where the Visual Index on page 281 comes in. There are sample photos for most of the recipes in this book, so that if you're ever still unsure on how best to serve something, check it out. Coupled with our tip boxes, you'll have the tools to feed your family with assurance.

One last note. We didn't include dietary indicators (such as Gluten-Free, Egg-Free, Dairy-Free, Vegetarian, or Vegan) because we didn't want to discourage anyone from trying a specific recipe before reading it through. When applicable, we've included substitutes for top allergens, to make these recipes more versatile and adaptable for different diet restrictions.

This book discusses feeding kids as early as six months of age, so safety is paramount. We offer numerous safety tips and information about choking hazards, but as the parent or caregiver it is imperative that you always supervise your child while eating and know how to step in if your child is choking. It is a risk with any food or liquid, so it's important to know basic first aid and CPR. If your child has any medical or developmental issues, work with your healthcare provider or feeding team before introducing solids. We recommend never leaving young children alone with food.

Overall, this cookbook is a celebration of one of life's greatest pleasures: eating. All three of us hope that the information we have shared will be tremendously helpful in your journey and that these simple and enjoyable recipes will inspire you to get in the kitchen and create some goodness for your family.

our family's food philosophies

Before we start with the basics, we wanted to share some Feeding Littles philosophies with you, as seen in this beautiful design by Jess Londeree. As you learn more about feeding your baby, toddler, or kid, we hope you'll keep the big picture in mind. Eating together. Low-stress meals. Listening to our bodies. Gratitude. We hope that you'll come to embrace these tenets as your own.

Our Family's FOOD Philosophies

1. WE EAT *together* WHENEVER POSSIBLE.
2. OUR MEALS ARE *fun*, LOW-STRESS, AND SOMETIMES SILLY. IT IS OK TO PLAY WITH OUR FOOD - WE ARE STILL LEARNING!
3. WE TURN OFF THE TV AND KEEP DEVICES OFF THE *table* WHEN WE EAT.
4. WE EAT WHEN WE ARE *hungry* AT REGULAR MEALS AND SNACKS, AND WE STOP EATING WHEN OUR BODIES SAY THEY'RE DONE.
5. WHEN FOOD IS SERVED, WE *choose* HOW MUCH TO EAT. WE CAN HAVE MORE OF ANY GIVEN FOOD WITHOUT EATING ANOTHER FOOD FIRST, AS LONG AS THERE'S *enough* FOOD FOR EVERYONE.
6. IF WE AREN'T HUNGRY FOR WHAT'S SERVED, THAT'S OK, BUT WE AREN'T SERVED ANYTHING DIFFERENT UNTIL THE NEXT *meal* OR SNACK. WE ARE *polite* WHEN WE DECLINE FOOD.
7. FOOD IS FOOD. OUR *self-worth* IS NOT DEFINED BY THE FOOD WE EAT.
8. WE SHOP FOR FOOD AND *cook* TOGETHER WHENEVER POSSIBLE. WE LOVE TO LEARN WHERE OUR FOOD COMES FROM.
9. WE *help* CLEAN UP AFTER MEALTIME.
10. WE HONOR OUR FAMILY'S TRADITIONS AROUND FOOD, HOLIDAYS, AND SPECIAL CELEBRATIONS. WE ARE *grateful* FOR THE FOOD WE EAT AND THE ABILITY TO SHARE IT WITH LOVED ONES.

FEEDING *littles*

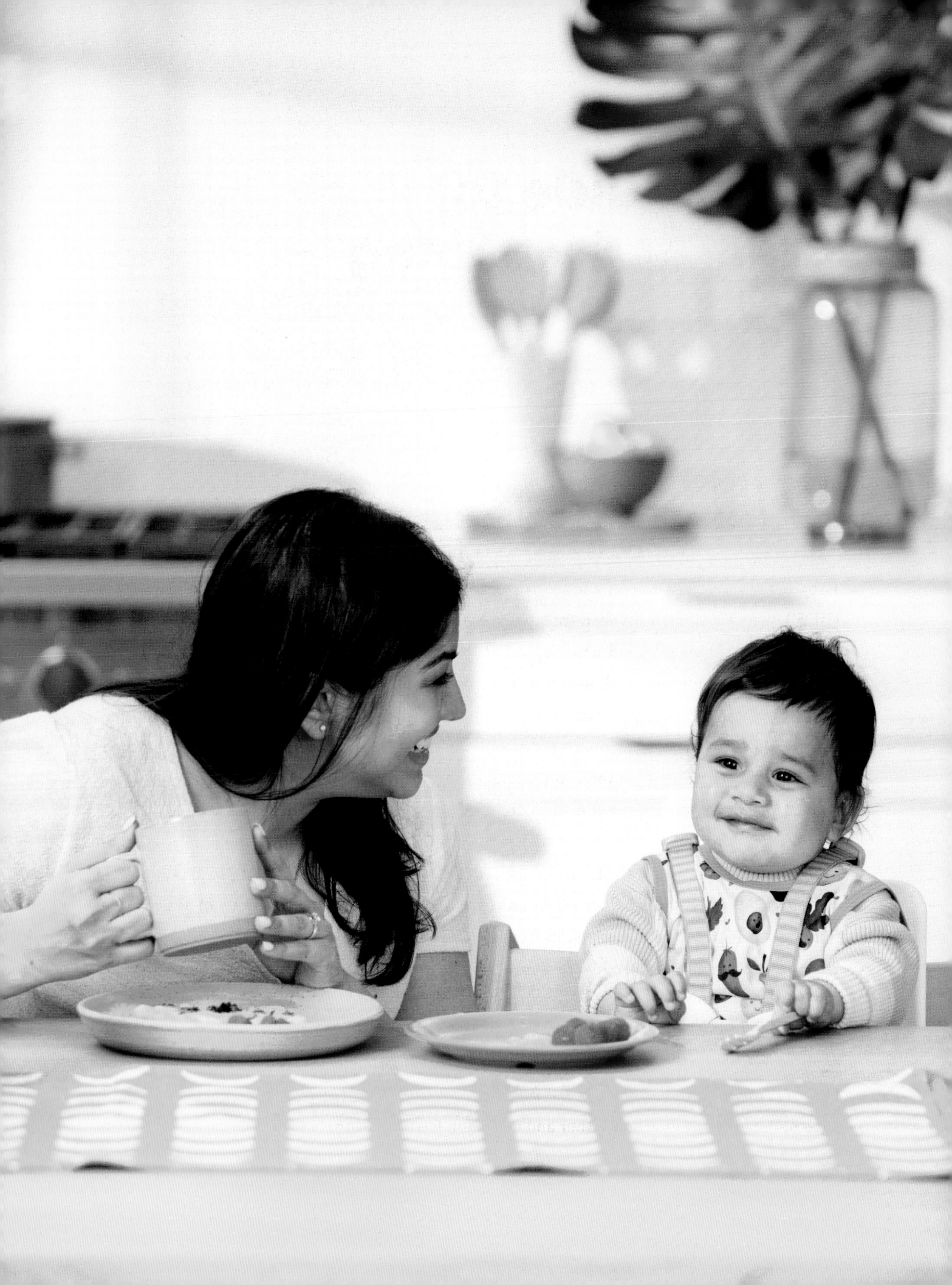

basic guide to baby-led weaning

what is baby-led weaning?

Baby-led weaning has gained a lot of popularity in recent years. Essentially, baby-led weaning (BLW) means letting a baby feed themself solid foods from the start. In much of the world, the term "weaning" means introduction of solid foods; in the United States, weaning means cessation of breastfeeding or bottle-feeding. Thus, when we say baby-led weaning, we also mean "infant self-feeding" (i.e., you don't have to stop nursing or bottle-feeding to start BLW).

Baby-led weaning involves offering whole strips or pieces of soft food a baby can put in their own mouth. They move the food to the side of their mouth with their tongue and chew with their strong back gums using the strength of their jaw. We also recommend letting babies use spoons and rounded forks preloaded with food like yogurt, hummus, mashed potatoes, or applesauce. This helps babies learn to use utensils and get familiar with various safe textures.

This may sound different than what you've heard about feeding babies. Many of us are more familiar with jarred foods and spoon-feeding. While BLW may seem like a new approach, it's what was always done before blenders and commercialized baby foods became available in the early twentieth century.

The baby food industry took off at a time when parents were advised to feed babies pureed foods very young—as early as a few days or weeks of age. Now that major governing bodies recommend waiting until around six months to introduce solids of any kind, many babies are old enough to skip baby food altogether and can begin feeding themselves.

Our philosophy is flexible and family-centered. What matters is following your baby's lead and feeling comfortable and confident in how you feed your child. You may want to use baby foods and spoon-feed your baby, and that's great, too. We always recommend doing what works best for your family. Our goal for our clients is to work toward their child self-feeding by twelve to fourteen months, no matter how they started, barring any medical or developmental issues. Talk to your provider before offering foods besides breast milk or formula.

WHY CONSIDER BABY-LED WEANING?

Many of the benefits of baby-led weaning come from practicing independent eating regularly. As feeding professionals who have worked with many clients on their BLW journeys, we have noticed the following benefits:

It's easier—one meal for everyone.

Promotes family meals.

Baby eats a wider variety of foods, textures, and flavors.

Baby chooses how much to eat—an important skill in connecting to their body.

Promotes hand-eye coordination, as well as oral-motor and fine-motor development.

Baby uses all of their senses to eat—great for sensory development!

Baby is able to model what they have been watching all along—people feeding themselves!

Might help prevent selective eating.

WHEN DO WE START?

We recommend introducing foods other than breast milk or formula starting around six months of age and when your baby shows readiness signs, including:

- Sitting well on the floor with minimal assistance.
- Bringing toys and hands to mouth.
- Showing interest in food. That could look like trying to grab

food as you eat it or watching the food go from your plate to your mouth. This can happen earlier than six months and is a good sign they're getting ready.
- Losing the tongue thrust reflex, which causes baby to push food out of their mouth.

WHY DO WE OFFER FOOD BESIDES MILK?

Breast milk and formula offer a host of amazing nutrients for your baby, but starting solids in the second half of infancy (six months and older) is important for:

- Obtaining critical nutrients like iron and zinc that don't transfer in large quantities through breast milk.
- Developing the muscles in their mouth that are necessary for speech, chewing, and swallowing.
- Introducing allergenic foods (dairy, peanuts, etc.), which the latest research suggests might help prevent food allergies.
- Building taste preferences and acceptance of diverse flavors and textures.

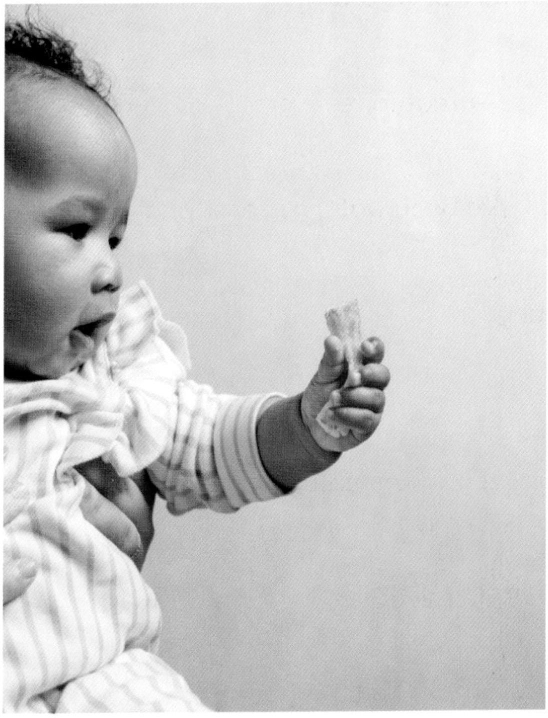

HOW TO START: THE BASICS

At six months of age, your baby can't pick up small pieces of food because they don't have a pincer grasp (tip of thumb and forefinger touch). That's why baby-led weaning is often associated with strips or sticks of food—your baby is able to hold that shape in the palm of their hand and bring it to their mouth. We recommend starting with any soft, fork-tender food that your family enjoys. As long as it passes the "squish test" between your fingers, it's good for baby: think avocado, roasted sweet potato, steamed broccoli, banana, or softly cooked chicken as first foods.

At the end of this book, you'll find a visual

index of images on how to serve our recipes to your baby. The index is just inspiration—you can modify the presentation of these meals depending on your comfort level and your baby's skills. For example, if your baby is developing a pincer grasp and can pick up smaller bits, try cutting their foods into little pieces.

The goal is for your baby to eat the foods you enjoy as a family. For example, if dinner is spaghetti, meatballs, and green beans, you can offer it to your baby as well. Quarter the meatballs so they're in wedges, and place a few pieces of the other food in front of your baby so they can pick it up. You can also hand it to them if they're struggling to grasp it from their high-chair tray.

Speaking of high chairs, positioning your baby is also important. We recommend that babies sit like adults for a meal:

- Upright or leaning slightly forward (not reclined)
- Ninety-degree bend at the hips, knees, and ankles
- Supported feet

When a baby feels stable under their feet, they can last longer in their high chair and will be more likely to try new foods.

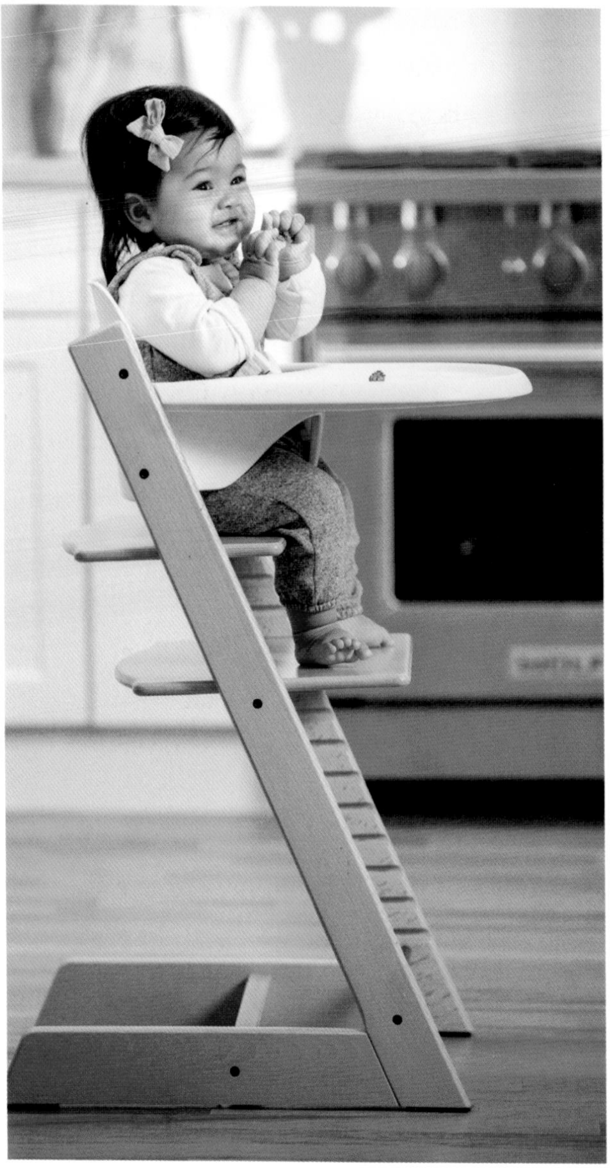

Can I Serve My Baby Everything?

Your baby can enjoy a lot of the same foods you eat, but we do recommend avoiding certain foods:

- Honey before age 1, as there's a small risk of infant botulism.
- Choking-hazard foods, which we discuss on page 15.
- Excess salt. The general guidance on sodium is no more than 400 mg per day because babies have immature kidneys, and high levels of sodium may be taxing to them. However, there is not a lot of science to support this recommendation, so we suggest offering mainly unsalted options and not worrying too much about sodium if your baby is eating a variety of foods.
- Soda. Babies need breast milk/formula as their main source of both nutrition and hydration. They can also have small amounts of water starting at age 6 months.
- Caffeine. Caffeine can interfere with your baby's sleep—we don't need that!
- "Diet" or very high-fiber foods. These can irritate the GI tract.
- Juice. Unless your baby is constipated, offer whole fruit over juice.

Scheduling

Many families start out with one meal a day to get used to the process. We recommend working up to three meals a day by around nine months. This allows your baby plenty of practice so that they build the skills needed to eventually feed themselves. It's a learning process, and it can take time for them to "get" it.

It's important for your baby to still drink plenty of breast milk or formula until around their first birthday. In general, aim for a minimum of 20 to 24 ounces of milk a day; some babies drink much more than this. As your baby starts to consume more food, their milk intake might slowly drop down, and that's expected.

Try to offer food within an hour after milk so your baby doesn't get too hungry by mealtime. They can easily become frustrated as they learn to self-feed. As they get older and more skilled, experiment with spacing out milk and solids a little more.

Six-month-olds don't usually consume a large amount of food when they're feeding themselves. With time and skill-building, we expect their food intake to improve. If your baby is struggling to self-feed, here are a few tips:

- Offer finger food more frequently. Bump it up to two or three meals a day if possible, and make sure to eat together.
- Try loaded spoons and forks. Put a small piece of food on the utensil and hand it to your baby.
- Try various textures. If a child is struggling with whole foods, try a smoother or pureed option on a loaded spoon. Then, gradually add more texture. For example, start with yogurt on spoons. Once they've got that down, add chopped bananas or crushed O's cereal to the yogurt. Try not to linger on smooth or pureed foods for too long; it's important for babies to practice chewing and trying different types of foods.
- Make sure your baby is using their hands and getting messy as they eat. Resist the urge to wipe down your baby throughout the meal—developmentally, the mess is a good thing for them to feel on their skin. More about mess below.
- Offer stick-shaped teething toys that help your baby learn where to put food in their mouth.

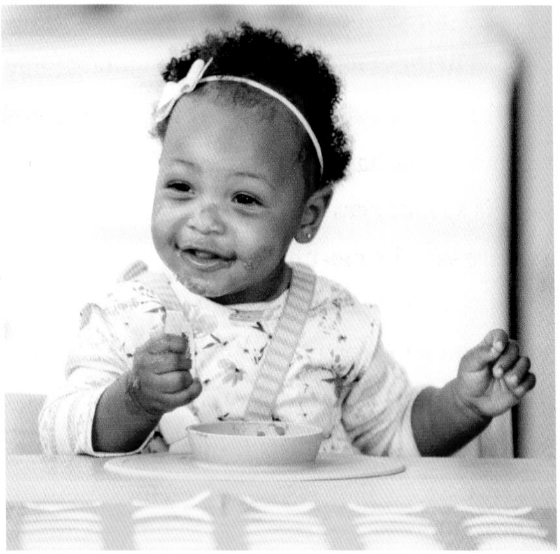

A WORD ON MESS

When babies and toddlers learn how to feed themselves with their hands and utensils, they are bound to get messy—*really* messy sometimes. While mess during mealtimes can be annoying, it's also important. Your child has to explore food with their hands to know how it will feel in their mouth. When they can't touch their meal, they're less likely to eat it.

If you're anxious about mess, here are some tips:

- Strip your child down to a diaper or use a bib.
- If you are feeding your child on carpet, protect the floor with a splash mat, towel, or shower curtain.
- You don't have to offer messy foods at each meal, but when you can, let your child get their hands and face messy. As they develop self-feeding skills, they become more tidy eaters and the mess subsides.
- Try to be gentle when cleaning up your child. Sometimes they avoid getting messy or dread mealtime because they don't want to get scrubbed down. Bring a bowl of warm water with a washcloth to their high chair and hold the bowl as they splash in the water; you can gently wipe them down while they play. Or, take your kiddo to the sink right after a meal and run the water so they can wash their hands as you softly wipe their face.
- Keep mess in perspective. Again, it's critical developmentally—if they can't feel it in their hands, they're more reluctant to put it in their mouths. As Judy says, it's a short-term investment with a long-term payout.

CHOKING HAZARDS, GAGGING, AND SAFETY

When parents learn about baby-led weaning, their biggest concern is safety. Most people are familiar with baby food and the concept of spoon-feeding, and they may not have seen a baby feeding themselves whole foods. The good news: the available data suggests that BLW is not any less safe than traditional feeding, as long as non-choking-hazard foods are provided. Plus, since finger foods have been recommended around this age for decades, we have significant history to help us understand that various soft textures are safe for most babies at six months.

When babies start eating whole foods, they may gag, and that can be scary to see. But gagging is not the same thing as choking—it's a normal oral protective mechanism that prevents babies from swallowing a piece of food that is too large. It might happen because your baby hasn't learned to move food to the side of their mouth with their tongue, chew, and effectively swallow. This is a process that takes time and practice.

When a child gags, we're paying attention to:

- Sound—if there's sound, there's breathing.
- Duration—gagging should be quick, and you should see the food come farther forward on your child's tongue. They will either spit it out or try to chew it again.
- Distress—your baby's face might turn red and their eyes might water, but they should never be in distress. If they are, it's time to intervene.
- Improvement—gagging improves with time and practice. It is most common in the first few weeks of BLW, but it should subside relatively quickly. If it doesn't, consider trying a smoother texture and talk to your provider.

Choking-hazard foods can pose a safety risk for children until age four. It's important to avoid or modify anything that can be considered choking hazards, and always supervise your child around food. Of course, if a food makes you uncomfortable, do not serve it to your child.

Modify:

- Grapes, cherries, cherry tomatoes, olives—quarter lengthwise
- Whole nuts—offer as thinly spread nut butter or ground
- Sausages, hotdogs—offer in small pieces
- Raw apples, hard pears—cook to soften, shred, or offer in very thin pieces
- Raw carrots—cook to soften, shred
- Small bones in meat, or skin—remove
- Hard dried fruit (raisins, cranberries)—soften by cooking or soaking in hot water

Avoid:

- Whole large seeds
- Popcorn
- Hard candy, gummy bears, sticky candy
- Gum
- Hard chips (tortilla chips, potato chips)

Kids can choke on anything, and they're more likely to choke on a non-food item. That's why it's so important to know how to help your child if they are choking. We encourage all parents and caregivers to take a first aid/CPR class so they can be prepared.

ALLERGENS

For years, pediatricians advised families to avoid allergenic foods like peanut butter and eggs in infancy. At the time, scientists thought it would help improve allergy risk. Recent research suggests otherwise. Delaying allergenic foods not only didn't help, but it actually *increased* the risk of developing a food allergy. For this reason, most providers now recommend early and frequent introduction of allergenic foods. We suggest starting them relatively soon after you begin solid foods, at around six months.

If your child has a higher risk of an allergy due to their family or medical history, make sure to work with your provider. You might be advised to do allergy testing or controlled, in-office exposures.

DINING OUT/TAKEOUT TIPS

Serving your baby what the family eats can make restaurant dining easy. Here are some things to consider:

- Offer your baby components of your meal. They probably do not need a separate meal.
- Avoid choking hazards and be mindful of spicy foods. Babies can have spicy foods, but some infants do not like or tolerate them well.
- If you aren't ready to serve your baby what you're eating, you can always order sides or serve them just one component of the meal. Often restaurants are more than willing to modify side dishes, especially if they know it's for a new eater.
- Babies can get messy when feeding themselves. Tipping a little extra is always appreciated if your baby makes a big mess at a restaurant.

For more help feeding your baby, head to feedinglittles.com to learn about our online Infant Course.

starter food

If you're thinking, "Which foods do I offer first?" that is totally up to you. From six months on, babies can enjoy all types of foods, from grains to meats to vegetables to fruits. Here's a small list of frequent first foods, along with a Starter Fruit and Vegetable Guide for more inspiration:

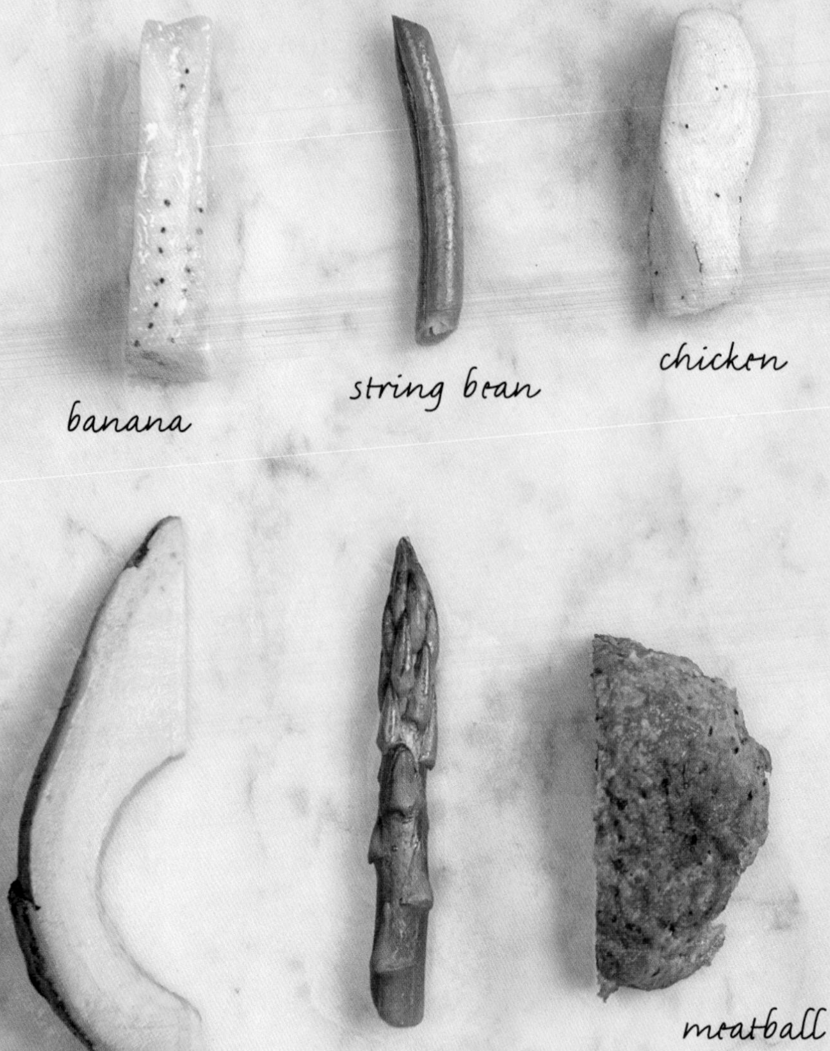

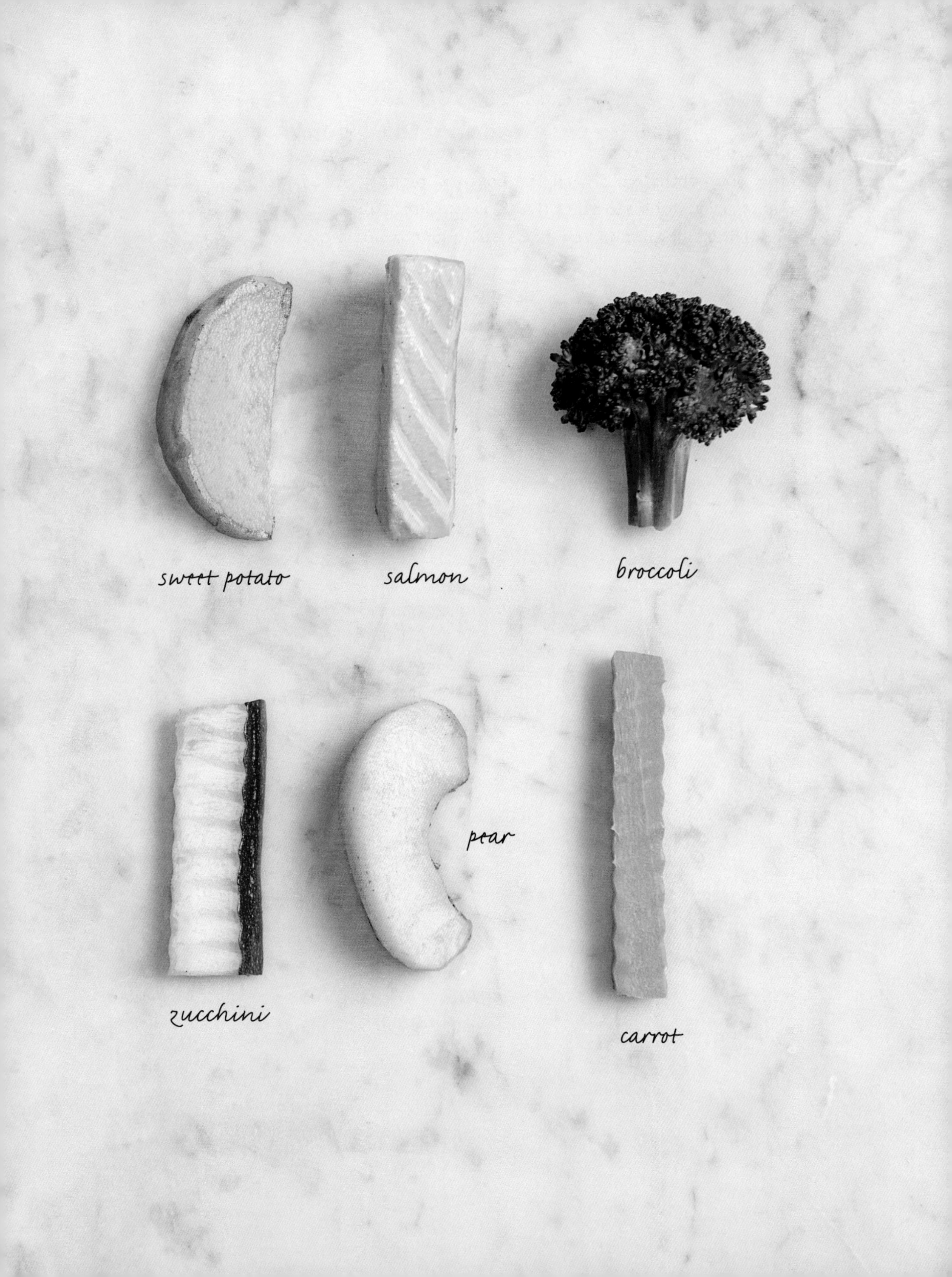
sweet potato
salmon
broccoli
zucchini
pear
carrot

starter fruit and vegetable guide

We generally recommend offering your baby whatever you are eating as a family. However, when you start this process, you might feel more comfortable with single-item foods like cooked cauliflower or a watermelon spear. If you do, here are some quick ideas to get you started. Cook them any way you like—steam, roast, sauté—just as long as they're soft enough to pass the squish test. You can cook with your favorite oils, whether that's olive, avocado, or coconut. In addition, we love using seasonings to expose your little one to different flavors, like dried oregano or curry powder, so spice it up before you roast or after you steam.

VEGETABLES	**PREPARATION AND SERVING (6-MONTH-OLDS)**
Broccoli, cauliflower	Cook until soft and serve as long stalks
Carrots, celery, bell peppers, eggplants, butternut squash, zucchini, yellow squash, sweet potatoes, etc.	Cook until soft and serve as strips
Tomatoes, mushrooms	Cook if desired to make softer and cut into strips Quarter if round (e.g., cherry tomatoes)
Asparagus, green beans, snow and snap peas	Cut ends, cook, and serve as sticks
FRUITS	**PREPARATION AND SERVING (6-MONTH-OLDS)**
Bananas	Cut into strips Can leave skin on the bottom for extra grip or roll into crushed cereal

Avocados, melons, peaches, nectarines, plums, pineapples, kiwis	Cut into wedges Can leave skin on the bottom for extra grip
Blueberries, raspberries, blackberries	Cut in half or squish Serve in yogurt or oatmeal so baby can pick up
Grapes, cherries	Remove skins and quarter
Strawberries	Remove stems and cut in half if large
Apples, hard pears, other hard fruits	Soften by baking or sautéing with coconut oil Shred with a cheese shredder (shredded fruit will require pincer grasp)

The most important thing about feeding your baby is eating together and trying to enjoy the process. We want our babies to see mealtime as a pleasant experience that everyone looks forward to. Each kiddo will follow their own timeline in learning how to eat—that's why it's "baby-led." Your job is to give them the opportunity to learn by exposing them to new foods and modeling how to eat them. We hope you have fun with it. It's a superb way to share the flavors, cultural foods, and traditions of your family.

feeding toddlers (and older kids)

If you have lived with a toddler, you might know that they are notoriously unpredictable and inconsistent when it comes to food. Those babies who try everything often become one-year-olds who turn their noses up at the cauliflower they loved yesterday. For toddlers, eating isn't as simple as sitting down to the table and putting food in their mouths. Their newly minted mobility allows them more independence and autonomy than they've ever had. Now they can make choices. Now they can say no. Furthermore, with toddlerhood comes food neophobia, or the fear of new foods. This is thought to be biologically driven, and understanding it may help you make sense of their maddening behavior. The idea is that they are hardwired to be skeptical of unknown foods because otherwise they might wander into the forest and try a poisonous berry or mushroom. This instinct protects them.

Regardless, picky or selective eating in toddlerhood is real for many families. The onset is generally between twelve and twenty-four months (or later), and it can ebb and flow as they get older. It often improves naturally around ages six to seven, but it depends on the child and how mealtimes are handled in your home. Try to think long-term. Yes, meals can be chaotic when your children are little, so imagine what you want it to *feel* like when they're older. When they're a teenager, what do you want them to remember about eating together? You're laying that foundation now, one brick by (kind of annoying) brick. Eventually the dinner table will be one of the few places you have an opportunity to connect with your kids.

If picky eating worsens or your child eats fewer than twenty total foods, talk with your provider. Sometimes private therapy is indicated for prolonged picky eating. The earlier you begin working with a feeding therapist, the faster you will see changes in your child's food journey. It is much easier to change a two-year-old's relationship with food than a ten-year-old's. Visit feedinglittles.com for a list of red flags and signs that it's time to reach out for hands-on, professional help.

Below are some basic tips for handling mealtimes with toddlers, preschoolers, and beyond.

FAMILY MEALS

One of the most simple, yet underrated, ways to help your child eat better is to eat together. In fact, it's the first thing we evaluate as feeding professionals. Why? Kids learn by imitation, and eating alone is actually pretty boring for them.

As parents, we know that sometimes all you want to do is get your kiddos fed so you can eat in peace. We get it. There's definitely room for this. However, we've found that when our clients start eating with their kids on a more regular basis, they start to look forward to it. Your child will learn that this is how meals work in your house, and they thrive on that routine. They also thrive on connecting with you—having conversations, telling jokes, and sharing about their day. Getting into the habit of eating together when you can is the first step toward more adventurous eating.

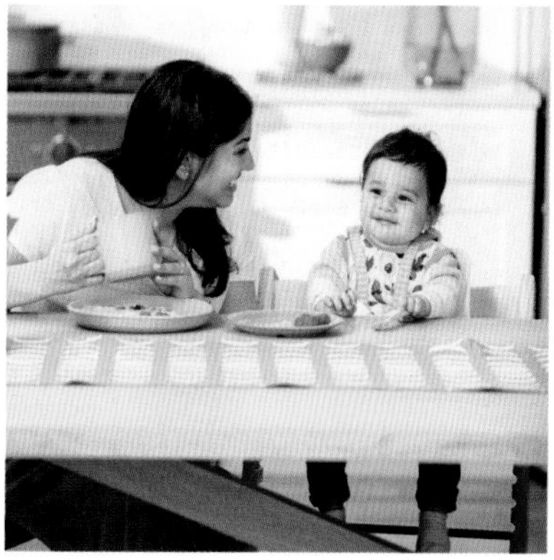

If you have an infant or toddler, try to avoid putting them in their high chair until the food is ready. But bring their high chair to the table, and invite them to the meal as early as possible. They have a limited tolerance for being confined, and the clock starts ticking the moment they're in the chair.

MINIMIZING DISTRACTIONS

Our busy world demands that our devices follow us wherever we go. Kids are drawn to screens and tend to tune out everything while in front of one. When the television, phone, or tablet are on during mealtime, they aren't mentally present with the rest of the family. That distraction might seem like it's helping your kids eat more, but they can become dependent on the screen to eat at all.

If possible, keep devices off during mealtimes. Our clients turn on music during meals for ambience and to signal the start of the meal. Of course, there's always room for flexibility—sometimes we turn the TV on during breakfast or eat during family movie night. Just try to make that the exception rather than the norm.

VARIETY

When kids become more selective about food, parents begin to worry. They start serving the foods they know their kid will eat. This limits the foods their child is used to seeing, and they begin to expect only a limited array on their tray. It makes sense that they become averse to anything new.

When kids are offered a wide variety of foods, even if they're not ready to eat them yet, they get used to their plate looking different every time. Even small changes like cutting a sandwich differently, swapping out the yogurt topping, or serving a bite on a toothpick (if age-appropriate) helps teach them to be more flexible.

When you can, try to add some more variety to your kiddo's meals. Try to pick one food from each color group when you go shopping, or serve a different fruit with lunch. We hope that this cookbook will help inspire you to try something new today and introduce fresh flavors to your family.

ONE FAMILIAR FOOD

One way to help your child come to any meal enthusiastically is by serving a familiar or preferred food. This may be something "beige" like bread, rice, or pasta, but it can also be a favorite fruit, veggie, or sauce or dip. Kids may need twenty or more exposures to a food to even give it a go, so try not to be discouraged if they don't reach for it at first. That familiar food will make sure they have something to eat in the meantime.

As Judy always says, "eating begets eating."

LOWER THE PRESSURE

It's so easy to carefully watch and evaluate our kids as they eat. We worry that they're not eating enough, or they're not eating the foods we want them to eat. Some families even count bites or dictate how much a child must eat before they can leave the table.

Here's the thing: kids don't do well with pressure—around food or otherwise. They're not comfortable being watched as they eat. It is one of the few things in their life that they can control, and when they sense pressure they tend to push back. Hard. Instead of laying on the pressure, think like a kid.

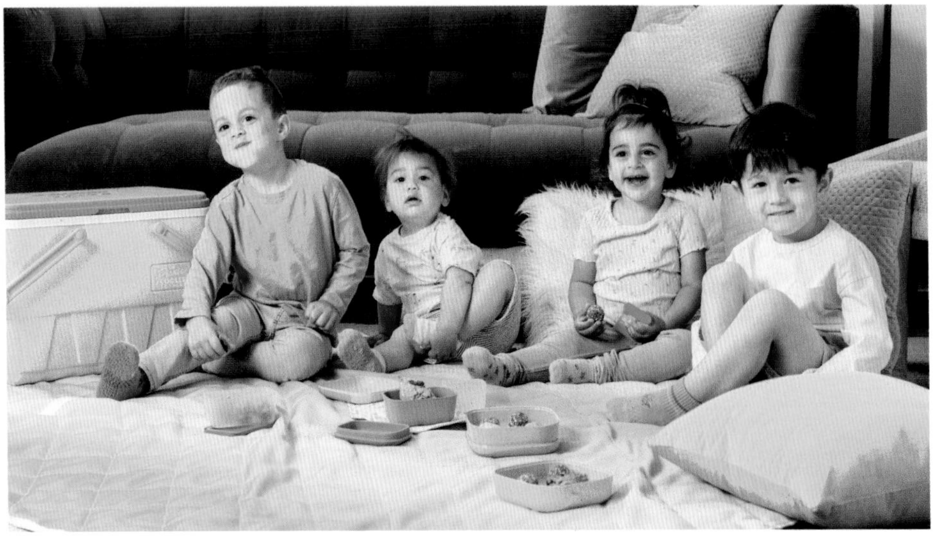

It's OK to play and pretend with food—it's how kids learn. It doesn't have to be a big production; just try eating like a dinosaur or sprinkling on Parmesan cheese "snow." Having fun can change the whole mood of the meal.

Language Matters

How you talk about food, eating, and bodies shapes how your child feels about themself and how they eat. Your language will have a lifelong impact—kids live up to the labels we place on them. When we say they "won't try anything new," they begin to believe that they indeed won't try anything new.

INSTEAD OF:	TRY:
"You're such a picky eater."	"You're still learning about new foods—we can learn together."
"He won't eat anything healthy."	"He has certain foods he prefers more than others right now."
"Why can't you eat all your food like your sister?"	"Is your tummy full? If so, it's OK to stop eating."

Kids also notice how we talk about our own bodies. Even when negative self-talk is not directed at our children, it can still influence how they feel about themselves. When we stand in front of the mirror and criticize how we look in a swimsuit, we teach our kids to do the same. When we associate health with weight, we teach them to prioritize weight as well.

Our kids will grow into the body that is genetically destined for them. They might be small or large. They might not fit societal standards for "ideal" body types. They might struggle to love their body, but it's important for us to help them learn to respect, love, and care for their body. One of the best ways we can do that is by what we say.

Of course, this can feel like a big undertaking. We all want our kids to be healthy, confident humans who love their body, and many of us did not grow up in a body-positive environment. We might struggle to find anything we love about our own bodies, and we might be scared to pass on body image issues or disordered eating patterns to our kids.

All we can do is try to keep our language weight-neutral. Try to be aware of how you talk about yourself, the food you serve, and the way your family eats. Know that you cannot control all of the messages your child will receive about food and their bodies—they're everywhere—but you can try to make small changes to how your family talks about these important topics.

Below are some examples of ways we can adjust our language to make it more positive.

INSTEAD OF:	TRY:
"These pants make me look fat."	"I'm going to try on something else that helps me feel more confident."
"I can't eat ice cream with you; I'm on a diet."	"Sure, I'd love to have some." or "No, thank you; I don't want any right now."
"If I don't work out, I won't fit into my clothes."	"Moving my body helps me when I'm stressed."
"You can eat anything; you're so lucky."	"We all eat different foods. Right now, I'm hungry for _____."
"I hate my thighs."	"I love how strong my legs are."

how to handle food waste

When feeding kids, there may be a lot that goes to waste. They drop it on the floor, rub it in their hair, or even chew it and spit it out. Sometimes we serve our kids a beautiful dinner, only to watch them eat rolls with butter as their entire meal.

Some parents assume that they'll waste less food if they only serve what they know their kid will eat, but kids are inconsistent creatures, even with their trusty "favorites." That's why we recommend offering a few components at each meal and letting kids choose how much to eat from what is being served.

HOW CAN WE MINIMIZE FOOD WASTE?

- Offer tiny portions to start. This also helps prevent your child from becoming overwhelmed, so they might be more likely to eat it. Remind them that they can always have more if they're hungry for it.
- Reuse what you can. If your kid didn't touch it, maybe it can go in your lunch the next day.
- Consider composting what's left.

In this cookbook, we feature many creative and delicious ways the whole family can enjoy fruits and vegetables. However, we understand that your child might not eat these foods—especially veggies—right now. Continue to serve them without pressure, ensuring there's always something familiar on your child's plate that they can eat. If you need to modify recipes to omit the veggies and want to serve them on the side instead, that's great, too. Veggies are great, but they're not the only way we get nutrition from food. Do what works for your family.

Feeding toddlers and school-age kids can be stressful, but we hope you can see it as a process. You'll have days when they'll eat everything and days when they'll eat very little. This is normal and expected. In fact, many toddlers eat only two decent meals (plus snacks) per day. Stay consistent, try to keep meals positive, and know that it gets better over time. If it doesn't, that's when you might want to talk to your provider.

For more help feeding your toddler or big kid, head to feedinglittles.com to check out our online courses.

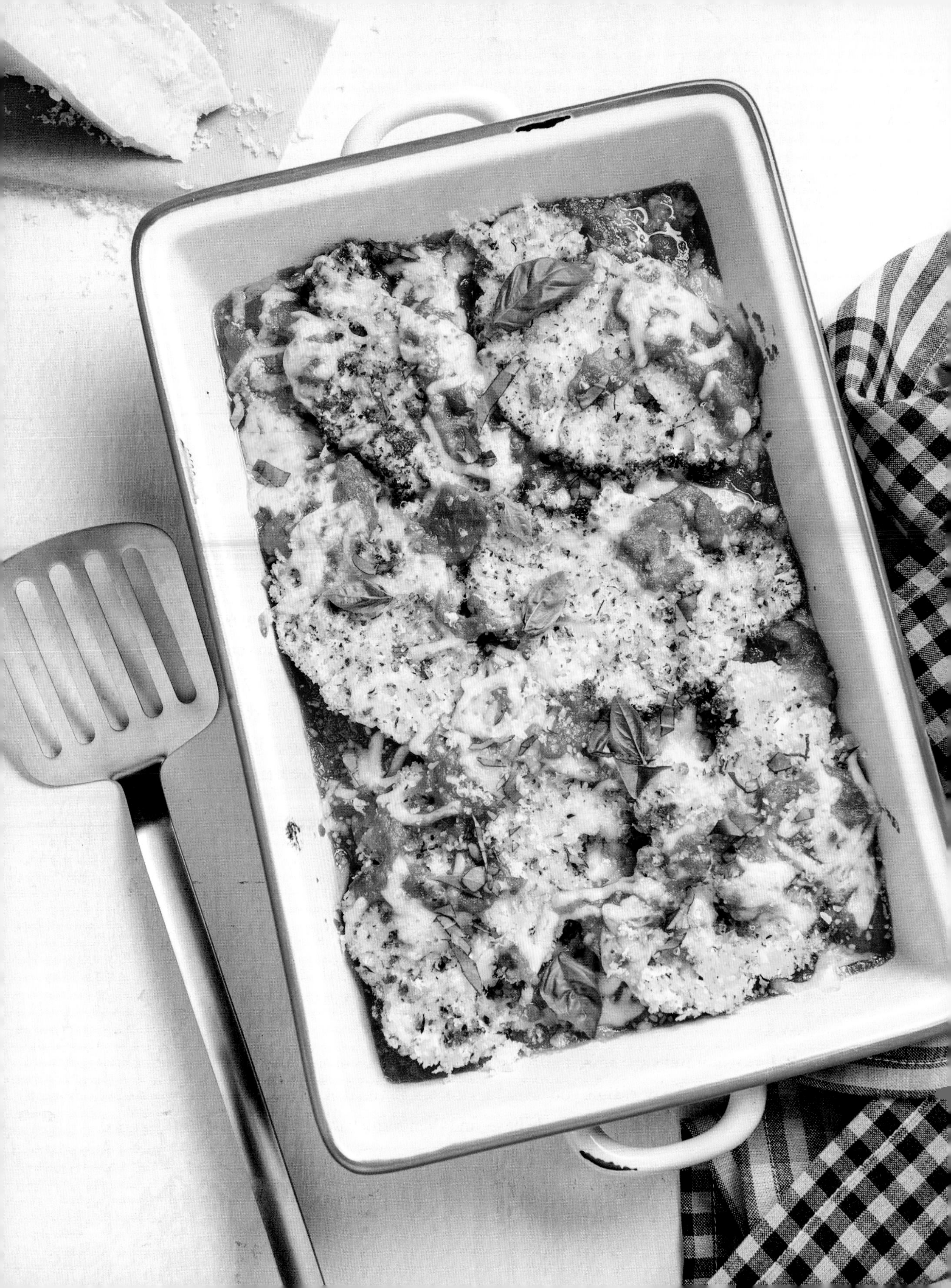

let's get in the kitchen

By the time you've reached this chapter, you're probably anxious to get cooking. You might be starting with lots of experience in the kitchen, or perhaps the thought of cooking regularly is intimidating. Know that this cookbook is for *you*, no matter your starting point. We want to help you discover new flavors and favorite recipes you can fit into your busy life.

One thing that can help with cooking is preparedness. It's easier to try a new recipe or throw something together if you have ingredients on hand. When you have a loose plan, even if it's just for one or two recipes a week, you're more likely to actually make that food and enjoy the experience.

In this chapter, we'll provide you with our suggestions on what to keep in your pantry, freezer, and fridge for easy throw-together meals, how to effectively (and pleasantly) involve your kiddos, and how to save time in the kitchen. We can't stress this enough: if cooking overwhelms you, start small. Buy ingredients for a few recipes to start. Know that you do not have to make a gourmet meal or anything fancy. Our Simple Staples (page 116) and I Can't Even (page 119) sections will be your go-tos on those nights when you, well, can't even.

kitchen essentials

First things first: shop your kitchen. You can often come up with delicious and nutritious meals without a trip to the store. It's like when you open your closet and say, "Ugh, I have nothing to wear"—but if you take inventory, you may surprise yourself. Turns out you have a lot to wear (and cook!).

If you have time and your budget allows, check in at the end of each week and restock pantry and freezer staples the next time you go to the grocery store. That way you can build your next week's meal plan from what you already have, and then restock those items. This has the added benefit of saving money, because you're not buying multiple cans of beans and letting them get lost in the back of the pantry. You're more likely to cook, too, if you know what you have. (Of course, if you find yourself winging it for whatever reason, that is no problem whatsoever. Each family will approach this process differently.)

When you open your refrigerator, maybe you only have some almost-expired bell peppers and a half-used jar of salsa. Well, if you also have a few pantry and freezer staples, dinner's on! You can make our Pressure Cooker Chicken Salsa Kinda-Chiladas (page 261) or our Southwestern Salsa Rice Bake with Chipotle Sauce (page 161).

Before we share our pantry and freezer staples, we want to acknowledge that having access to enough food and adequate storage for that food is a privilege not afforded to everyone. Additionally, these pantry staples are items we like to have on hand, but they don't necessarily reflect everyone's preferences, needs, or culture. You might not need or even like everything on this list; it's simply a starting point.

Pantry Essentials

- Garlic and onions: the key to every great meal.
- Oils for cooking and baking: olive, coconut, sesame, grapeseed, and avocado. Also, one in a spray format.
- Flours for baking and cooking: whole wheat, all-purpose, almond, coconut, oat, and tapioca.
- Arrowroot powder or cornstarch: for thickening sauces.
- Rolled oats: for breakfast foods, baking, and cooking. Note: if a recipe calls for oat flour, blend oats in a high-speed blender until fine.
- Ground flaxseed: an easy ingredient to add to baked goods for extra omega-3s and fiber.
- Chia seeds: for binding meatballs, making pudding, and tossing into baked goods for a bonus burst of nutrients.
- Rice and other grains: Whether it's brown, white, or legume, rice is an absolute necessity for easy stir-fries, casseroles, soups,

and burrito bowls. We also love farro as a readily available, hearty option.

- Quinoa: a complete protein, this powerhouse food is handy for stirring into chilis, soups, stir-fries, salads, and more.
- Dry and cooked/canned lentils: a versatile food that is a rich source of protein (try our Lentil Gyro Wraps on page 215).
- Spices and seasonings: There's nothing more important than an adequate spice drawer to transform simple foods and vegetables into delicious meals. We recommend having the following on hand: garlic powder, dried oregano/parsley/basil/thyme/rosemary, bay leaves, ground ginger, cinnamon, curry powder, ground cumin, chili powder, and paprika.
- Curry paste: red is a great starter paste for making Thai curries.
- Nut butters (or sun butter, if there's an allergy).
- Canned tomatoes: diced, crushed, and whole peeled.
- Jarred pasta sauce: tomato basil, marinara, and any of your favorite go-tos.
- Pasta, pasta, pasta: You can never have enough penne, rotini, lasagna, orzo, spaghetti—any and all. Always keep lasagna noodles on hand, as lasagna is the ultimate family meal as a soup, roll-ups, or the classic version. For extra nutrient power, try legume-based pastas (like lentil or chickpea).
- Boxed mac and cheese: if you know, you know.
- Broth (vegetable, beef, and chicken): for soups and cooking.
- Canned beans: cannellini (white), chickpeas, black, and pinto to start.
- Canned coconut milk: light and full-fat, always unsweetened, great for curries or for thickening sauces without dairy.
- Canned vegetables: These are handy in case you can't make it to the grocery store (maybe you're sick; maybe you're dealing with a newborn and can't leave the house)—canned vegetables

are still highly nutritious, so keep 'em in the back of the pantry. They're also useful for easy stir-fries. Start with green beans, corn, peas, and sliced carrots.

- Canned sweet potato, pumpkin, and butternut squash: For baking and making pasta sauces, these pureed vegetables are some of the most versatile items you can have. Try our Butternut Squash Sage Baked Ziti (page 153).
- Sauces and condiments: teriyaki, soy sauce (low sodium) or tamari (if gluten-free), balsamic vinegar, red wine vinegar, apple cider vinegar, tahini, maple syrup, honey, ketchup, Dijon mustard, hot sauce, and barbecue sauce.
- Breakfast essentials: we love keeping instant oatmeal and pancake and waffle mix around.
- Canned tuna and salmon: for green salads and mayo-based salads or cakes.

Freezer Essentials

- Vegetables: any and all, especially peas, carrots, bell peppers, broccoli, edamame, green beans, corn, and mixes (for example, "mixed vegetables" or "peas and carrots").
- Fruit: any and all for smoothies, for baking, or for homemade jams.
- Pizza crusts.
- French fries and sweet potato fries: What burger night is complete without fries?
- Tortillas: any day can be Taco Tuesday.
- Waffles: for snacks and breakfasts . . . and breakfast for dinner.
- Proteins: bacon, chicken, seafood, ground meats, sausage.
- Bread, burger and hot dog buns, and English muffins.
- Meat burgers and veggie burgers.

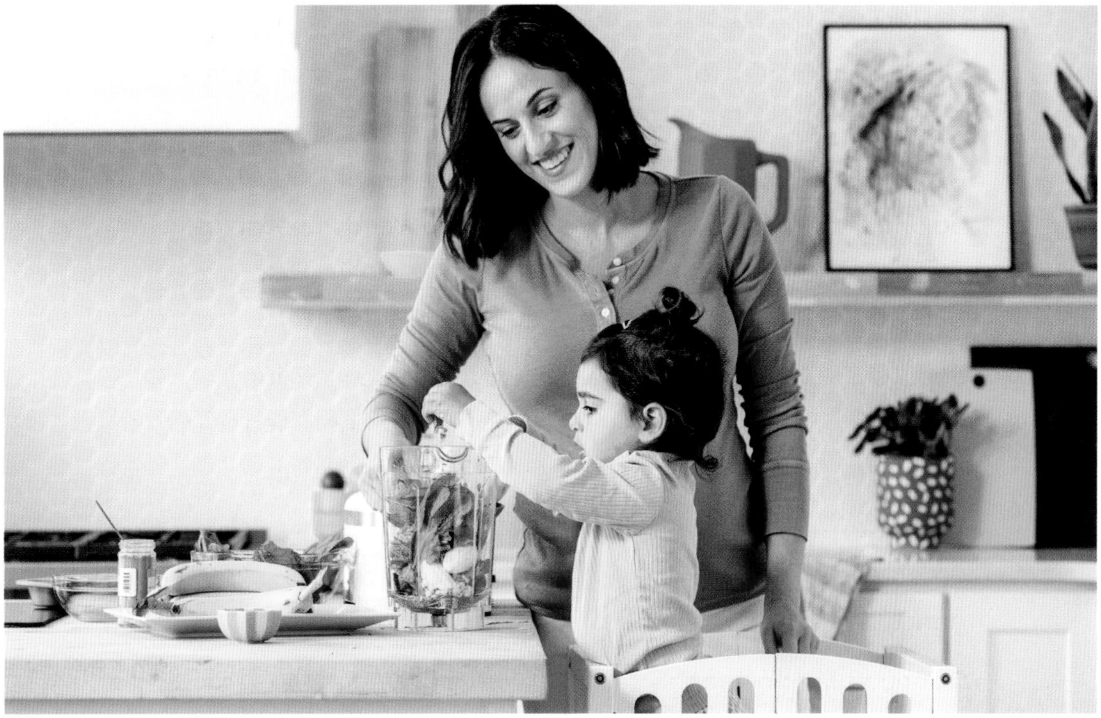

cooking with kids

You might have noticed that your child is more likely to eat a food they have helped prepare themself. They're proud of their creation, and they feel more comfortable with it because they have been interacting with it during prep time. However, cooking with kids is also messy and can be overwhelming. How can you make it a positive experience for everyone?

1. Safety is key.

First and foremost, be careful with anything sharp or hot. Teach your toddler that the stove is hot—"We don't ever touch the stove; ouch, hot!" As they get older, you can demonstrate how to use oven mitts and pull something out of the oven safely. Of course, hand hygiene is a safety issue as well. Wash your hands together before handling any food.

2. Start early, but keep it small.

As soon as your child can stand, they can start helping in the kitchen. It may feel overwhelming to have your child in the kitchen as you cook, so instead of having them around the whole time, focus on one or two short tasks. They don't need to complete every step with you—less is more here.

Young children can help with:

- Finding bowls or utensils
- Pouring
- Scooping
- Stirring
- Greasing a pan
- Tearing lettuce
- Washing food
- Squeezing lemons
- Setting the table (start with napkins or other non-breakable items)

As your child gets older and practices more, their kitchen skills will improve and they will be able to use gadgets and appliances safely.

3. Lower your expectations.

When kids "help," odds are things won't go as planned. They might spill, spatter, or smear ingredients everywhere. It might not be the idyllic moment you had hoped for, but try to remember that you're building memories and creating experiences, too. And it's OK if the food you made together isn't quite as beautiful as you expected. Try to keep your expectations low and focus on spending time together.

Tips for Saving Time in the Kitchen

We all want to make our family home-cooked meals, but we don't want to spend all day and night in the kitchen. With the following tips, you'll save time and still feed your loved ones deliciously.

1. Meal plan and meal prep: Easier said than done, but this is the #1 way to save time—and avoid the last-minute question "What's for dinner?" By meal planning, you know exactly what your family will be eating that week. Of course, it's important to leave room for exhausted nights and unexpected events (or celebrations!), but a mostly set meal plan can be tremendously helpful in saving time. Once you know what's cookin', you can prep parts of that meal so that when you go to put everything together, vegetables are presliced, sauces are premade, and so forth. Preparation is the key to success.
2. Wash fruits and vegetables after grocery shopping: Between properly washing your produce and drying it, meal prep time can add up. Your family is also more likely to snack on fruits and veggies if they're ready to go.
3. Prep your space: Before you start a recipe, skim it and gather all of the necessary tools, from sheet pans to skillets. This way, you won't burn the garlic while you're looking for a spatula.
4. Prep your ingredients: This is the most surefire way to a seamless cooking experience—it's why restaurant chefs always have what they call mise en place before they turn on the stove. If you're a parent, you know that unexpected things come up, and the last thing you need is to fumble with chopping onions while your toddler is asking to use the potty. Have everything prepared so that even if you're pulled in a different direction, you can pick up where you left off.
5. Have a trash bowl or compost bowl nearby: Instead of taking multiple trips to the garbage or sink to dump garbage, place a large bowl next to your workspace for trash, and when you're done, you can simply toss it all in the garbage or compost. Plus, when our spaces are more clean and organized, we tend to feel more relaxed and efficient.
6. Invest in a quality set of knives: If just slicing a vegetable seems like it takes forever or requires a lot of elbow grease, it's probably time to upgrade those knives, or at least get them sharpened. You'll be amazed by how much time you save with a quality set of knives.

Throughout the book, you'll see tips to speed up and simplify our recipes in the I Can't Even boxes. Easy swaps such as microwavable grains or premade sauces will help you cut corners without sacrificing flavor or quality.

Now that you're prepared to start feeding your family, let's get cooking.

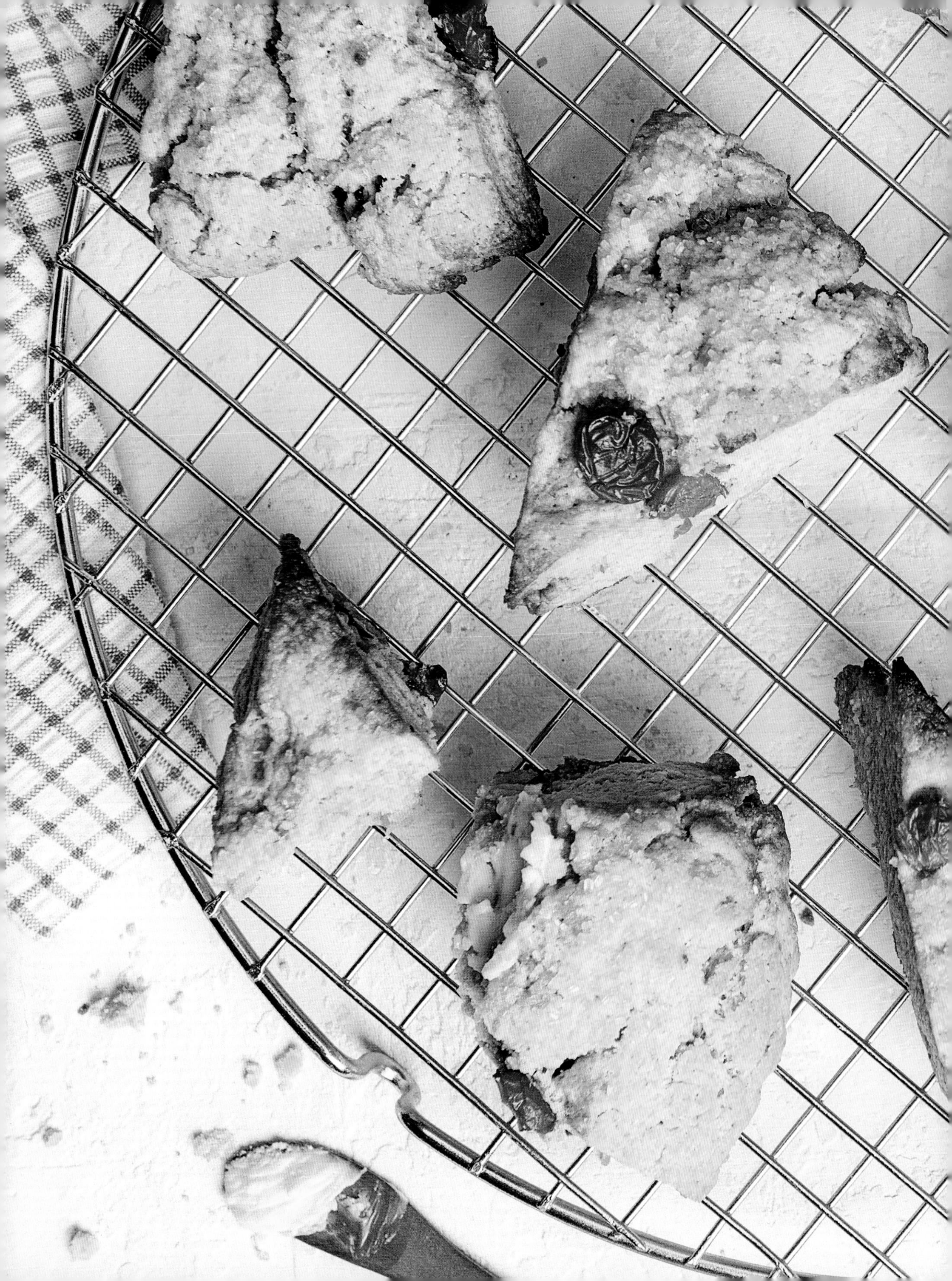

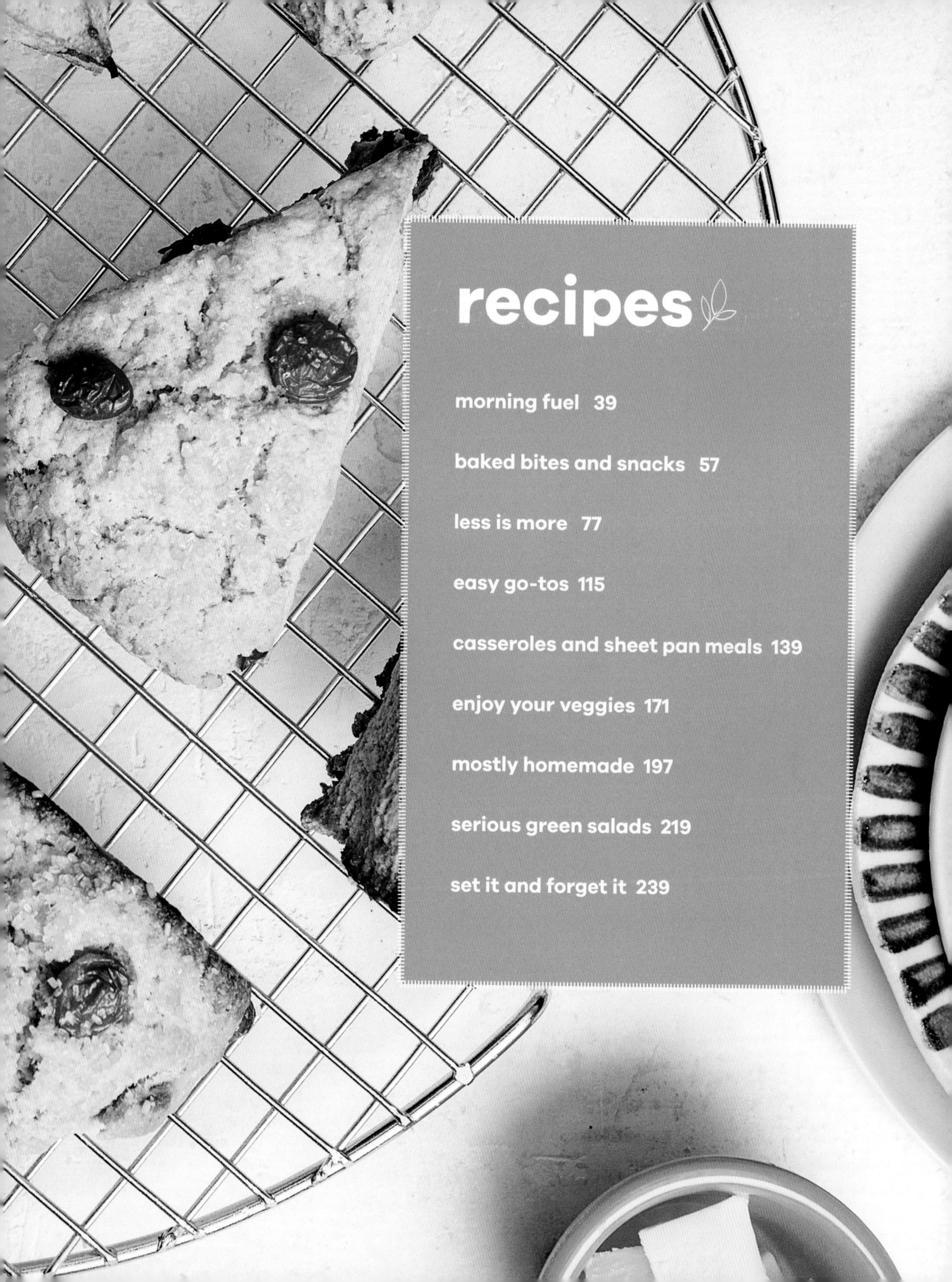

recipes

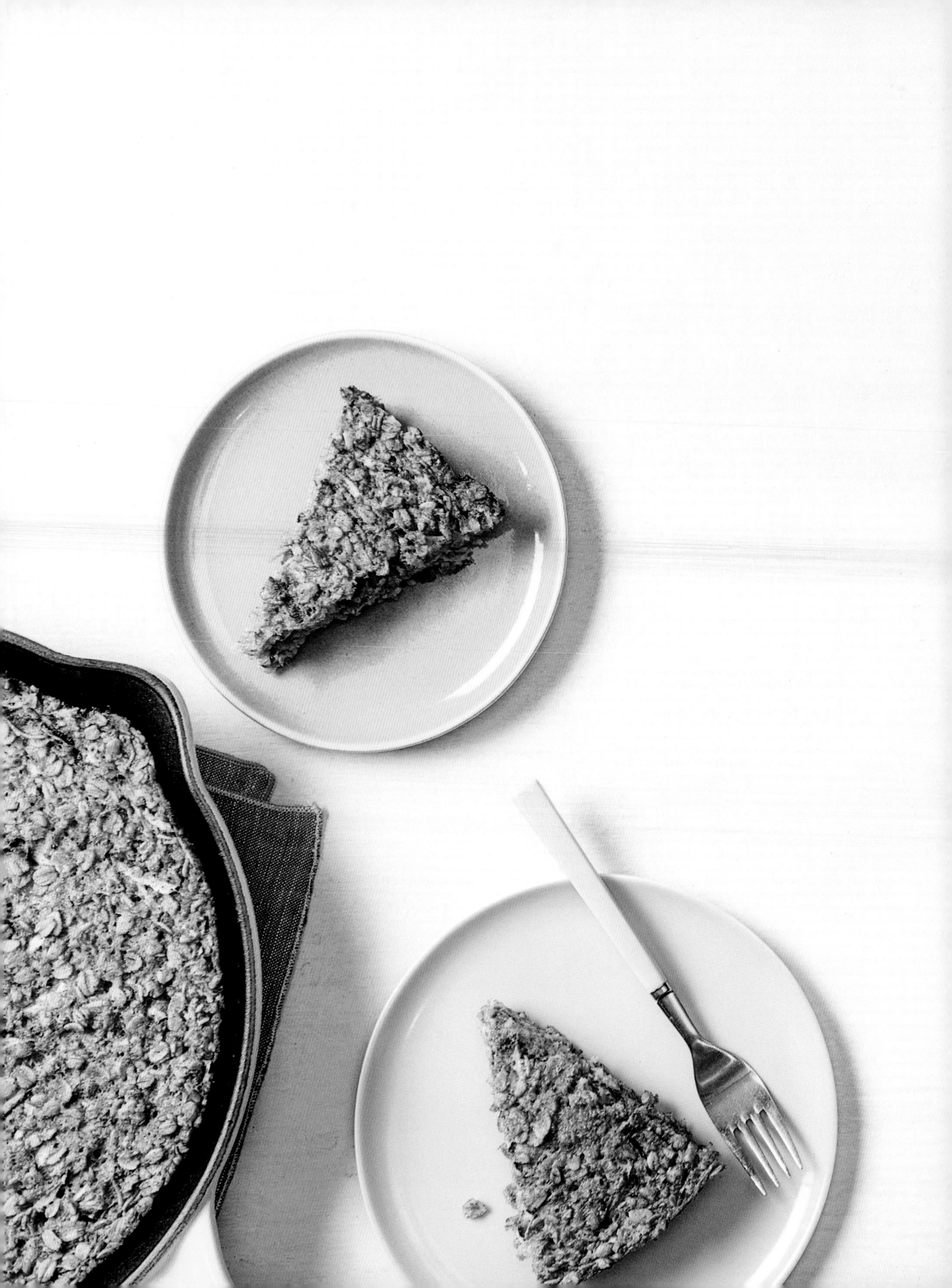

morning fuel

We all know the cliché "Breakfast is the most important meal of the day." Well, it's a cliché for a reason: it's true for most of us. When we wake up, it's time to nourish our bodies, setting the pace for the rest of the day. But when life is hectic, breakfast can feel like an afterthought. That's OK. Not every meal has to be a production, and cereal or toaster waffles are great options for busy mornings. But on the weekends or those mornings when you happen to wake up ten minutes early, your whole family will run to the table for these recipes—we promise.

Whether you want to break your eggs-and-toast rut or are looking for ways to incorporate more vegetables into your diet, you'll find something fresh and fun here, in yummy options like Zucchini Bread Oatmeal Bake (page 41) or Everything Bagel Broccoli and Cheddar Egg Donuts (page 55). If you have an egg sensitivity in the family, there are plenty of egg-free recipes, too, like our AB&J Chia Seed Pudding (page 45) or Vegan Pumpkin Waffles (page 49). And if you do have ten minutes the night before, you'll love our Carrot Cake Overnight Oats (see page 44), which is a delectable balance of sweet and savory.

We've also noted hacks that make breakfast a breeze, to help you get something on the table that everyone will love, so you're not standing at the stovetop making five different dishes, scarfing down handfuls of dry cereal while your family eats happily at the table. That's when our Build Your Own Sheet Pan Eggs (page 47) and our Sheet Pan Blueberry and Butternut Squash Pancakes (page 50) really come through. These recipes are designed to give you more time to enjoy a meal with your family—and less time cooking and cleaning.

There are so many easy ways to enjoy breakfast and not feel like you're running a diner. And if you just truly can't even, pop some waffles in the toaster, grab a yogurt, and enjoy your coffee—you're doing great.

INSPIRALIZED TIP

If you omit the zucchini and walnuts, you'll have the recipe for a basic oatmeal bake that you can jazz up to your liking. Try shredded carrots, raisins, well-chopped pecans, and a pinch of nutmeg for a carrot cake flavor, or keep it simple by stirring in chopped strawberries or blueberries.

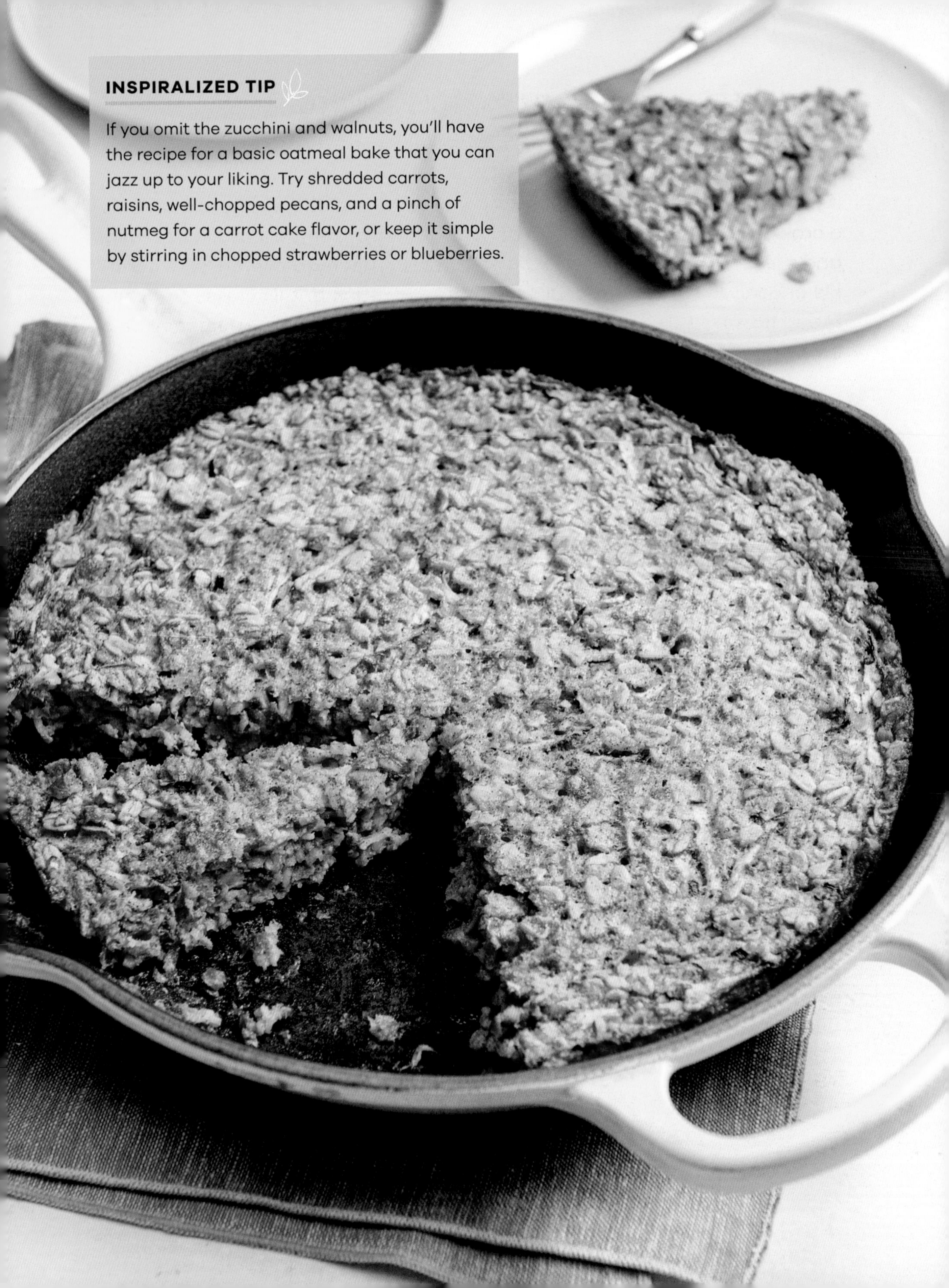

zucchini bread oatmeal bake

time to prep: 20 minutes / time to cook: 45 minutes / makes: 6 to 12 pieces

If you're new to oatmeal bakes, welcome to the revolution. They are not only a crowd-pleaser, they're easy to throw together, are enjoyable all week long, and are a fun way to break up the oatmeal monotony. Sometimes we sprinkle chocolate chips on top, but most days we stick to this classic zucchini bread flavor. Just like in a traditional zucchini bread, the walnuts provide a lovely crunch that keeps you coming back, bite after bite.

Cooking spray, for greasing the skillet

½ cup shredded zucchini

1¾ cups plain unsweetened almond milk (or milk of choice)

⅓ cup maple syrup

2 large eggs, whisked

3 tablespoons melted coconut oil, cooled slightly

1 teaspoon vanilla extract

2 cups rolled oats

½ cup finely chopped walnuts

1 teaspoon ground cinnamon

1 teaspoon baking powder

¼ teaspoon fine-grain sea salt

Preheat the oven to 375°F. Grease a 10-inch oven-safe skillet or an 8 x 8-inch pan with cooking spray.

Place the zucchini in the middle of a cheesecloth or paper towel, wrap it up, and squeeze any excess moisture out. Place the zucchini in a large mixing bowl with the milk, maple syrup, eggs, coconut oil, and vanilla. Whisk until blended.

Combine the oats, walnuts, cinnamon, baking powder, and salt in a medium mixing bowl. Stir to combine.

Pour the dry oat mixture into the prepared skillet. Pour the wet ingredients over the dry mixture. Using a spatula, stir together the ingredients and gently pat down any remaining dry oats on top to submerge in the wet ingredients.

Bake for 45 minutes, or until the top is firm and the edges are golden brown. Remove the pan from the oven and let it cool for a few minutes. Slice into 6 large or 12 small triangles. Serve warm.

FEEDING LITTLES TIP

Oats offer soluble fiber, which keeps us full and satisfied. It also can help kiddos struggling with constipation.

egg-adilla with pepper confetti

time to prep: 5 minutes / time to cook: 10 minutes / serves: 1

Egg + quesadilla = egg-adilla. These will become an absolute staple meal in your home, and they are so easy that you'll wonder how you didn't come up with them yourself. Add whatever fillings you want, like this pepper confetti (chopped bell peppers in various colors)—or just stick to cheese! Your child can help sprinkle in the confetti before you cook it.

1 (8-inch) tortilla

1 teaspoon extra-virgin olive oil

2 tablespoons diced bell peppers, various colors

1 tablespoon diced onion

Salt and pepper

1 large egg, whisked

2 tablespoons shredded Mexican cheese blend

Place an 8-inch skillet over medium heat. Once the pan is warm, put in the tortilla and let it cook for 30 seconds per side to warm up. Set the tortilla aside and immediately add the oil to the pan. When the oil is shimmering, add the peppers and onion, season with salt and pepper, and cook until soft, about 5 minutes. Pour the egg over the peppers and onion mixture and let set, tilting the pan and pushing in the edges to cook any raw egg. Cook until the egg is set, except for a little bit of egg on top. However, if you tilt the pan, there should be no raw egg running off. Top with the tortilla and then flip. On one half of the egg, sprinkle evenly with cheese. Fold the tortilla over like a quesadilla and press down. Cook for 30 seconds, flip, and cook another 30 seconds, until the cheese is melted. Transfer the egg-adilla to a plate and serve.

INSPIRALIZED TIP

When I make this for myself or a fellow adult, I use two eggs instead of one—and I slather it with hot sauce.

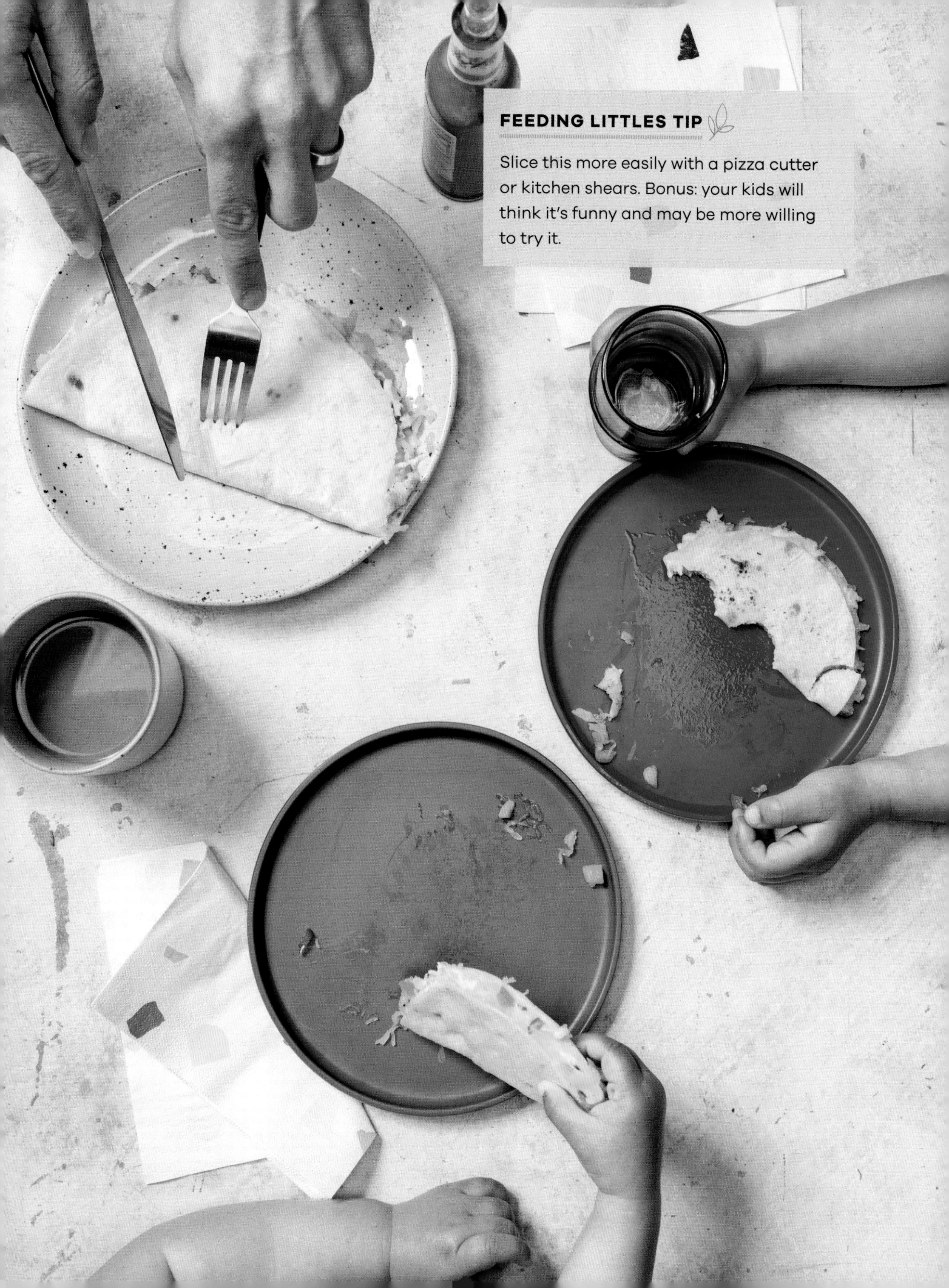

FEEDING LITTLES TIP

Slice this more easily with a pizza cutter or kitchen shears. Bonus: your kids will think it's funny and may be more willing to try it.

carrot cake overnight oats

time to prep: 20 minutes + overnight for soaking / serves: 4

After I've fed, bathed, and put the kids down for sleep and tidied up, all I want to do is hit the couch. It's tough to rally after a long day, but by taking fifteen minutes out of your (much-needed) mindless watching or scrolling, you can get that time back in the morning by throwing together overnight oats. When you wake up and have this nutrient- and veggie-packed breakfast to feed to your whole family, you'll be glad you put in the time. Overnight oats can be made in so many different varieties and flavors, but I love a classic carrot cake because it reminds me of one of my favorite desserts.

2 cups rolled oats

1 cup finely grated carrots or about 2 medium carrots, peeled and finely grated

3 Medjool dates, pitted and finely chopped

1 teaspoon ground cinnamon

⅛ teaspoon ground nutmeg

1½ tablespoons ground flaxseed

1 tablespoon chia seeds

2¼ cups unsweetened almond milk

3 tablespoons maple syrup

1 teaspoon vanilla extract

Mix together the oats, carrots, dates, cinnamon, nutmeg, flaxseed, and chia seeds in a large mixing bowl. Add the almond milk, maple syrup, and vanilla and mix to thoroughly combine. Cover and refrigerate overnight. Uncover and serve.

INSPIRALIZED TIP

For a more traditional carrot cake flavor, or if you can't find dates, swap the dates for ½ cup raisins.

FEEDING LITTLES TIP

Many toddlers love overnight oats, but babies might struggle to chew this dish. Before serving to a baby, briefly cook on the stove to soften the raw carrots and oats. You can also pop it in the microwave for 30 to 90 seconds, testing to make sure the heat level is correct. (Psst: this dish is amazing warm for adults, too.)

ab&j chia seed pudding

time to prep: 10 minutes + at least 2 hours or overnight, preferably / serves: 1

Chia seeds are versatile energy boosters that absorb ten to twelve times their weight in water and gel up. These little seeds can be enjoyed as a nutrient-packed snack or breakfast when combined with the right ingredients to make a sweet and flavorful pudding. Drawing inspiration from a universally beloved combo, this AB&J will undoubtedly hit the spot, but you can go totally traditional with peanut butter if you prefer it over almond.

If you're a parent, you probably are familiar with water beads, which are tiny beads that expand when you put them in water. This pudding has a similar wow factor, so be sure to include your little ones in making it.

1 cup almond milk (or milk of choice or full-fat canned coconut milk, for creamier consistency)

1 teaspoon maple syrup

3 tablespoons smooth almond butter

½ teaspoon vanilla extract

¼ cup chia seeds

¼ cup preferred jelly

Stir together the milk, maple syrup, 1 tablespoon of almond butter, and vanilla in a cereal or soup bowl. Stir in the chia seeds, cover, and refrigerate overnight or for at least 2 hours.

To assemble, add the jelly and remaining 2 tablespoons of almond butter and, using a spoon, swirl slightly to combine or create your own fancy design. Serve.

INSPIRALIZED TIP

If you're packing this for on the go, put it in a small mason jar with the almond butter on the bottom, then the chia pudding, and the jelly on top. Seal the jar and don't forget a spoon. Mix before serving.

FEEDING LITTLES TIP

This recipe is a good way for babies and toddlers to enjoy chia seeds, which are packed with fiber and omega-3 fatty acids. You can omit the jelly or maple syrup if you're not ready to serve it to your child, but we recommend adding some smashed fruit for sweetness. Save this recipe for when your child struggles to "go"—it's a constipation remedy, too.

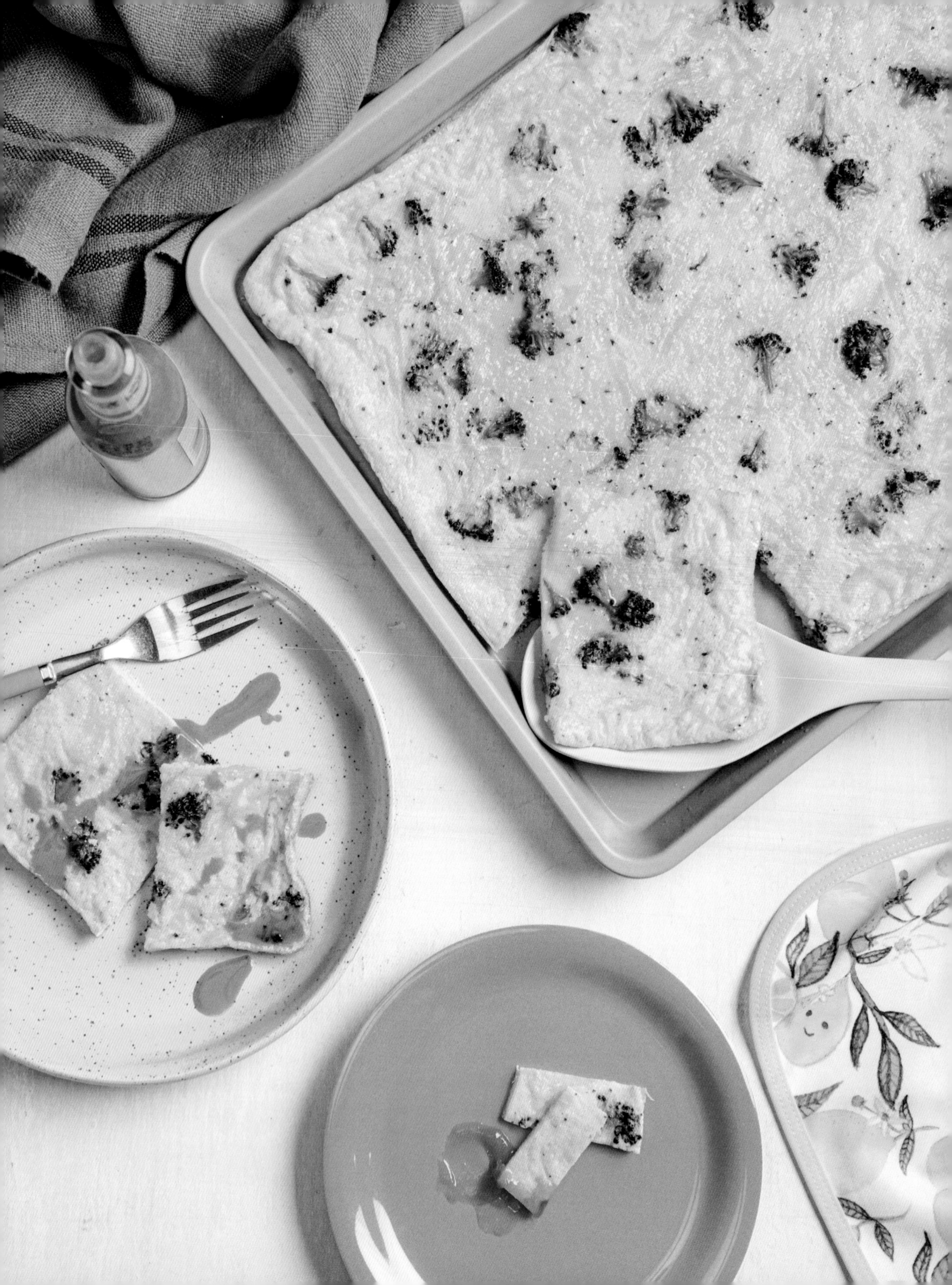

build your own sheet pan eggs

time to prep: 5 minutes / time to cook: 10 to 13 minutes / makes: 8 squares (1 square per serving = 8 servings)

Have you ever looked longingly at your partner sitting on the couch soaking up all the groggy morning snuggles with your kids while you're monotonously scrambling eggs? Here's your solution: sheet pan eggs, which are baked for easy slicing and serving. And don't forget to grab your cookie cutters around the holidays or other special occasions to make fun shapes and themes.

Speaking of holidays, these eggs are perfect for feeding large groups with different taste preferences. Simply pour the whisked eggs into the baking pan, let guests choose their toppings, and sprinkle in different sections. Bake, cut, and serve!

Olive oil or cooking spray, for greasing the pan

16 large eggs

Salt and pepper

Preheat the oven to 350°F. Thoroughly grease a large sheet pan by brushing with olive oil.

In a large bowl, beat the eggs and then add your desired fillings (see Suggested Filling Combos below). Season with salt and black pepper. Pour the mixture into the prepared pan, making sure the eggs are distributed evenly.

Bake for 10 to 13 minutes, until the eggs are just set. Remove from the oven and slice into 8 squares or however you would prefer to serve.

Suggested Filling Combos

Southwestern: ½ cup diced ham + ½ cup diced green and red bell peppers. Heat a tablespoon of oil in a large skillet over medium heat, cook the peppers until soft, about 7 minutes, and add to the eggs with the ham.

Broccoli and Cheddar: ½ cup finely chopped broccoli florets + ¼ cup shredded cheddar cheese. Heat a tablespoon of oil in a large skillet over medium heat and

(recipe continues)

cook the broccoli until bright green, about 3 minutes, then add to the eggs. Once the eggs are in the sheet pan, sprinkle evenly with the cheese.

Pizza: ¼ cup sliced pepperoni + ½ cup quartered cherry tomatoes + ½ cup shredded mozzarella cheese. After pouring the eggs into the sheet pan, top evenly with pepperoni, tomatoes, and mozzarella.

Pesto Zucchini: 1 small zucchini, sliced into ⅛-inch-thick rounds + 3 tablespoons pesto sauce. After pouring the eggs into the sheet pan, scatter the zucchini slices around the eggs. When serving, place a teaspoon of pesto on each slice of your cooked eggs, so that all slices get some pesto.

INSPIRALIZED TIP

When cut into squares, these eggs are ideal for egg sandwiches, on toast or a bagel. Stack two slices or make a thinner sandwich with just one slice. Top with cheese or cream cheese and enjoy.

FEEDING LITTLES TIP

This is a great way to serve eggs to babies, as traditional scrambled eggs can be hard to pick up if we push them around the pan too much. These sheet pan eggs cut perfectly into strips and can be a more inviting texture for babies and kids who don't love eggs . . . yet.

vegan pumpkin waffles

time to prep: 20 minutes / time to cook: 15 to 45 minutes / makes: 8 waffles, serves 2 to 4 (2 to 4 waffles per serving)

I'll be honest. I'm a boxed mix kind of mom. Rarely do I make pancakes or waffles from scratch, but every once in a while, when I'm feeling ambitious, I make a big batch and freeze them. I like the flexibility to add in the ingredients I want, easily switch up the flavors, and in this case, make an egg- and dairy-free version for any guests that have allergies. I'm also a fan of anything pumpkin, but if you're not, you can easily swap in canned sweet potato.

Cooking spray or coconut oil, for greasing the waffle iron

1 cup whole wheat flour

1 teaspoon ground cinnamon

1 tablespoon baking powder

¼ teaspoon salt

1 cup non-dairy milk

½ cup pumpkin puree

2 tablespoons maple syrup, plus more for serving

2 tablespoons melted coconut oil

1 tablespoon apple cider vinegar

1 teaspoon vanilla extract

Fresh berries, for serving

Preheat the waffle iron. Grease the waffle iron with cooking spray or brush with coconut oil.

Place the flour, cinnamon, baking powder, and salt in a medium bowl, and stir to combine.

Place the milk, pumpkin, maple syrup, coconut oil, apple cider vinegar, and vanilla in another medium bowl, and whisk to combine.

Pour the wet ingredients into the bowl with the dry ingredients and whisk until smooth.

Pour the batter into the heated waffle iron and cook until the waffle is browned and firm to your preference, 5 to 7 minutes per waffle batch. Serve the waffles with fresh berries and maple syrup.

INSPIRALIZED TIP

If you want to give these waffles a seasonal taste, add 1 teaspoon pumpkin pie spice to the batter.

FEEDING LITTLES TIP

Slice these waffles into sticks for easy dipping into nut butter mixed with yogurt or maple syrup. There's something so satisfying about dunking, even as an adult. The dips are a great way to introduce a new food or allergen in a small and approachable manner.

sheet pan blueberry and butternut squash pancakes

time to prep: 10 minutes / time to cook: 15 to 17 minutes / makes: 12 pancakes squares (3 squares per serving = 4 servings)

After a few failed attempts at making heart-shaped pancakes, I decided to take matters into my own hands, turn my Choose Your Own Adventure Blender Muffins (page 61) into pancakes, bake them in a sheet pan, and grab my cookie cutters. I call that working smarter, not harder. Plus, if you have two kids who like their pancakes differently (*"Blueberry!" or "No, chocolate!"*), they can have it their way, without the extra time at the stovetop. And don't forget a generous drizzling of maple syrup.

Cooking spray, for greasing the sheet pan

½ cup cooked cubed butternut squash

2 ripe bananas

4 large eggs

½ cup rolled oats

2 tablespoons ground flaxseed

½ teaspoon ground cinnamon

½ cup blueberries

Maple syrup, for serving

Preheat the oven to 350°F. Grease a 10 x 12½ -inch sheet pan with cooking spray.

Blend the squash, bananas, eggs, oats, flaxseed, and cinnamon together in a blender until smooth. Pour the batter onto the prepared sheet pan. Shake the pan until the batter is evenly spread. Top evenly with the blueberries.

Bake for 15 to 17 minutes or until the pancake is firm and the edges have browned.

Slice into 12 square pieces or other shapes and serve with maple syrup.

INSPIRALIZED TIP

If you have it, grease the sheet pan with unrefined coconut oil for a sweet coconut flavor.

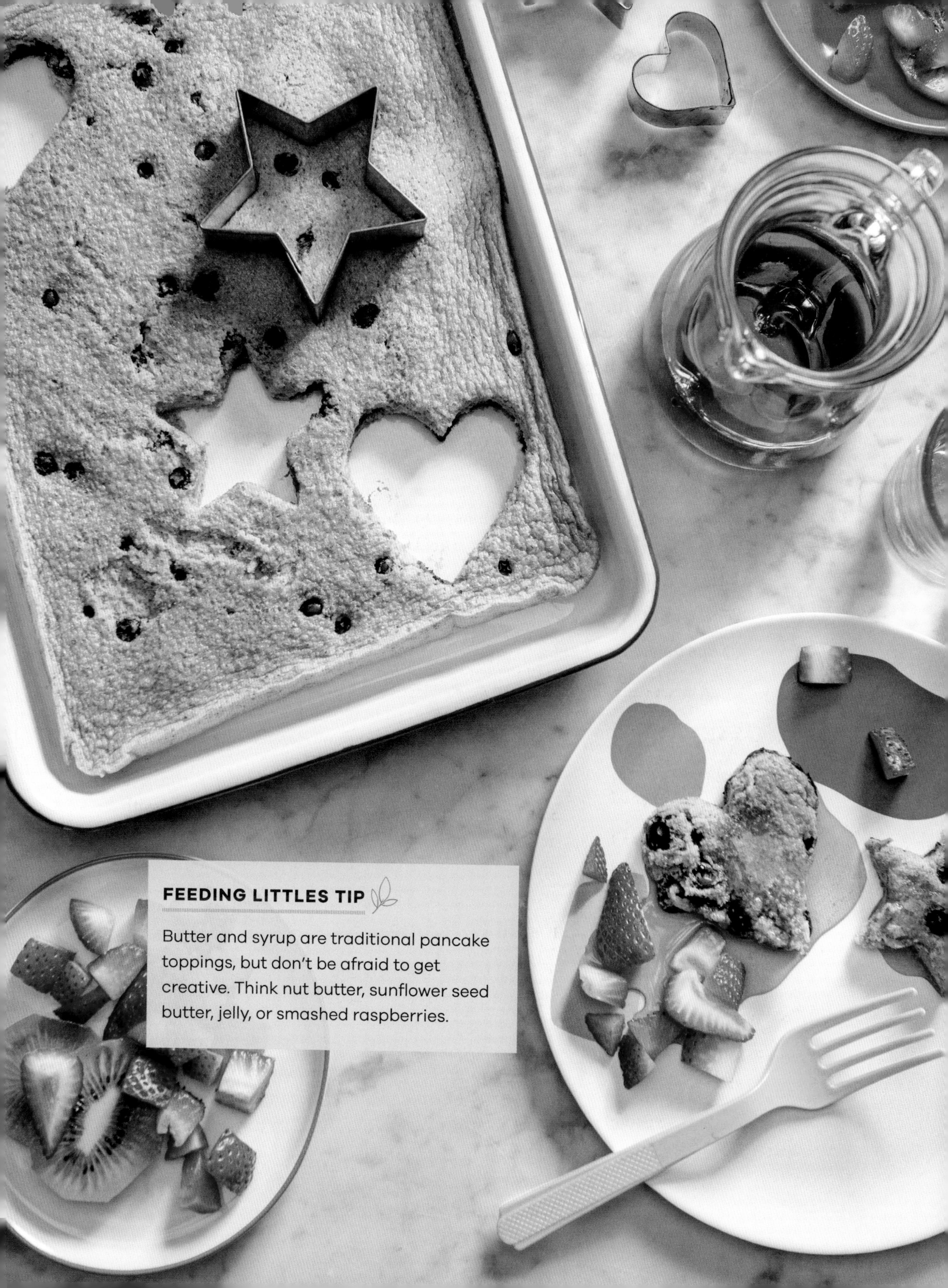

FEEDING LITTLES TIP

Butter and syrup are traditional pancake toppings, but don't be afraid to get creative. Think nut butter, sunflower seed butter, jelly, or smashed raspberries.

overnight french toast casserole with coconut whipped cream

time to prep: 15 minutes + overnight / time to cook: 35 to 40 minutes / serves: 6 to 8

I remember my mother making French toast on holidays and birthdays, but it always took so much preparation and time. If she had only known about this version, we would have gotten to enjoy it more often. If you love French toast but don't want to deal with the mess, the dishes, and the stovetop time, try this casserole. It has the delightful consistency of bread pudding, topped with a quick coconut whipped cream for extra sweetness. Something tells me more French toast is in your future.

For the casserole

Cooking spray, for greasing the baking dish

1 loaf (1 pound) unsliced sourdough bread

8 large eggs

3 cups non-dairy milk of choice (if not dairy-free, substitute cow's milk if desired)

½ cup maple syrup

1 tablespoon vanilla extract

1 teaspoon ground cinnamon

For the coconut whipped cream

1 can (14 ounces) full-fat coconut milk, refrigerated overnight placed upside down

½ teaspoon vanilla extract

2 teaspoons maple syrup (optional to sweeten)

Grease a 9 x 13-inch baking dish with cooking spray and set aside.

Slice or tear the bread into bite-sized cubed pieces. Arrange in an even layer in the prepared baking dish.

Whisk the eggs together in a large bowl. Add the milk, maple syrup, and vanilla, and whisk thoroughly to combine. Add the cinnamon and whisk again. Pour the mixture over the bread in the baking dish. Cover tightly with foil or plastic wrap and refrigerate overnight.

When ready to bake, preheat the oven to 350°F. Uncover the casserole and push down any pieces of bread that may be poking out so they are mostly submerged. Bake for 35 to 40 minutes or until the top is browned and slightly crispy.

While the casserole bakes, prepare the coconut whipped cream. Open the upside-down can of coconut milk carefully (don't shake!) and scoop out the thickened cream at the top. Place in a medium mixing bowl, and discard the liquids (or save for future use). Add the vanilla and maple syrup (if using) and, using a hand mixer, beat until creamy and smooth, about 1 minute. Once the whipped coconut cream is prepared, place in the refrigerator until ready to use, so it hardens further.

Once it has cooled slightly, serve the casserole with the whipped cream.

INSPIRALIZED TIP

Challah French toast is also amazing; if you decide to use it, toast the challah slightly before soaking overnight so it's not mushy.

FEEDING LITTLES TIP

If serving this to a baby, try unsweetened yogurt on the side instead of the coconut whipped cream.

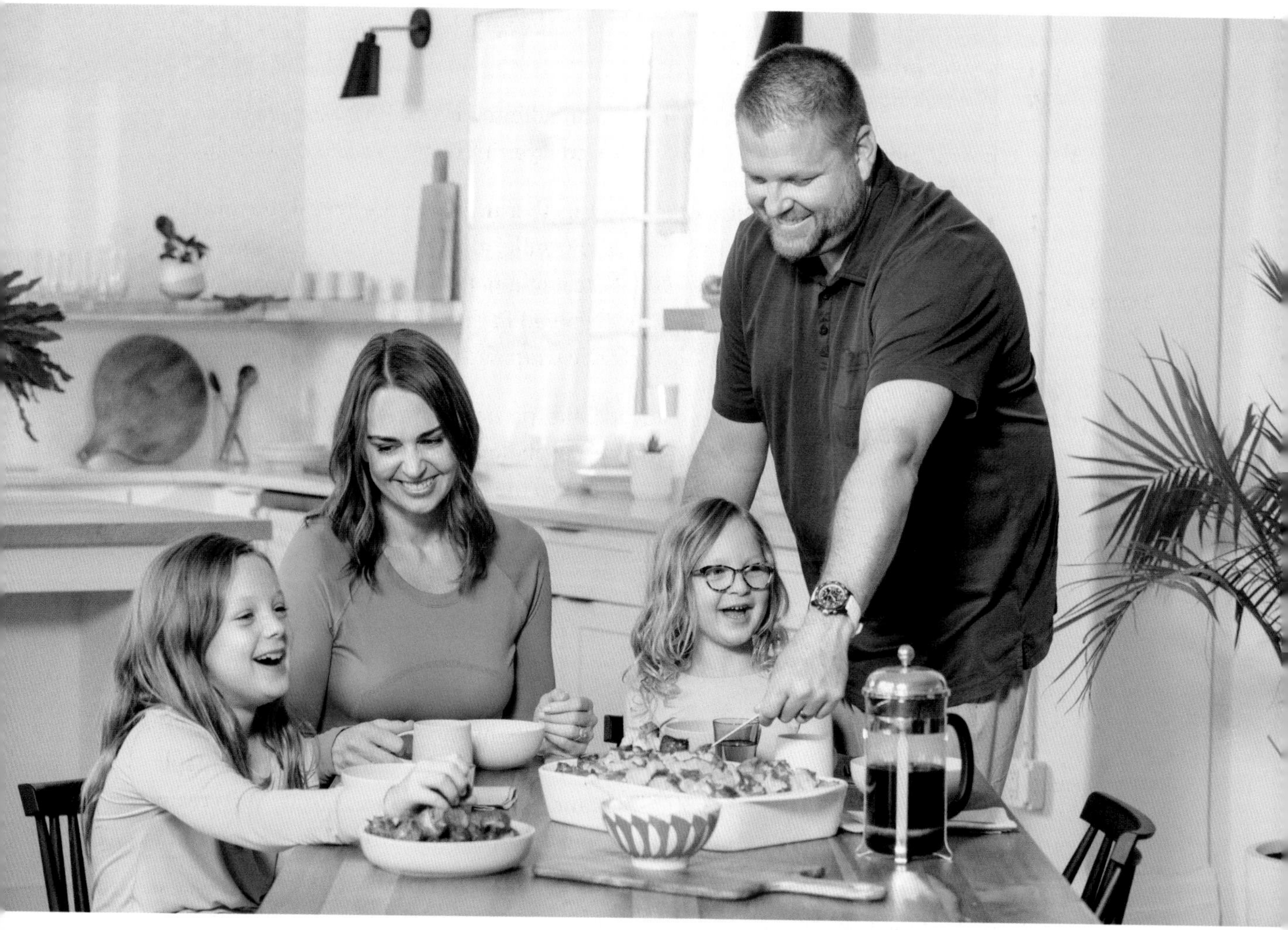

beach vacation breakfast smoothie

time to prep: 10 minutes / makes: 2 smoothies

During the COVID pandemic, there were a lot of endless days at home. Somewhere along the way, we started having picnics. We'd gather stuffed animals, blankets, books, and snacks, and set up in the living room. It's funny how something so simple can thrill little kids (and liven up the day for parents, too), but it worked. One time my son asked for a beach picnic, and we pulled out the beach toys from the basement, put our suits on, grabbed towels, and made this Beach Vacation Breakfast Smoothie. It is a non-alcoholic, nutrition-packed version of a piña colada with that nostalgic coconut flavor.

1 cup frozen pineapple

1 frozen banana

1 cup canned unsweetened full-fat coconut milk

½ cup shredded carrot

1 tablespoon shredded coconut, plus more for garnish

Pineapple wedges, for serving (optional)

Place the pineapple, banana, coconut milk, carrot, and shredded coconut in a large high-speed blender. Blend until creamy. Garnish with shredded coconut and a pineapple wedge, if desired. Serve.

INSPIRALIZED TIP

This is a family cookbook, so I'm not sure if I should be saying this, but if you drink alcohol, add a 2-ounce rum floater on top of your smoothie. A nourishing beverage indeed.

FEEDING LITTLES TIP

This smoothie is great as a snack or served on the side of a meal. For more staying power, serve it with food with protein, like peanut butter toast or an egg.

everything bagel broccoli and cheddar egg donuts

time to prep: 15 minutes / time to cook: 20 minutes / makes: 6 donuts

I'm always looking for new ways to serve up eggs, and these savory donuts are extra grabbable for tiny hands. I also love that they are shallow, so the whole donut turns golden brown. We serve these with buttered toast, fruit, and ketchup or hot sauce.

- **Cooking spray, for greasing the donut pan**
- **1 teaspoon extra-virgin olive oil**
- **1 cup chopped broccoli florets**
- **¼ teaspoon garlic powder**
- **Salt and pepper**
- **5 large eggs**
- **1 tablespoon everything bagel seasoning**
- **6 tablespoons shredded cheddar cheese**

FEEDING LITTLES TIP

These egg donuts really pop with most vegetables. Experiment with mixing in chopped bell peppers, onions, or mushrooms.

Preheat the oven to 400°F. Grease 6 cavities of a donut pan with cooking spray.

Heat the oil in a small skillet until shimmering, then add the broccoli. Season with the garlic powder and salt and pepper, and cook until fork-tender and browned, about 5 minutes. To speed up the process, add a few tablespoons of water to steam-cook in the pan. Remove from the heat.

While the broccoli cooks, whisk the eggs in a medium bowl. Set aside.

In each donut cavity, add just enough broccoli florets to cover the bottom. Sprinkle with a pinch of everything bagel seasoning. Using a ladle or the bowl directly, pour in the whisked eggs to fill a little more than halfway to the top. Sprinkle with another pinch of everything bagel seasoning and cheese, about a tablespoon of cheese per donut.

Bake for 10 to 15 minutes or until the eggs are completely set. Remove from the oven and let cool until the pan is ready to handle to pop the donuts out. Serve immediately or freeze for future use (they last about 3 months in the freezer).

INSPIRALIZED TIP

These donuts can easily be turned into muffins by pouring the batter into a muffin pan instead and baking 3 to 5 minutes longer. Double the recipe to get 6 large muffins.

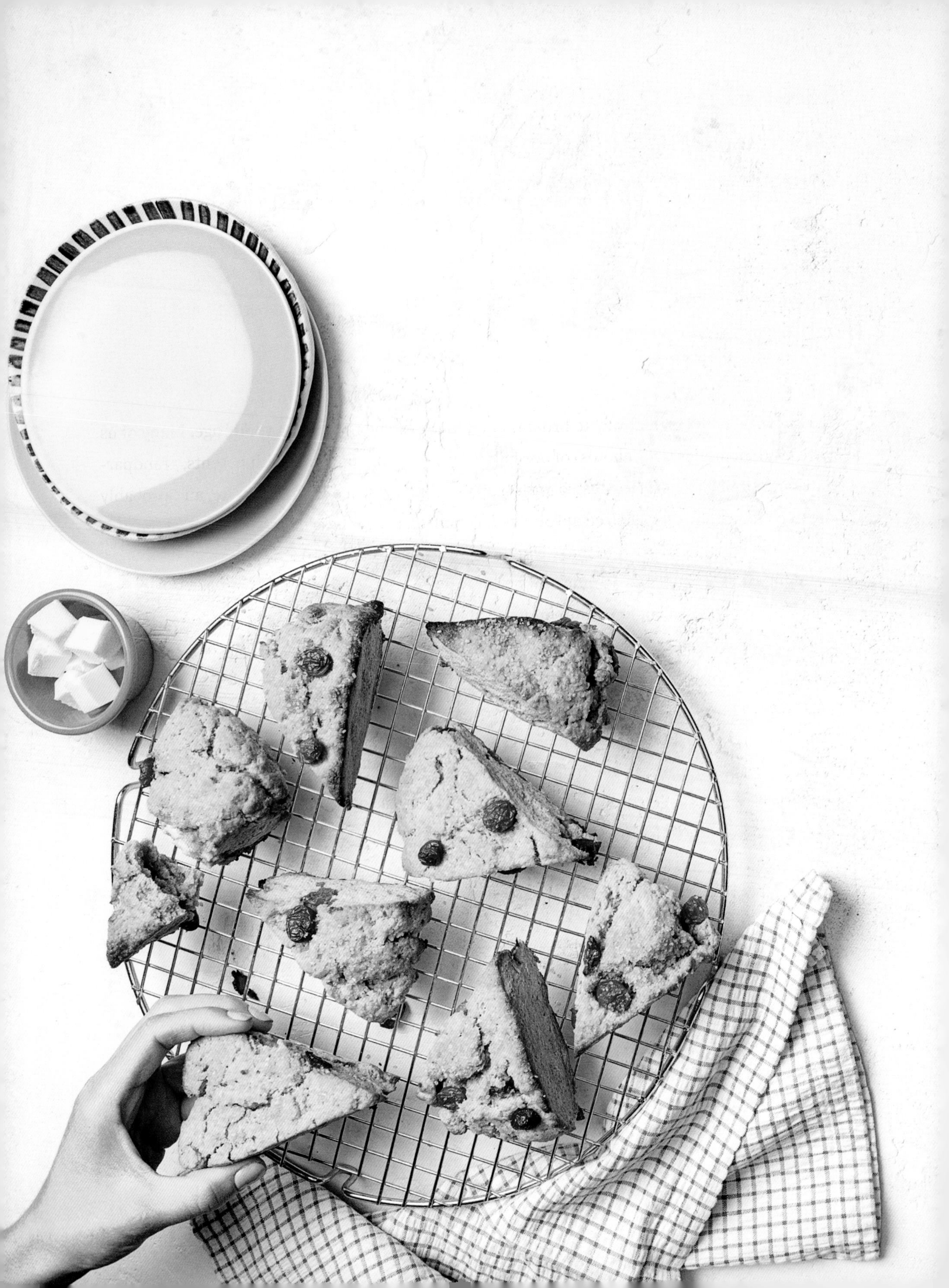

baked bites and snacks

Baking with kids is a great way to bring them into the kitchen, even at a young age. Many of us have fond memories (and photos) of our baking and cooking moments with parents, grandparents, and siblings. Our faces dusted with flour, our lips smudged with chocolate, and probably dressed in an adorably oversized apron. Even if you don't have these memories from your childhood, hopefully you're ready to make them with your own family.

Baking teaches our littles so much more than motor skills. Kids learn early math (measuring ingredients, talking about measurements, halving and doubling recipes), nutrition (talking about the benefits of all the ingredients), following directions and learning the order of things, sensory awareness (textures, colors, odors, and more), and even art. Baking is also a great opportunity to encourage language development by talking through every step and asking questions like, "Is this dough sticky or smooth?"

And frankly, many of us need to learn a little P-A-T-I-E-N-C-E. Cooking with kids definitely requires it, and it's a good quality to model in front of our children, especially when all we're thinking about is the mess afterwards.

While we encourage you to bring your kiddo into the kitchen, many of us are mess-averse or don't love to bake. If that sounds like you, here are some tips to get started:

- Prepare, prepare, prepare. Sometimes we don't have the luxury of prepping ahead of time, but if you can swing it, preparation is the key to success. Especially for smaller children, measure everything out and place in developmentally appropriate bowls, cups, and containers. Mugs with handles work great for little hands. And, of course, use age-appropriate utensils (you may want to invest in toddler baking utensils). Make sure you have all needed utensils and appliances nearby.

- Consider using a learning tower for children eighteen months and older. It is a great way to bring your child up to counter height, and helps keep your kiddo engaged (instead of wandering around the kitchen as you bake). You can use step stools for older kids, or clip-on high chairs for your younger kiddos, so they can play around with ingredients and utensils while you do the heavy lifting.

- Start small. Perhaps simply ask your child to crack eggs into a bowl every time you're baking something that calls for eggs. Then, when you're having your child help you with the full recipe and they go to crack eggs, their muscle memory will kick in and your child will feel more confident. They don't have to help with every step, and it's important to set safety boundaries along the way.

- Embrace the mess (and try not to stress). We know that's easier said than done, but when you expect a mess it's easier to focus on being present and having fun. Don't bake when you're pressed for time. Clean as you go or place a plastic tablecloth over the work area, but remember that getting messy is part of the fun for your kiddos. If an egg drops and breaks on the floor, just go with it.

- Ahead of time, give your toddler a choice so they feel empowered. Let them look at pictures in a cookbook (like this one!) or a magazine and point to what they want to make, which might ultimately encourage them to have a taste, as they are more involved in the process.

- Make it official with a toddler chef's hat and apron. Once they put it on, they'll be in baking mode and it'll make the experience that much more special.

- If you're making something that you want to be "perfect" (like a cake for a special occasion) and you don't want your kiddo dumping a full jar of sprinkles on top, make a little extra on the side and let your child have at it.

- Explain the joyful experience of sharing food with your littles, encouraging them by saying something like, "We'll make sure to save one or two muffins for Grandma and Grandpa; they would love some!"

Whether you decide to make these recipes with your kids or not, this section is meant mostly for snack-type baked goods. While some of them can certainly be enjoyed as desserts (such as our Glazed Chocolate-Zucchini Donuts, on page 65), they're meant more for snack-time enjoyment (like our Peanut Butter and Blueberry Muffins with chia, on page 67) or food for on-the-go (like Chickpea and Coconut Bites, on page 69). Many of these recipes can even be enjoyed as full meals, such as the Choose Your Own Adventure Blender Muffins (page 61), served at breakfast with a side of bright berries.

Some of the baked goods and desserts in this section contain added sugars. While some current guidelines recommend waiting until age two to introduce added sugars, every family approaches it differently. Some families will wait until their children are one to two years of age to serve added sugars, while others start in infancy, especially if there are older siblings at home. This is an individual choice, as sugar eventually becomes a part of most kids' eating landscapes and can be part of a balanced diet. It's up to you when you decide to introduce it.

Please note: Avoid any honey with infants younger than twelve months of age. It can increase their risk of infant botulism (although the risk is very low), so omit the honey for any recipe that calls for it.

strawberry oatmeal squares

time to prep: 30 minutes / time to cook: 40 to 45 minutes / makes: 12 squares

There's nothing better than a recipe that is portable, prepable, and can double as a meal and a snack. These oatmeal squares are ready to enjoy all week long for breakfast, in your kid's lunch box, or as a three p.m. pick-me-up. And the sweeter your strawberries, the more their natural sugars release in the oven and pack an even sweeter punch. Next time you're in peak season, hit the strawberry fields with your little ones and make these oatmeal squares together.

Cooking spray, for greasing the dish

2 cups rolled oats

1 teaspoon ground cinnamon

1 teaspoon baking powder

¼ teaspoon fine-grain sea salt

¾ cup sliced strawberries

1 cup non-dairy milk

⅓ cup unsweetened applesauce

2 tablespoons maple syrup

2 flax eggs*

1½ tablespoons coconut oil, melted and cooled

1 teaspoon vanilla extract

Preheat the oven to 375°F. Grease an 8 x 8-inch baking dish with cooking spray.

Place the oats, cinnamon, baking powder, and salt in a large mixing bowl. Whisk to combine.

Mash half of the strawberries and place in a smaller mixing bowl along with the milk, applesauce, maple syrup, flax eggs, coconut oil, and vanilla. Stir until blended.

Pour the wet ingredients into the dry mixture and stir well to combine. Pour into the baking dish. Top with the remaining strawberry slices, pushing down into the mixture.

Bake for 40 to 45 minutes, until the top is nice and golden. Remove your baked oatmeal from the oven and let it cool completely before cutting into squares, as it will firm up as it cools.

* To make a flax egg, stir together 1 tablespoon of ground flaxseed with 2 tablespoons of water and let it sit in the refrigerator for 10 minutes or until thickened.

FEEDING LITTLES TIP

To add extra protein and brain-boosting fats, top the squares with smooth almond or peanut butter for a PB&J flavor.

INSPIRALIZED TIP

Add extra nutrition without changing the look or flavor of these oatmeal squares by stirring a tablespoon of chia seeds into the dry ingredients.

choose your own adventure blender muffins

time to prep: 10 minutes / time to cook: 22 to 25 minutes / makes: about 6 muffins (varies)

Welcome to the ultimate family muffin that is truly BYO: build your own! The equation is easy: banana + oats + eggs + flaxseed + shredded vegetable + seasonings. I love adding cinnamon and vanilla extract to keep it simple, but you can stir in chocolate chips, pumpkin pie or chai spice, or berries. These muffins are packed with nutrition and are an easy way to use up leftover vegetables and reduce food waste. And since this is a blender recipe, it's perfect for safely making with your kids. Be warned: you may want to make a double or triple batch—these are so yummy and portable, they'll be gone before you know it.

The Basic Blender Muffin Recipe

Cooking spray, for greasing the muffin pan

2 large eggs

4 ounces raw vegetable (for example, shredded carrots, spinach, shredded beets)

1 large, ripe banana

¼ cup rolled oats

1 tablespoon ground flaxseed

¼ teaspoon vanilla extract

⅛ teaspoon ground cinnamon

Preheat the oven to 350°F. Grease a muffin pan with cooking spray or place silicone muffin liners on a baking sheet.

Place the eggs, vegetable, banana, oats, flaxseed, vanilla, and cinnamon in a high-speed blender. Blend until creamy.

Pour the batter into the muffin cups and bake for 22 to 25 minutes or until the edges are golden brown and the muffins are firm. Serve immediately. To store, refrigerate for 3 to 5 days or freeze for up to 3 months.

(recipe continues)

Other Flavor Equations

Blueberry

Base recipe using parsnips or butternut squash, raw or roasted until fork-tender + ⅓ cup blueberries (fold blueberries in after blending base recipe)

Pumpkin Spice

Base recipe minus the vegetable + ⅓ cup pumpkin puree + ½ teaspoon pumpkin pie spice

Banana Nut

Base recipe using ⅓ cup cooked butternut squash + ¼ cup finely chopped pecans (stir pecans in after blending base recipe) + ¼ banana thinly sliced (place 1 banana slice in each batter-filled muffin cup)

Carrot Cake

Base recipe using ⅔ cup shredded carrot + ¼ teaspoon ground ginger + ¼ cup finely chopped pecans (sprinkle the pecans on top of the muffin batter)

INSPIRALIZED TIP

There are a few nuances to keep in mind, especially when you're creating your own flavor combinations. Most of all, the banana size and ripeness is important—you want a large banana that's ripe but not browned and overripe. For extra-large bananas, adjust by using more oats (and vice versa—a smaller banana means less oats). Keep trying your own combinations of banana, oats, and vegetables until you reach your family's desired consistency.

FEEDING LITTLES TIP

Banana allergy? Try ½ cup applesauce instead. If your child is easily constipated when eating banana or applesauce, try ½ cup pumpkin puree and a sweetener of choice to taste, like a date, maple syrup, or honey (for children over one).

pumpkin and chocolate snacking loaf with chia

time to prep: 15 minutes / time to cook: 40 minutes / makes: 1 loaf

Whether you're serving this vegetable-packed snack warmed with butter, drizzled with a creamy nut butter, or alongside yogurt and fruit, this loaf is for all occasions. It is dense—making it ideal for slicing into special shapes or strips that fit nicely in small hands—and thick enough to be served with utensils if desired. The chocolate chips are a welcome ingredient for many picky eaters, but don't be afraid to omit them—it's still sweet enough thanks to the banana and applesauce.

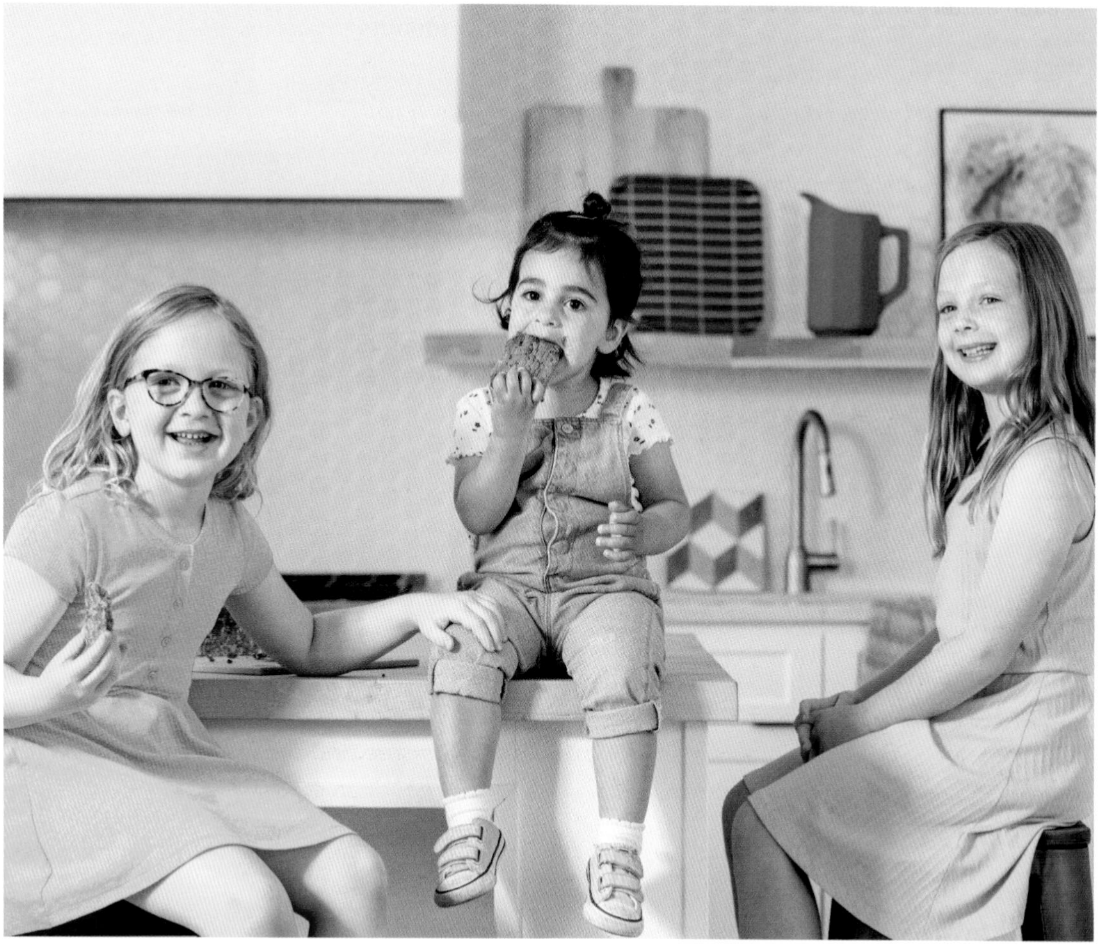

(recipe continues)

Coconut oil or cooking spray, for greasing the pan

1¼ cups plus 2 tablespoons whole wheat flour or gluten-free all-purpose flour

1 cup rolled oats

1 teaspoon baking powder

½ teaspoon baking soda

1 teaspoon ground cinnamon

1 tablespoon chia seeds

1 large banana, mashed (you can replace with ¼ cup of applesauce, but the bread will be a bit mushy—make sure to bake for an extra 5 minutes and let it cool completely before slicing for best results)

1 can (15 ounces) pumpkin puree

1 teaspoon vanilla extract

1 cup unsweetened applesauce

½ cup non-dairy chocolate chips

Preheat the oven to 350°F. Grease a standard loaf pan with coconut oil or cooking spray.

Mix together the flour, oats, baking powder, baking soda, cinnamon, and chia seeds in a large bowl. Add the banana, pumpkin, vanilla, applesauce, and ¼ cup of the chocolate chips and stir together until combined.

Pour the mixture into the loaf pan and smooth with the back of a spoon. Sprinkle the remaining ¼ cup of chocolate chips over the top and press them into the batter. Bake for 40 minutes or until browned on the outside and a toothpick comes out clean. The loaf firms up substantially during the cooling process.

For best results, let it cool for 20 minutes. Slice and serve or freeze for up to 3 months.

FEEDING LITTLES TIP

This is a perfect recipe to bake with your toddler or older child. The ingredients are simple for younger kids, and older kids can strengthen their measuring and math skills.

INSPIRALIZED TIP

To get the most out of this recipe, switch up the vegetable puree. Canned butternut squash or sweet potato work equally well.

glazed chocolate-zucchini donuts

time to prep: 20 minutes / time to cook: 20 to 25 minutes / makes: 12 donuts

One of my fondest childhood memories is staring out at our driveway from the dining room windows every Sunday morning, waiting for my father to round the corner, because Sunday mornings meant Dunkin' Donuts. If you're looking for an at-home alternative to the donut shop, we're here for you. Kids love the novelty of a homemade donut, and chocolate pairs surprisingly well with zucchini. If you have a child that can't stand zucchini, omit it and enjoy these as classic chocolate donuts. You just may be inspired to start your own weekend tradition.

Cooking spray, for greasing the donut pan

½ cup coconut flour

¼ cup tapioca flour

¾ teaspoon baking soda

¼ teaspoon salt

1 teaspoon ground cinnamon

1½ tablespoons cacao powder

3 large eggs

3 tablespoons maple syrup

2 teaspoons vanilla extract

2 tablespoons unsweetened plain almond milk

1 tablespoon coconut oil, melted and slightly cooled

1 ripe banana, very well mashed

½ cup finely grated zucchini

½ cup chocolate chips

Preheat the oven to 350°F. Grease a 12-cavity donut pan with cooking spray. Set aside.

Mix the coconut flour, tapioca flour, baking soda, salt, cinnamon, and cacao powder together in a medium bowl.

Mix the eggs, maple syrup, vanilla, almond milk, coconut oil, and banana together in another medium bowl.

Add the dry ingredients to the bowl with the wet ingredients. Place the zucchini in a cheesecloth or paper towel and squeeze out any excess moisture. Add the zucchini to the batter mixture and stir until the batter is combined.

Fill the donut cavities halfway with the batter, making sure to leave the centers open to create the donut hole when baking. Bake for 20 to 25 minutes or until a toothpick comes out clean when you pierce the center of a donut, and the donut is firm on the outside. Pop the donuts out carefully and set aside on a sheet of parchment paper.

Place a small saucepan over medium-high heat and add in the chocolate chips. Let the pan heat, stirring frequently, until the chocolate chips are fully melted.

Drizzle the chocolate over the donuts. Enjoy immediately, or wait 20 minutes for the chocolate to harden.

(recipe continues)

INSPIRALIZED TIP

For those with allergies or dietary restrictions, substitute ½ cup of applesauce for the banana.

FEEDING LITTLES TIP

If your child is reluctant to try these donuts but loves milk, encourage them to dunk the donut so they can become more comfortable with this new texture.

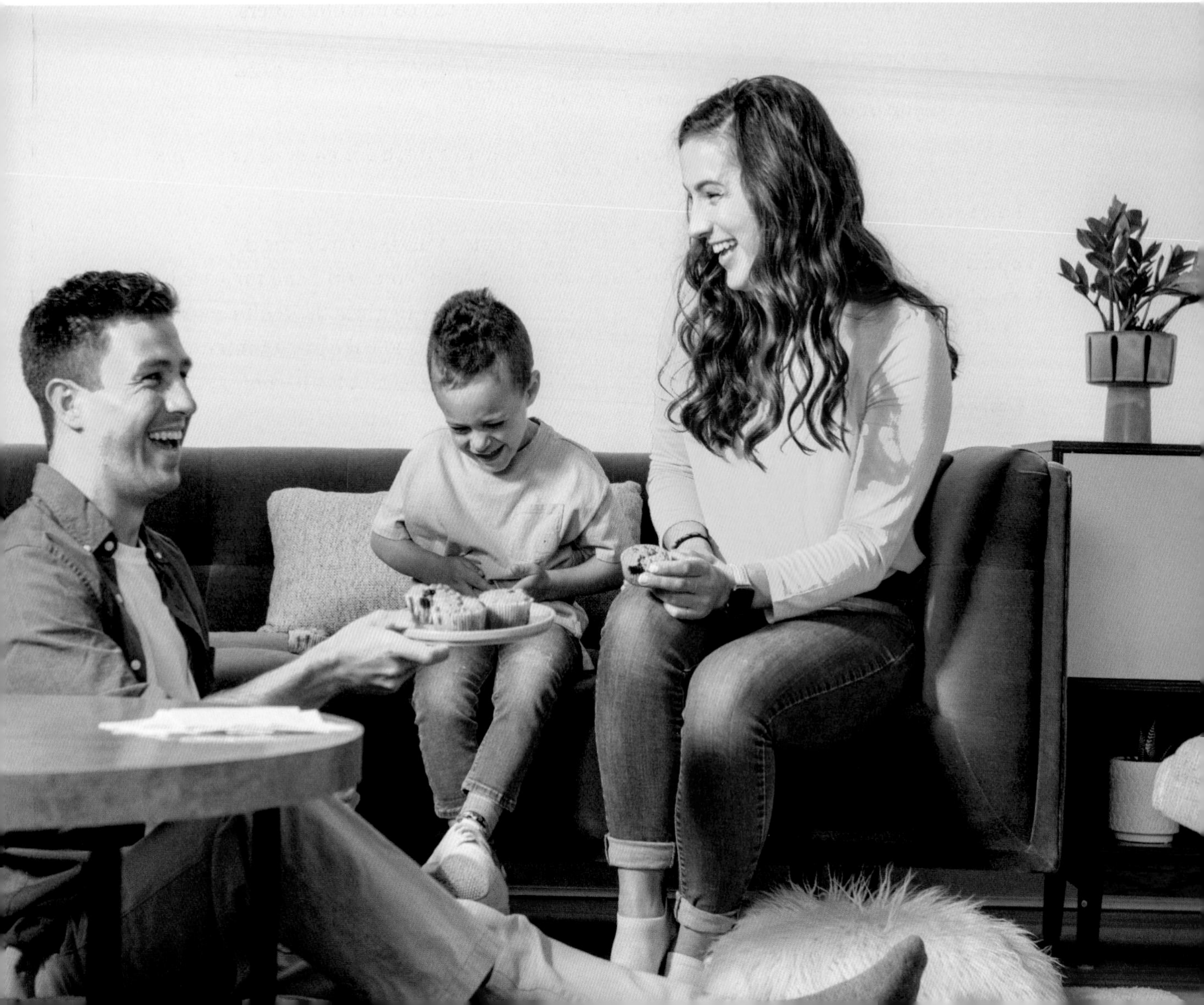

peanut butter and blueberry muffins

time to prep: 10 minutes / time to cook: 20 minutes / makes: 10 to 12 muffins

Every baker should have a solid blueberry muffin in their repertoire. Thanks to ingredients that are naturally sweet, these muffins don't need added sugar, making them great for babies six months and older. These are the kinds of easy meals that you'll pack for snacks and lunches and want to have in your freezer for last-minute breakfasts. Pro tip—if you eat these fresh out of the oven while the blueberries are freshly burst, you'll get a peanut-butter-and-jelly vibe in each bite—just be careful not to burn the roof of your mouth.

Cooking spray, for greasing the muffin pan

½ cup peanut butter

½ cup applesauce

2 large eggs

1 teaspoon vanilla extract

1 cup almond flour (regular whole wheat flour works, too, but the muffins won't be as fluffy)

1½ teaspoons baking powder

1 tablespoon chia seeds

½ cup blueberries (frozen work well, too)

Preheat the oven to 350°F. Grease a 12-cup muffin pan with cooking spray or use silicone muffin liners.

Mix together the peanut butter, applesauce, eggs, and vanilla in a medium bowl.

Mix together the almond flour, baking powder, and chia seeds in a large bowl.

Add the wet ingredients to the bowl with the dry ingredients, stir to combine thoroughly, and then stir in the blueberries. Spoon the batter into the muffin cups, filling two-thirds of the way, and bake for 20 minutes or until firm and golden brown. Let sit for 10 minutes to cool and then serve.

INSPIRALIZED TIP

If you have a nut allergy, substitute sun butter. If you prefer another nut butter, both almond and cashew work and give the muffins a slightly different flavor.

FEEDING LITTLES TIP

This recipe is a great way to serve allergenic foods like peanut butter, eggs, and almond flour to babies and toddlers.

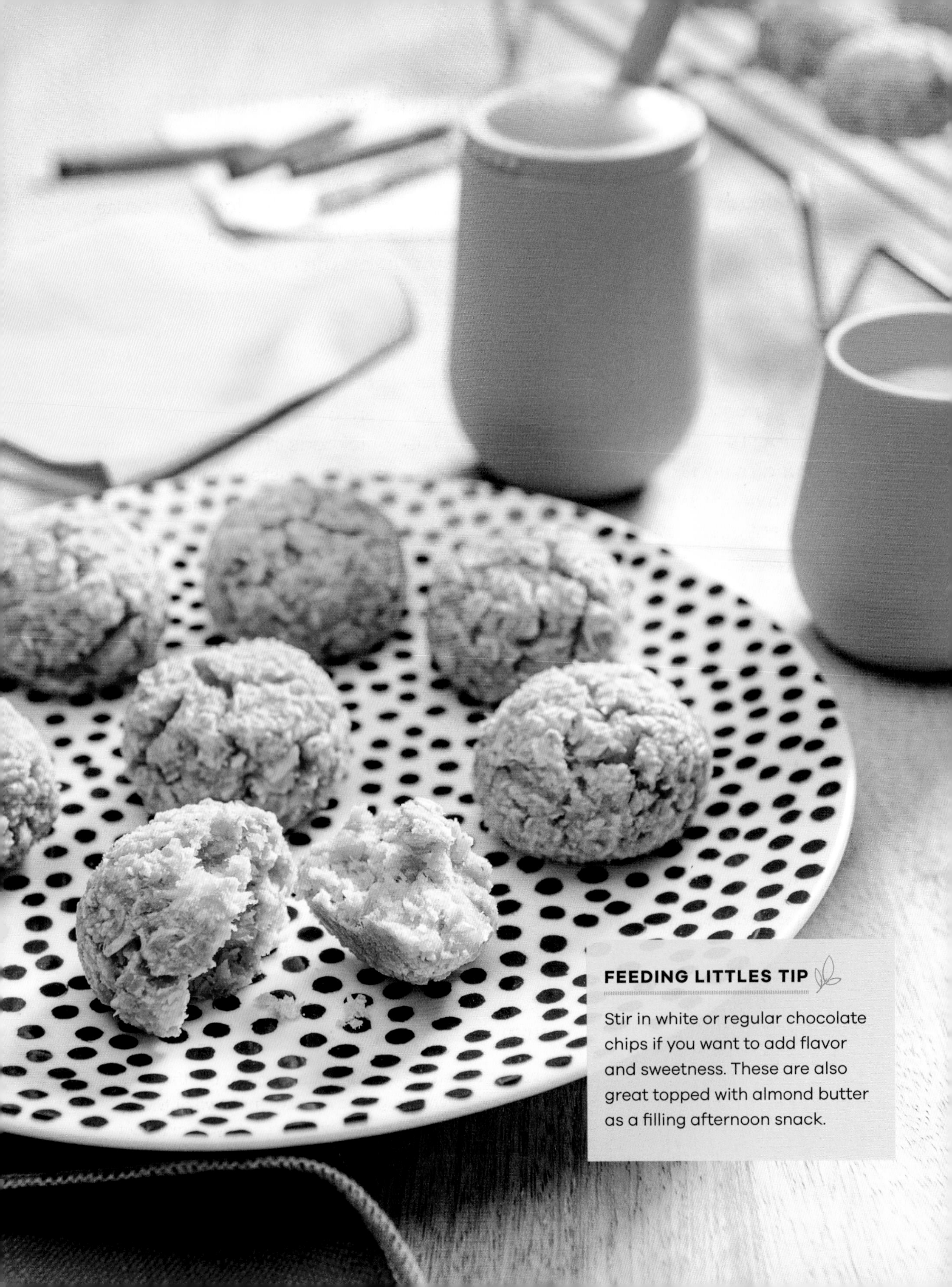

FEEDING LITTLES TIP

Stir in white or regular chocolate chips if you want to add flavor and sweetness. These are also great topped with almond butter as a filling afternoon snack.

chickpea and coconut bites

time to prep: 15 minutes / time to cook: 15 to 20 minutes / makes: 20 cookies

Chickpeas (aka garbanzo beans) are one of my favorite foods because they're so versatile; I always have them on hand—batch cooked and stored in the freezer or a can of them in the pantry. If you end up cooking with a lot of chickpeas as well, you may find it more economical to cook them yourself (from dry) and keep them in the freezer for up to 3 months. There are many methods, but I love to place a pound of dry chickpeas in a slow cooker with 7 cups of water and cook on high for 3 to 4 hours or low for 6 to 8 hours. Cooking your own chickpeas also preserves more of their nutritional integrity! You'll see throughout this book that I use chickpeas in many ways, from a "tuna" salad to curries, and even in a cookie. Their taste is mild enough that they absorb the flavors of whatever you're making. Plus, they are an excellent source of protein and fiber, so they'll keep you and your little ones satiated. How many snacks can say that?

1 can (15½ ounces) chickpeas, drained and rinsed

1 cup rolled oats

2 large eggs

½ cup unsweetened shredded coconut

¼ cup maple syrup

1 teaspoon vanilla extract

1 teaspoon baking powder

Preheat the oven to 350°F. Line a baking sheet with parchment paper.

Place the chickpeas, oats, eggs, coconut, maple syrup, vanilla, and baking powder into a food processor or high-speed blender and pulse until no whole chickpeas remain.

Using a tablespoon, place spoonfuls of the blended mixture onto the prepared baking sheet and use the tablespoon to smooth into circular (cookie) shapes.

Transfer the bites to the oven and bake for 15 to 20 minutes or until golden brown at the edges and bottom. Let cool before serving. Freeze for up to 3 months.

INSPIRALIZED TIP

If you've baked these bites for 20 minutes but they still seem soft (even though they're golden brown at the edges), don't worry—they'll harden as they sit and cool.

megan's favorite peanut butter cookies

time to prep: 5 minutes / time to cook: 11 to 13 minutes / makes: 30 to 40 cookies (depends on amount of sugar used)

True story: Megan tested these cookies six times to get them just right. She wanted an easily adaptable recipe that was completely allergy-friendly, and now people ask for her "famous" cookies. Depending on how long you bake them and how much sugar you use, they can go from soft to crispy, so this recipe is truly one-size-fits-all.

2 cups peanut butter (modify with almond butter or sun butter, if desired)

2 cups coconut sugar or brown sugar (modify with 1 cup for less sweetness)

2 large eggs (modify with 4 egg replacers)

1 teaspoon baking soda

1 (10-ounce) bag chocolate chips (modify with dairy-free chocolate chips)

Preheat the oven to 350°F. Line two baking sheets with parchment paper.

Combine the peanut butter, sugar, eggs, and baking soda in a large mixing bowl. Using an electric mixer or spoon, mix together until combined. Fold in the chocolate chips and stir to combine thoroughly.

Using a tablespoon, scoop out tablespoons of the dough and form into balls. Place 1 inch apart onto the prepared baking sheets. Bake for 11 to 13 minutes or until the cookies are set and lightly golden brown. Allow to cool for at least 5 minutes to harden up before serving.

INSPIRALIZED TIP

Tolerance for sweetness varies greatly. If you like a sweet cookie, go for the full 2 cups of sugar. If not, try 1 cup, or anywhere in between. And remember that the chocolate chips also add a sweet kick. Sugar makes up a significant volume of the dough, so be aware that you might want to use the full 2 cups of sugar to stick closer to 40 cookies.

FEEDING LITTLES TIP

Since these cookies don't contain flour, they tend to burn more easily on the bottom if you bake them too long. Watch for a somewhat firm, slightly browned top.

nut-free apple pie energy balls

time to prep: 20 minutes / makes: 12 balls

Apple pie is nostalgia in a bite, which is why I had to include it here. Energy balls are exactly as they sound: a ball of protein, fiber, and brain-boosting fats, typically derived from nuts and fruit. Here, we use apples, dates, chia seeds, and flaxseed, which are all energy-enhancing foods that help keep you satiated and provide that midday boost. These apple pie balls have gotten my family through long road trips and hangry moods (both for adults and toddlers), and you'll want to keep them around, too.

1 cup freeze-dried apples (the crunchy ones, not the soft ones)

½ cup rolled oats

2 tablespoons ground flaxseed

1 tablespoon chia seeds

¼ teaspoon ground cinnamon

1 cup soft Medjool dates, pitted

Place the apples in a food processor and pulse until no large pieces remain. Add the oats, flaxseed, chia seeds, and cinnamon, and pulse until medium-coarse. Transfer to a medium mixing bowl and wipe out the food processor.

Place the dates in the food processor and process until the dates stick together into a ball. Add the dates to the apple mixture and knead the ingredients together until combined evenly. Roll the mixture into balls, and store in an airtight container in the refrigerator for a week or in the freezer for up to a month.

INSPIRALIZED TIP

The two most important ingredients here are the apples and the dates. If you use soft dried apples, it won't work, so make sure you use the crunchy, chip-like freeze-dried apples. As for the dates, you should be able to mush them with your fingers to check for softness. If they don't have give, soak them for 15 minutes in hot water, and make sure you pat them completely dry before using them in the recipe.

FEEDING LITTLES TIP

Crumble into pieces and serve as a topping for yogurt when you need a convenient breakfast option.

chia seed banana bread

time to prep: 15 minutes / time to cook: 30 to 35 minutes / serves: 8

In our household, we call this "nanny bread," because "nanny" (for banana) was one of my son's first words, and I never want to forget how cute he sounded saying it. This perfectly sweet, nutrient-packed banana bread includes ingredients that will nourish your family while not sacrificing that classic flavor.

Cooking spray, for greasing the loaf pan

¼ cup coconut flour

1½ cups almond flour

2 tablespoons chia seeds

1 teaspoon baking soda

1 teaspoon baking powder

1 teaspoon ground cinnamon

¼ teaspoon ground nutmeg

¼ teaspoon salt

3 large eggs

¼ cup maple syrup

1 teaspoon vanilla extract

2 tablespoons almond milk

1 tablespoon coconut oil, melted and slightly cooled

2 ripe bananas, well mashed, and 1 ripe banana, sliced into ¼-inch-thick rounds

½ cup walnuts, well chopped

Preheat the oven to 350°F. Grease a loaf pan with cooking spray (preferably coconut oil spray) and set aside.

Combine the coconut flour, almond flour, chia seeds, baking soda, baking powder, cinnamon, nutmeg, and salt in a large mixing bowl.

Combine the eggs, maple syrup, vanilla, almond milk, coconut oil, and the mashed bananas together in another large mixing bowl.

Add the dry ingredients to the bowl with the wet ingredients and stir well until smooth. Fold in the walnuts. Transfer the batter into the loaf pan. Set the banana slices on top, pressing into the batter slightly. Bake for 30 to 35 minutes or until a toothpick comes out clean when you pierce the center of the loaf and the edges are golden brown.

Remove the loaf from the oven and let cool for 10 to 15 minutes before slicing, for best results. Serve.

INSPIRALIZED TIP

For an extra nutritious boost, finely shred zucchini to yield ½ cup and then drain the excess water by wringing it in a paper towel or cheesecloth. Fold into the wet ingredients.

FEEDING LITTLES TIP

Make sure to finely chop the nuts if serving this to kids younger than four.

cranberry greek yogurt scones with orange zest

time to prep: 30 minutes / time to cook: 20 to 25 minutes / makes: 8 scones

Scones: what a classic! Scones are typically made with flour, sugar, cold butter, and cream or milk and have savory or sweet flavors. When brainstorming a baked recipe that could work as either a savory breakfast or a sweet snack, I landed on a cranberry scone with a simplified preparation method and a secret ingredient: Greek yogurt. There's no flouring of surfaces or kneading, just mixing and slicing, so even a kitchen novice can nail this recipe, and it is fun to make with our little bakers, without the mess.

2 cups whole wheat pastry flour

½ cup coconut sugar (or granulated sugar), plus more to sprinkle

2 teaspoons baking powder

½ teaspoon salt

⅔ cup plain Greek whole milk yogurt

1 teaspoon orange zest

1 teaspoon vanilla extract

⅔ cup coconut oil (or ½ cup unsalted butter), melted and slightly cooled

1 large egg

½ cup dried (or frozen) cranberries

Combine the flour, sugar, baking powder, and salt in a large bowl.

Combine the Greek yogurt, orange zest, vanilla, coconut oil, and egg in a medium bowl. Pour the mixture into the bowl with the dry ingredients and stir. The mixture should be doughlike, but not wet. Carefully fold in the cranberries.

On a piece of parchment paper, form the dough into a ball. Press the ball into an 8-inch disc and with a sharp knife, cut into 8 wedges. Sprinkle the wedges with extra sugar to make a crunchy top.

Transfer the scones on the parchment paper to a plate and refrigerate for 15 minutes. Meanwhile, preheat the oven to 400°F.

Place the scones (still on the piece of parchment paper) on a large baking sheet and arrange the scones 2 inches apart. Bake for 20 to 25 minutes or until the scones are golden brown around the edges. Remove from the oven and let cool slightly before serving.

(recipe continues)

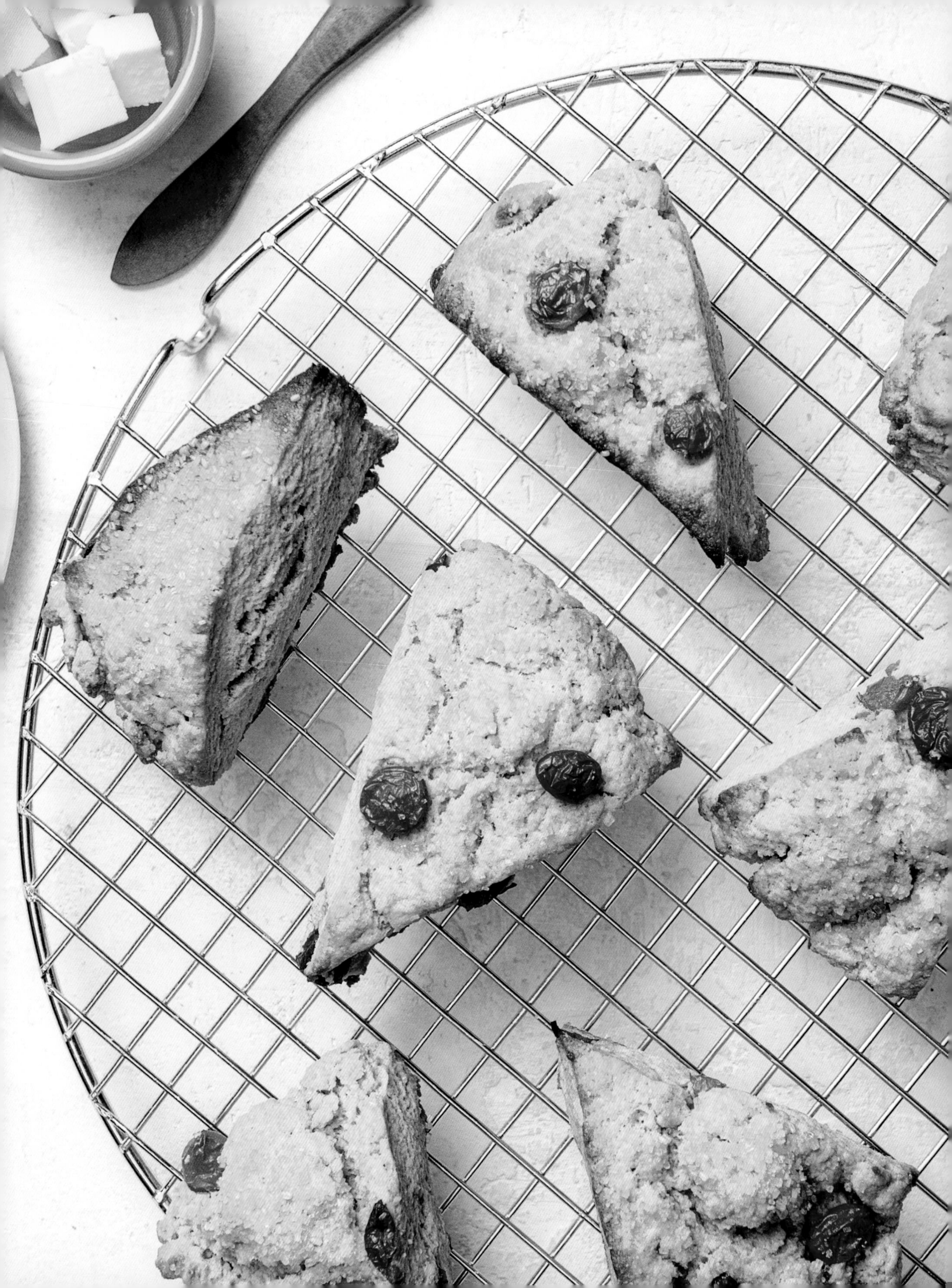

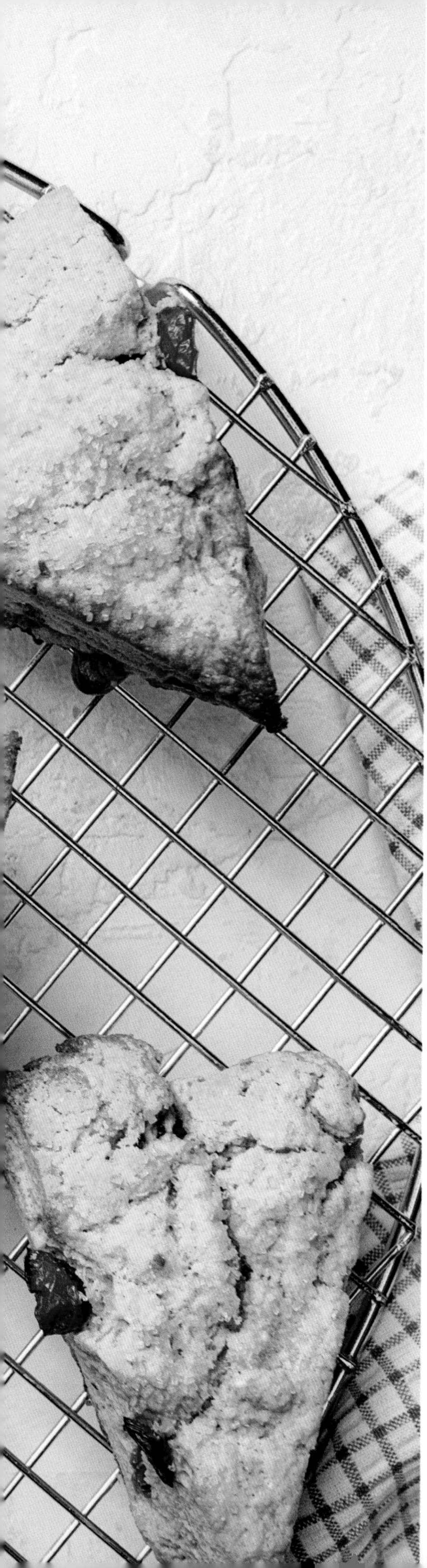

INSPIRALIZED TIP

Add variety by switching up the fruit from cranberry to blueberry, strawberry, or raspberry. For example, swap the orange zest for lemon and the cranberry for blueberry to make a blueberry-lemon scone. The tarter fruits won't be as sweet, so keep that in mind. Also, chocolate is always fair game. Alternately, skip the fruit altogether and serve with jam.

FEEDING LITTLES TIP

Scones are really fun for "afternoon tea" with your toddler. Put water or milk in little teacups, sit on the floor or at a kid table, and enjoy your snack together.

PREP AHEAD

These scones can be prepped ahead and store well in the refrigerator for 3 days or in the freezer for 3 months.

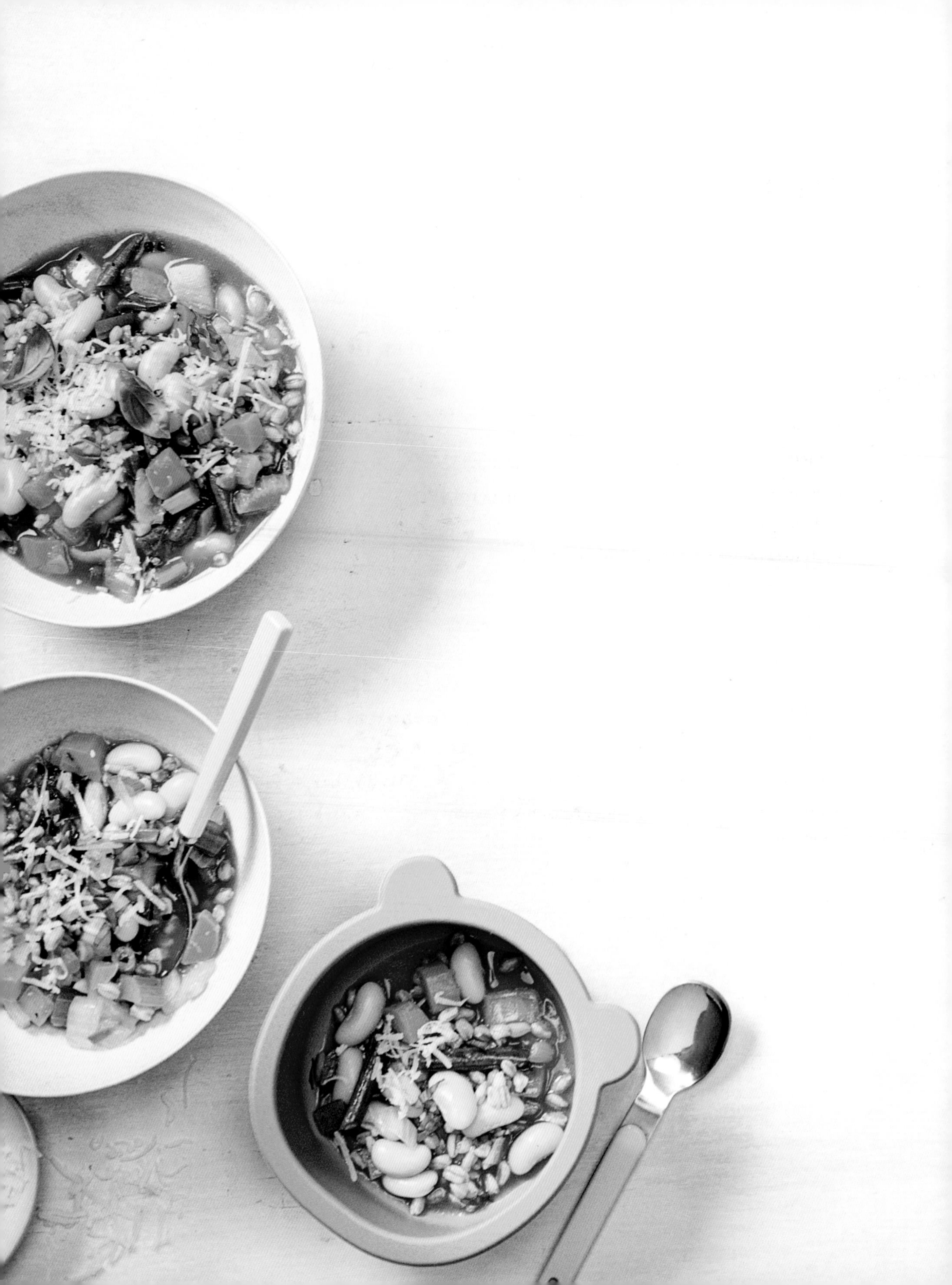

less is more

We originally planned for this chapter to be named "Five Ingredients or Less," but we ultimately landed on "Less Is More" so we could include low-ingredient recipes and ones that take less time, less preparation, or use simple cooking methods.

While other recipes in this book fit that bill, these are built for those times when you don't want to spend a lot of time cooking or just want to swing by the farmers market or grocery store and pick up a few ingredients to make dinner. Many of these recipes utilize pantry ingredients, so you can cook a nutritious dinner with staples you already have on hand like seasonings, broths, canned goods, and grains. Find out more about our pantry favorites on page 30.

Our goal is to try to incorporate nourishing ingredients and increase exposure to a wide variety of flavors and foods. Almost all of these recipes have ten ingredients or less (including pantry staples like olive oil and garlic) but deliver robust tastes.

Cooking a nourishing, satisfying meal for your family doesn't have to be a big production or require fancy or exotic ingredients. And remember, any food we put on the table is fuel for our loved ones.

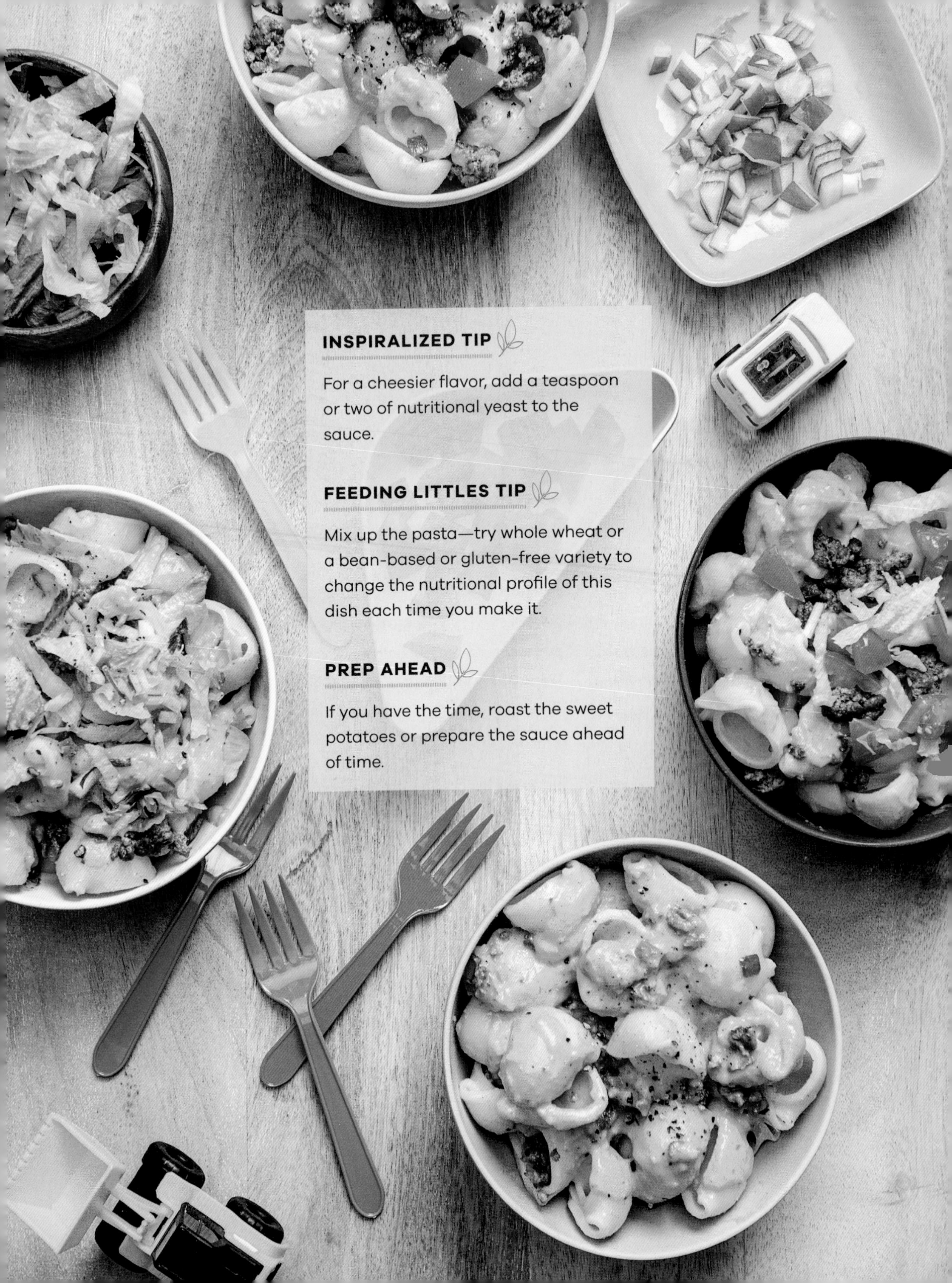

INSPIRALIZED TIP

For a cheesier flavor, add a teaspoon or two of nutritional yeast to the sauce.

FEEDING LITTLES TIP

Mix up the pasta—try whole wheat or a bean-based or gluten-free variety to change the nutritional profile of this dish each time you make it.

PREP AHEAD

If you have the time, roast the sweet potatoes or prepare the sauce ahead of time.

cheesy cheeseless hamburger pasta

time to prep: 15 minutes / time to cook: about 35 minutes / serves: 4

This recipe isn't just a plain old pasta; it's a full-on pasta *night*, because this is the kind of meal that's an interactive experience. Chop up your favorite burger toppings, place them in little bowls, and serve the pasta alongside the fixings. Are you a lettuce, tomato, onion, and pickle purist? Prefer yours with avocado, bacon, and jalapeños? Chop it all up and build your own burger bar. This pasta is dairy-free, and while you can certainly add shredded cheddar on top, it's delightfully creamy and cheesy—without any cheese!

1 medium sweet potato, peeled and cubed

2 tablespoons extra-virgin olive oil

4 garlic cloves, minced

1 red onion, diced

1 pound 93% lean ground beef

1½ teaspoons paprika

1 teaspoon dried oregano

½ teaspoon salt, plus more to taste

Pepper

1 cup canned unsweetened full-fat coconut milk

¼ teaspoon dried thyme

1 box (8 ounces) shellbows or similar pasta

In a small skillet over high heat, place the sweet potato and cover with water. Bring to a boil. Once boiling, reduce the heat to medium-high and let simmer until the sweet potato is fork-tender, about 10 minutes. Drain, pat dry, and set aside.

Meanwhile, heat 1 tablespoon of the oil in a large skillet over medium heat. Once the oil is shimmering, add half of the garlic and half of the onion and cook for 3 minutes or until the onion is translucent. Push the vegetables to the side, add in the beef, and crumble using a silicone spatula or spoon. Once crumbled, season with 1 teaspoon of the paprika, the oregano, ½ teaspoon salt, and pepper to taste. Cook the beef until browned and no longer raw, about 10 minutes. Remove from the heat, set aside, and carefully wipe down the skillet. Immediately add the remaining 1 tablespoon oil and remaining garlic and onion and let cook until translucent, about 5 minutes. Transfer to a blender along with the sweet potato, coconut milk, the remaining ½ teaspoon paprika, the thyme, and salt and pepper to taste, and blend until smooth. Taste and adjust to your preference.

Fill a medium pot halfway with water and bring to a boil. Once boiling, add the pasta and cook until al dente. Drain into a colander.

Combine the sauce and cooked pasta back into the pot and stir in the beef. Serve.

pesto orzo with crispy beans and brussels sprouts

time to prep: 15 minutes / time to cook: 25 minutes / serves: 4 adults

You may have already noticed that I add beans to many meals. I love beans because they're a rich, plant-based source of protein and fiber. I must've eaten a gallon during my pregnancies, since they're a solid source of folate, which is an essential nutrient for fetal development. Plus, roasting beans makes them taste like potatoes, and you can quote me on that. If you've never tried it, let this recipe be your motivation—you won't believe how roasting a can of beans elevates their flavor and consistency. Tossed with Brussels sprouts that are roasted until crispy and pesto, there's plenty to love in this simple dish.

1 pound Brussels sprouts, shredded

1 can (15 ounces) cannellini beans, drained, rinsed, and patted dry

Extra-virgin olive oil, to drizzle (about 2 tablespoons)

½ teaspoon garlic powder

Salt and pepper

1¼ cups orzo pasta

2½ cups water

¼ cup pesto sauce

Preheat the oven to 400°F. Line a large baking sheet with parchment paper and lay out the Brussels sprouts and beans. You may need to use two baking sheets for this if you don't have a large one, as the more crowded the vegetables are, the less they crisp up. Drizzle with the olive oil and toss to coat. Season with the garlic powder and salt and pepper. Roast for 20 to 25 minutes or until the sprouts are fork-tender and some leaves have crisped.

Meanwhile, prepare the orzo. Combine the orzo and water in a medium pot and bring to a boil. Once boiling, reduce to a simmer and let it cook until all of the liquid is absorbed, about 15 minutes.

Toss the cooked Brussels sprouts, beans, orzo, and pesto in a large mixing bowl. Divide among plates or bowls and serve.

INSPIRALIZED TIP

To switch it up and add more nutrients, sub the orzo for a legume-based lookalike, such as Banza, which makes "rice" out of chickpeas. Trader Joe's also has a Risoni that is amazing.

FEEDING LITTLES TIP

This is an easy meal to deconstruct if your child is overwhelmed by combination foods. Serve the pesto as a dip. You can also have them build their pasta with you—they might be more interested in trying it if they assembled it themselves.

I CAN'T EVEN

Buy pre-shredded Brussels sprouts.

PREP AHEAD

This entire dish can be prepped ahead of time.

egg salad pitas with carrots

time to prep: 10 minutes / serves: 4

Egg salad: pretty basic, right? Sometimes we're so focused on trying new things that we forget about the recipes that are classics for a reason—namely, they're easy and great. I adore nothing more than elevating the classics, in this case with shredded carrot, which adds a crunch that kids love.

4 pitas, halved

8 hard-boiled eggs, peeled and diced

1 tablespoon Dijon mustard

2 tablespoons mayonnaise (vegan mayonnaise works, too)

Salt and pepper, to taste

½ cup shredded carrot

4 romaine or butter lettuce leaves, lightly chopped

Warm the pitas in the oven or toaster.

Meanwhile, in a large bowl, toss the eggs, mustard, mayonnaise, salt, pepper, and carrots together until combined. Open a pita half, spoon in about ¼ heaping cup of egg salad, and top with some lettuce. Repeat with the remaining pita, egg salad, and lettuce until all sandwiches are made. Serve.

INSPIRALIZED TIP

I love curried egg salad and if your family does, too, stir in ½ tablespoon of curry powder (or more).

FEEDING LITTLES TIP

Raw carrots can be a choking hazard, so shredding them is a safer way to serve them. However, if your baby is still working on their chewing skills, you might want to omit the carrots entirely or steam or sauté the shreds until softened. This recipe is an excellent way to expose baby to eggs, a common allergen.

I CAN'T EVEN

Buy premade hard-boiled eggs.

PREP AHEAD

This egg salad lasts up to 3 days in the refrigerator.

creamy BLAT pasta salad with bowties

time to prep: 10 minutes / time to cook: 20 minutes / serves: 4

Love creamy pasta sauces, but hate the labor behind them? You're in luck, because this pasta salad uses just two ingredients to form a sauce that coats the bowties: pasta water and cheese. It's that easy. Not only that, you'll switch up your meal game by taking a classic sandwich and turning it into this pasta salad. BLTs may be great, but BLATs are even better, adding in heart-healthy avocados, with the lettuce adding the right amount of crunch.

8 ounces farfalle/bowtie pasta

6 strips bacon

1 cup cherry tomatoes, halved

2 avocados, peeled, pitted, and cubed

¼ teaspoon garlic powder

Salt and pepper

1 cup shredded Mexican cheese blend

2 cups chopped romaine lettuce

In a large pot of boiling water, cook the pasta according to the package directions until al dente.

While the pasta cooks, place the bacon in a large skillet and set over medium heat. Cook the bacon until crispy, flipping as the edges curl, and set it aside on a paper towel–lined plate. Break the bacon up into ½-inch pieces and set it aside. You may need to cook the bacon in batches.

Drain the pasta into a colander, reserving ½ cup of the pasta water (very important—don't forget this step!). Place the pasta back into the large pot and stir in the bacon, tomatoes, and avocados. Season with the garlic powder and salt and pepper, and toss to combine. Add the cheese and stir to combine thoroughly. Immediately pour in the reserved pasta water, stirring as you pour, until the cheese melts and a creamy sauce comes together. You may or may not use all of the pasta water.

Stir in the romaine until combined and serve immediately.

(recipe continues)

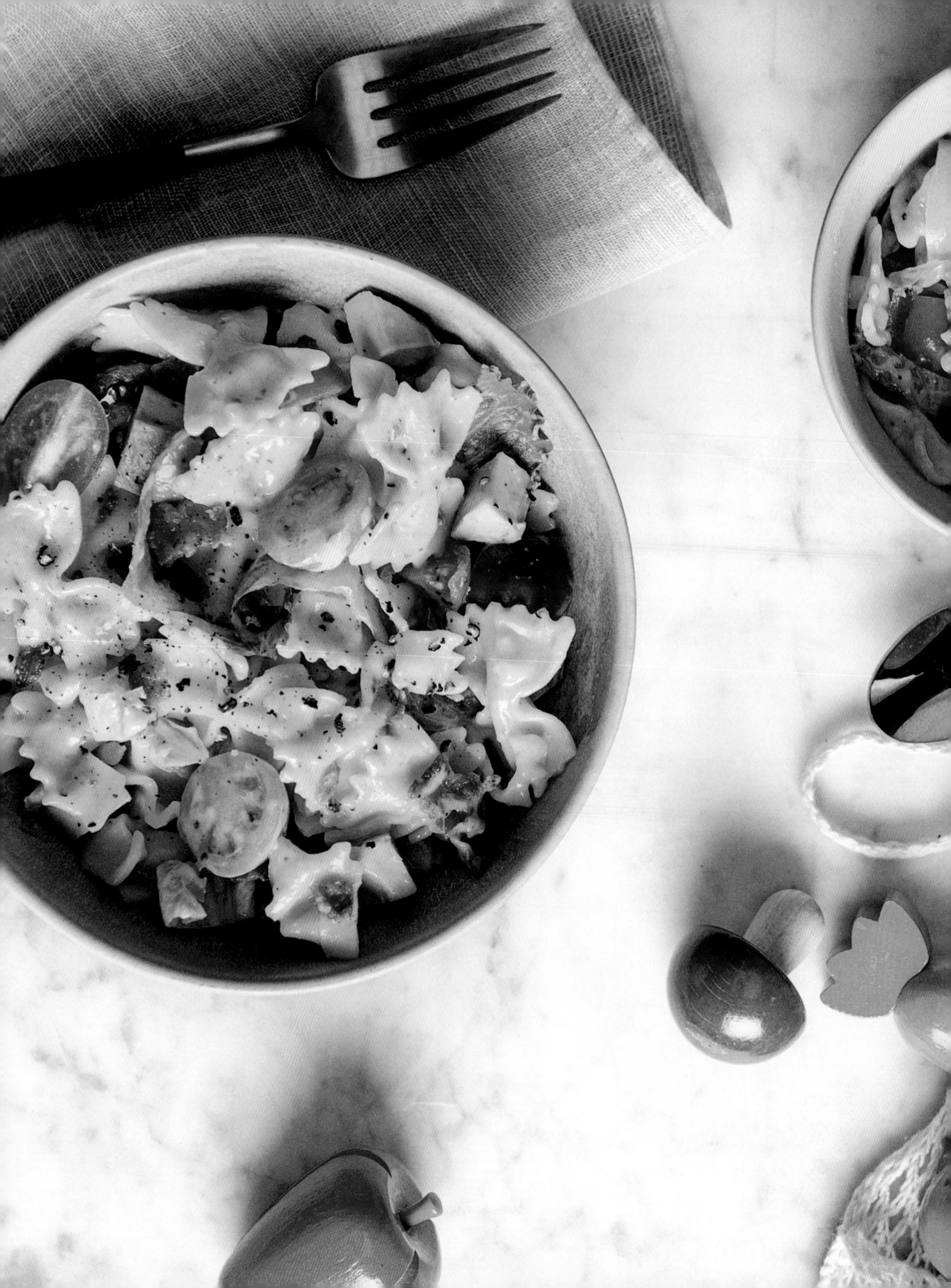

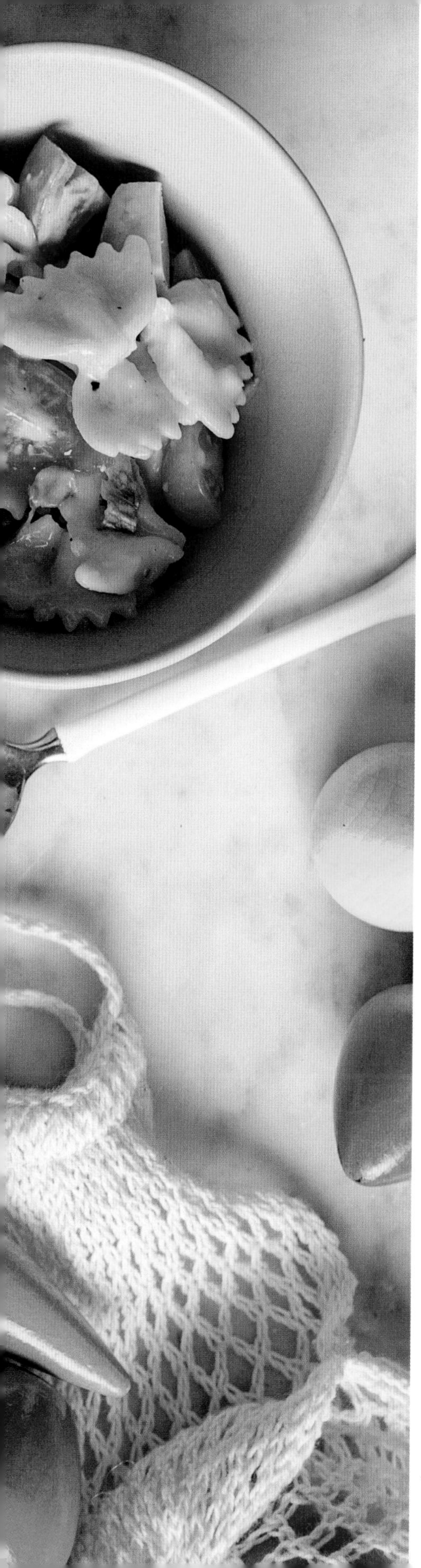

INSPIRALIZED TIP

The pasta shapes that work best here (aside from farfalle/bowties) are rigatoni, macaroni, and rotini.

FEEDING LITTLES TIP

This is a fun way to introduce your toddler to raw lettuce, especially if they aren't interested in green salads yet. Crunchy greens like romaine tend to be easier to chew, and you can offer them starting at around fourteen to sixteen months.

PREP AHEAD

This dish can be prepared ahead of time, but when you go to reheat, add some olive oil or a splash of water to add moisture back into the sauce.

sesame ginger steak, pepper, and string bean stir-fry

time to prep: 10 minutes / time to cook: 35 minutes / serves: 4

Everyone needs a go-to stir-fry for those days when meal planning just seems overwhelming. We always put a stir-fry on our meal plan because you can use whatever vegetables you have in your refrigerator. Even an onion, carrot, and egg stir-fry can be great with the right sauce, so that the vegetables and proteins are flavorful and the rice soaks up some liquid. Peppers and string beans are classic stir-fry veggies that can be cooked crisp or tender, making this a customizable dish you'll revisit over and over.

1¼ cups dry white rice

10 ounces trimmed string beans

2 red bell peppers, seeded and sliced

1 tablespoon sesame oil

1 tablespoon rice vinegar

3 tablespoons low-sodium soy sauce

½ tablespoon sriracha

2 garlic cloves, minced

1-inch knob ginger, peeled and minced

1 teaspoon arrowroot powder

2 teaspoons extra-virgin olive oil

1 pound beef sirloin, cut into strips

Salt and pepper

White sesame seeds, for garnish

Cook the rice according to the package instructions.

Meanwhile, fill a medium pot one-third of the way with water and bring to a boil. Top with a colander or steamer basket and once boiling, add the string beans and peppers and cook until fork-tender, about 5 minutes. Set aside.

Meanwhile, prepare the sauce. Whisk together the sesame oil, rice vinegar, soy sauce, sriracha, half of the garlic, and half of the ginger in a small bowl. Separately, whisk together 1 teaspoon of water with the arrowroot powder to make a slurry. Pour into the sauce and whisk to combine. Set aside.

Heat the olive oil in a large skillet over medium-high heat. Once the oil is shimmering, add the beef, remaining garlic, and remaining ginger, and season with salt and pepper. Cook until the beef is browned, about 5 minutes. Add the cooked string beans and bell peppers and toss. Pour the prepared sauce into the skillet and let cook until the sauce is thickened, about 2 minutes.

Divide the cooked rice into bowls and top with the beef and vegetable mixture. Garnish with the sesame seeds and serve.

INSPIRALIZED TIP

This stir-fry works well with shrimp, chicken, tofu, and pork, so swap out the protein for your favorites.

FEEDING LITTLES TIP

This is a fun dish to eat with chopsticks if your family doesn't usually use them. Trainer chopsticks can help kids as early as two years of age. Also, ensure the meat is fork-tender if serving this to a baby or young toddler.

I CAN'T EVEN

Use microwavable rice.

PREP AHEAD

Prep the vegetables ahead of time and place in an airtight bag or container. Prepare the rice. When it's time to cook, most of the work will be done and this recipe will take less than 20 minutes.

lamb chops with curried tahini couscous and chickpeas

time to prep: 20 minutes / time to cook: about 25 minutes / serves: 4 (2 lamb chops per person)

Some of my most beloved videos of my children are of them eating meat with "bone" handles, where they're holding the bone of a chicken drumstick or a lamb chop and gnawing on it. It's a hilarious reminder of their early food experiences, when they were just excited to try new things. This dairy-free couscous has a wonderful creamy taste, thanks to nutty tahini, which is a tasty way to introduce sesame to your young eater. The curry powder brings in a little spice, while the raisins add a sweetness that levels out that heat. The couscous is flavorful and filling on its own, but the lamb chops bring the flavors together and make this a special meal that's suitable for eaters of all ages.

8 lamb rib chops, about ¾ inch thick

1 cup traditional pearl couscous

½ cup peeled and diced carrot

2 tablespoons tahini

2 tablespoons water

1 lemon, juiced

¼ teaspoon garlic powder

½ tablespoon curry powder, plus more as needed

Salt and pepper

2 tablespoons avocado oil

1 can (15½ ounces) chickpeas, drained and rinsed

⅓ cup raisins

Take the lamb chops out of the refrigerator and let them rest on the counter to bring up to room temperature, about 10 minutes.

Bring 2 cups of water to a boil in a saucepan. Once boiling, add the couscous and carrots, bring to a boil again, and reduce the heat to a simmer. Cover and cook until tender, about 15 minutes. Drain any remaining water.

Meanwhile, prepare the curry dressing. In a large bowl, whisk together the tahini, water, lemon juice, garlic powder, and curry powder, and season generously with salt and pepper. Taste, and if you'd like, add more curry powder by the teaspoon until your heat threshold is met.

As the couscous cooks, cook the lamb chops. Season them generously with salt and pepper. Heat the oil in a large cast-iron skillet over medium heat. Once the oil is shimmering, add the lamb chops. Sear for about 3 minutes, flip the chops, and cook for another 3 to 5 minutes, depending on your doneness preference—4 more minutes is medium, 5 minutes is well-done.

Once the couscous is cooked, add to the bowl with the tahini dressing along with the chickpeas and raisins, season with salt and pepper, and toss to coat thoroughly.

Serve the couscous with the lamb chops.

FEEDING LITTLES TIP

Lamb and couscous might be new to your child. If so, pair this dish with a few familiar sides like roasted veggies and crusty bread with butter. If serving lamb on the bone to your child (and it's too big for them to hold), cut off some of the meat.

PREP AHEAD

The curried couscous can be prepared ahead of time and lasts in the refrigerator for up to 3 days for optimal freshness.

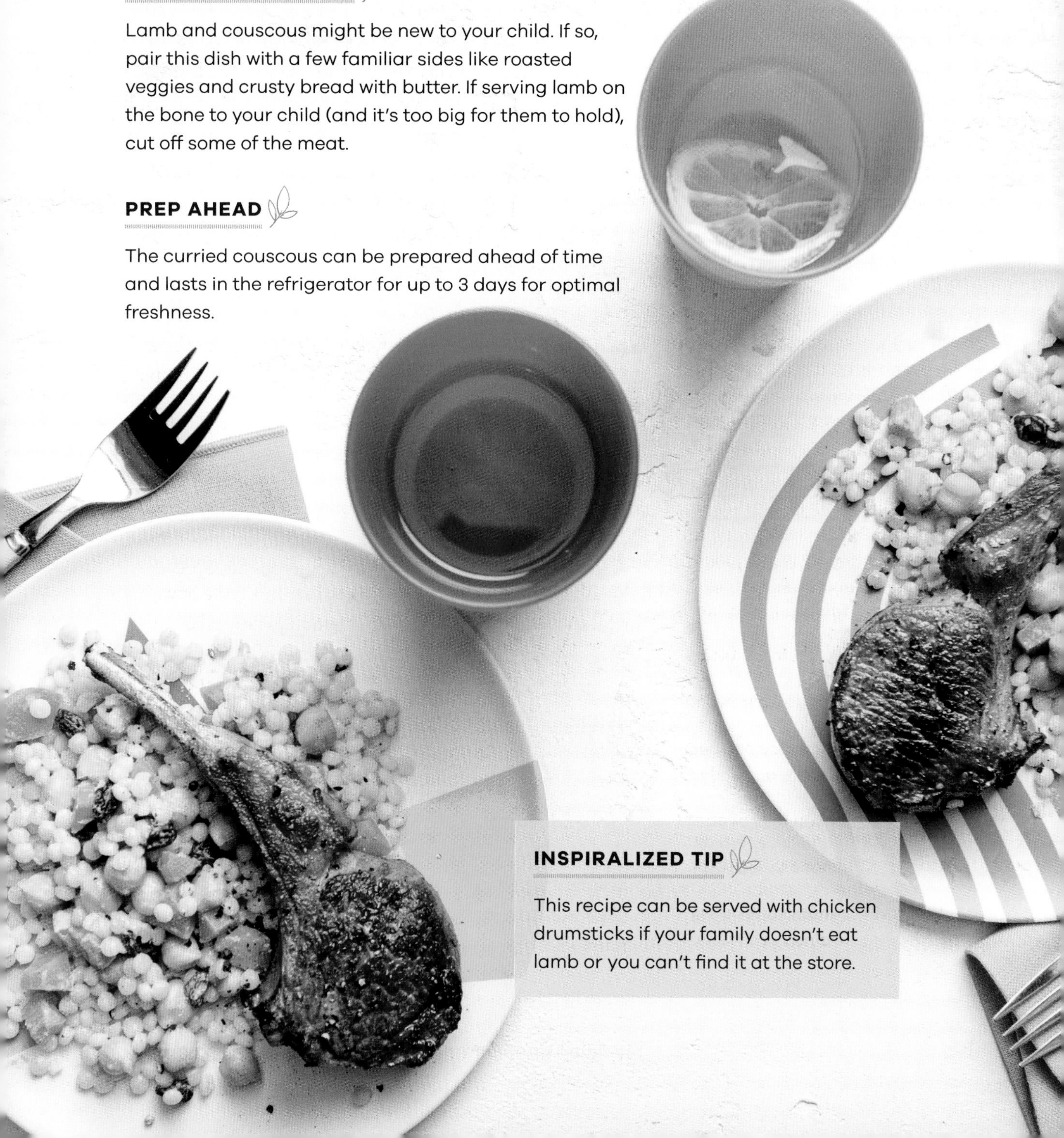

INSPIRALIZED TIP

This recipe can be served with chicken drumsticks if your family doesn't eat lamb or you can't find it at the store.

chickpea "tuna" melts

time to prep: 15 minutes / time to cook: 3 to 5 minutes / serves: 4

I have been making chickpea "tuna" salads since 2008, after I feverishly read a book about veganism and hours later decided to go fully vegan. About three years later, I started adding fish back into my diet, and then slowly but surely, the other proteins as well. Now I try to listen to how my body feels and what it's telling me it needs. I've always felt my best when I eat a primarily plant-based diet, but I also strongly believe that your body craves different nutrients and foods during different seasons of life (I ate so many beef meatballs when I was pregnant with my daughter Roma!). What I most appreciate about my vegan days is how they inspired me to get creative. One of the dishes that has stuck with me over the years was this vegan tuna salad, using chickpeas, which mimics a tuna melt when topped with cheddar cheese and sliced tomato.

2 cans (15½ ounces each) chickpeas, drained and rinsed

3½ tablespoons mayonnaise

1½ tablespoons Dijon mustard

3 tablespoons minced celery

1 tablespoon Old Bay seasoning

Salt and pepper

8 slices multigrain bread

4 slices cheddar cheese

8 thin slices beefsteak tomato

Lettuce, for serving

Set the oven to broil or, if you have a toaster oven, the toaster oven method is best.

Smash the chickpeas in a medium bowl (I like to use the bottom of the mayonnaise jar or a potato masher) until mostly crushed, but still a bit chunky. Add the mayonnaise, Dijon mustard, celery, and Old Bay seasoning, season with salt and pepper, and stir to combine thoroughly. Spread the mixture onto 4 slices of bread, top each with a slice of cheese, and set on a baking sheet along with the other 4 slices of bread, which will be used to top the sandwiches. Put the baking sheet in the oven and let cook for 3 to 5 minutes or until the cheese melts. Immediately place 2 tomato slices on top of the slices of bread with the melted cheese, then top with lettuce and the remaining 4 slices of toast.

INSPIRALIZED TIP

Tuna melts are great on English muffins, a kid-friendly bread. Serve them open-faced or close the sandwiches up.

FEEDING LITTLES TIP

A whole sandwich is probably too difficult for a baby to eat, so deconstructing the components can really help. Try the chickpea salad on loaded spoons first, then spread it on some toast for your baby. If they do well with that, serve it with melted cheese on top as we show in the visual index (page 284). Remember, our recommendations in the index are simply ideas, so modify them as needed.

PREP AHEAD

The chickpea salad (without the cheese, tomato, lettuce, and bread) saves well in the refrigerator for up to 3 days.

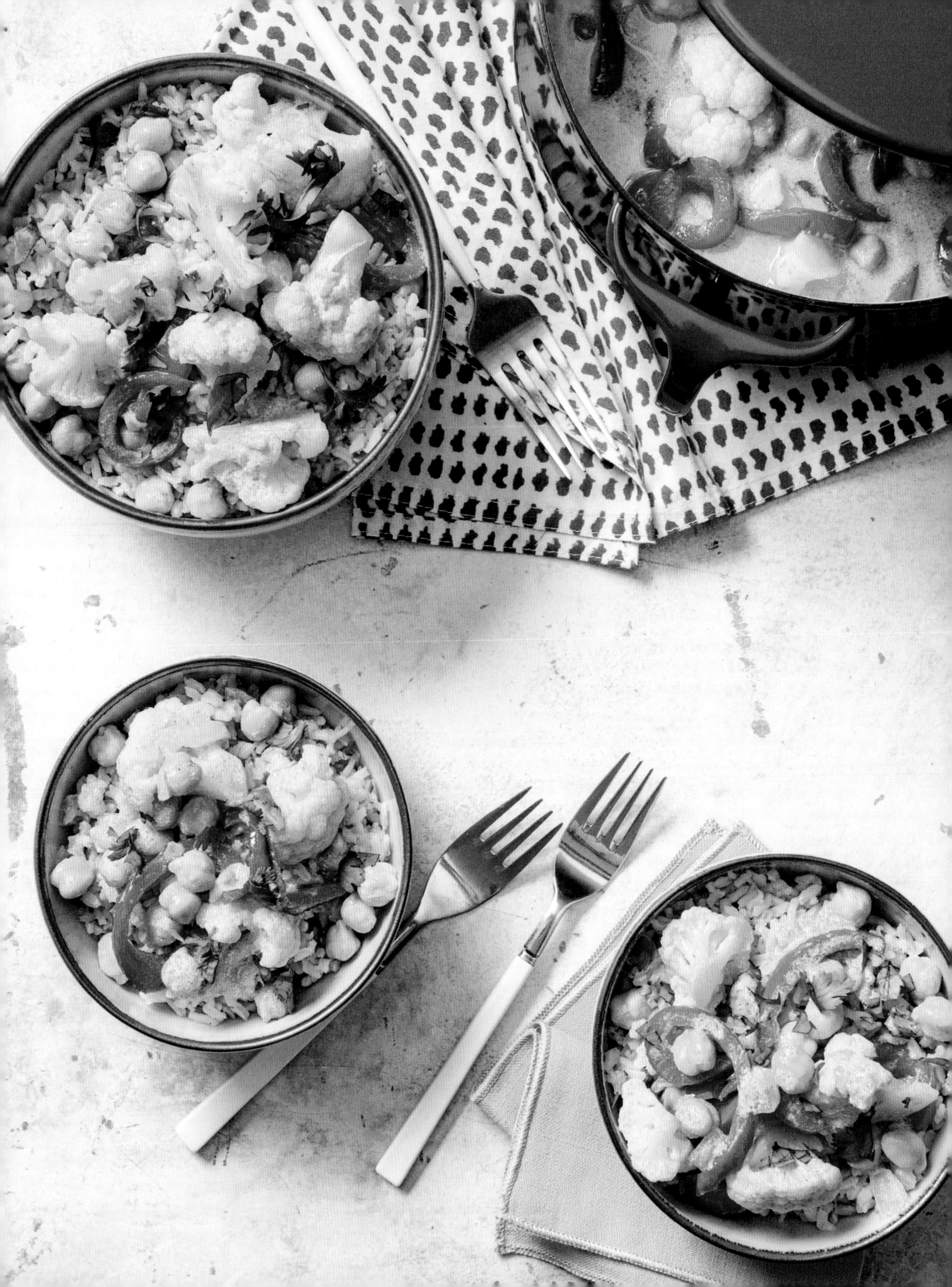

one pot cauliflower and chickpea coconut curry

time to prep: 15 minutes / time to cook: about 25 minutes / serves: 6

If I had to guess, I have probably made about twenty-five different versions of this curry. I knew I had to include one in this book, because it's a staple in our home as a customizable go-to that everyone loves. The curry paste is light and mild enough to introduce beginner eaters to the flavor, and the ingredients are basic. Cauliflower, chickpeas, and bell peppers soak up the flavors as they soften, and the dish serves well over rice or quinoa, making it easy for preloaded utensils. Plus, it's one pot, so I never dread the cleanup afterwards. It *is* a bit of a messy dish for little eaters, but it's well worth it.

1 tablespoon extra-virgin olive oil

1-inch knob ginger, peeled and minced

2 garlic cloves, minced

1 small onion, diced

1½ to 2 tablespoons red curry paste

Cauliflower florets from 1 large head

2 red bell peppers, seeded and sliced

Salt and pepper

1 can (15½ ounces) chickpeas, drained and rinsed

2 cans (14 ounces each) lite coconut milk (if you only have full-fat, use 1 can full-fat and 1 can water)

(ingredients continue)

Heat the oil in a large pot over medium-high heat. Once the oil is shimmering, add the ginger, garlic, and onion and cook for 3 to 5 minutes or until the onion is mostly soft. Add the curry paste and stir continually until the vegetables are coated in the paste. Add the cauliflower and bell peppers, season generously with salt and pepper, and stir well to combine. Add the chickpeas, coconut milk, and broth, and season with salt and pepper. Stir well to combine and raise the heat to high and bring to a boil. Once the pot is boiling, reduce the heat to medium-low and let it simmer for 20 minutes or until the cauliflower is fork-tender.

Serve with brown rice or quinoa and garnish with cilantro.

INSPIRALIZED TIP

If you've never used red curry paste before, start with 1 tablespoon. Then, after you add in the coconut milk and broth, taste. If the curry is not flavorful enough, spoon a little of the liquid from the curry into a small bowl and whisk in another ½ to 1 tablespoon of curry paste. Add the curry paste back into the curry, stir well, and taste again.

(recipe continues)

½ cup low-sodium vegetable broth

3 cups cooked brown rice or quinoa, for serving

Cilantro leaves, for garnish

FEEDING LITTLES TIP

If curry is a new flavor for your family, make sure to have a few familiar side dishes for your young eater. Naan and fruit will pair well with this.

I CAN'T EVEN

To save prep time and perhaps an extra trip to the grocery store, swap the fresh ginger for ½ teaspoon of ginger powder. Use microwavable rice or quinoa.

PREP AHEAD

This dish can be entirely prepped ahead of time. It saves well in the refrigerator for up to 3 days and up to 3 months in the freezer.

pizza rolls with spinach

time to prep: 20 minutes / time to cook: 15 minutes / makes: 8 rolls

When I first tested this recipe, my husband was the only one around to be a taste tester, and he was on a work call. I handed him the batch thinking he'd eat just one and deliver his review, but when I came back to grab the leftovers, the plate was empty. These pizza rolls are a delicious way to introduce spinach while also presenting a flavor that's familiar to many kids. Consider yourself warned: these go quickly, so make sure you save some for the kids before the adults devour them, and vice versa.

For the pizza rolls

1 container (8 ounces) crescent rolls

1 cup marinara sauce or tomato basil sauce

½ cup shredded mozzarella cheese, plus more as needed

Cooking spray, for baking the rolls

For the pesto

½ cup packed fresh basil leaves

½ cup packed baby spinach

¼ cup freshly grated Parmesan cheese

¼ cup extra-virgin olive oil

2 tablespoons pine nuts

2 small garlic cloves, minced

Salt and pepper, to taste

Preheat the oven to 350°F. Line a large baking sheet with parchment paper.

Roll the crescent rolls out and manipulate the dough so they are rectangles. To do this, roll out the dough with the pointed triangle end at the top. Slice off part of the left side and place that piece on the top to form a rectangle. Press the seam together to join the two pieces together. Spread the marinara sauce evenly over the dough, all the way to the edges, about 2 tablespoons per roll. Top with mozzarella cheese, about a tablespoon.

Roll the dough from top to bottom and seal the edge. Place the rolls on the baking sheet, about 2 inches apart. Spritz the tops with cooking spray, and bake for 15 minutes or until the tops are golden brown.

While the rolls are baking, prepare the pesto. Place the basil, spinach, cheese, oil, pine nuts, garlic, and salt and pepper in a food processor. Process until smooth.

Drizzle the pesto over the baked rolls and serve.

(recipe continues)

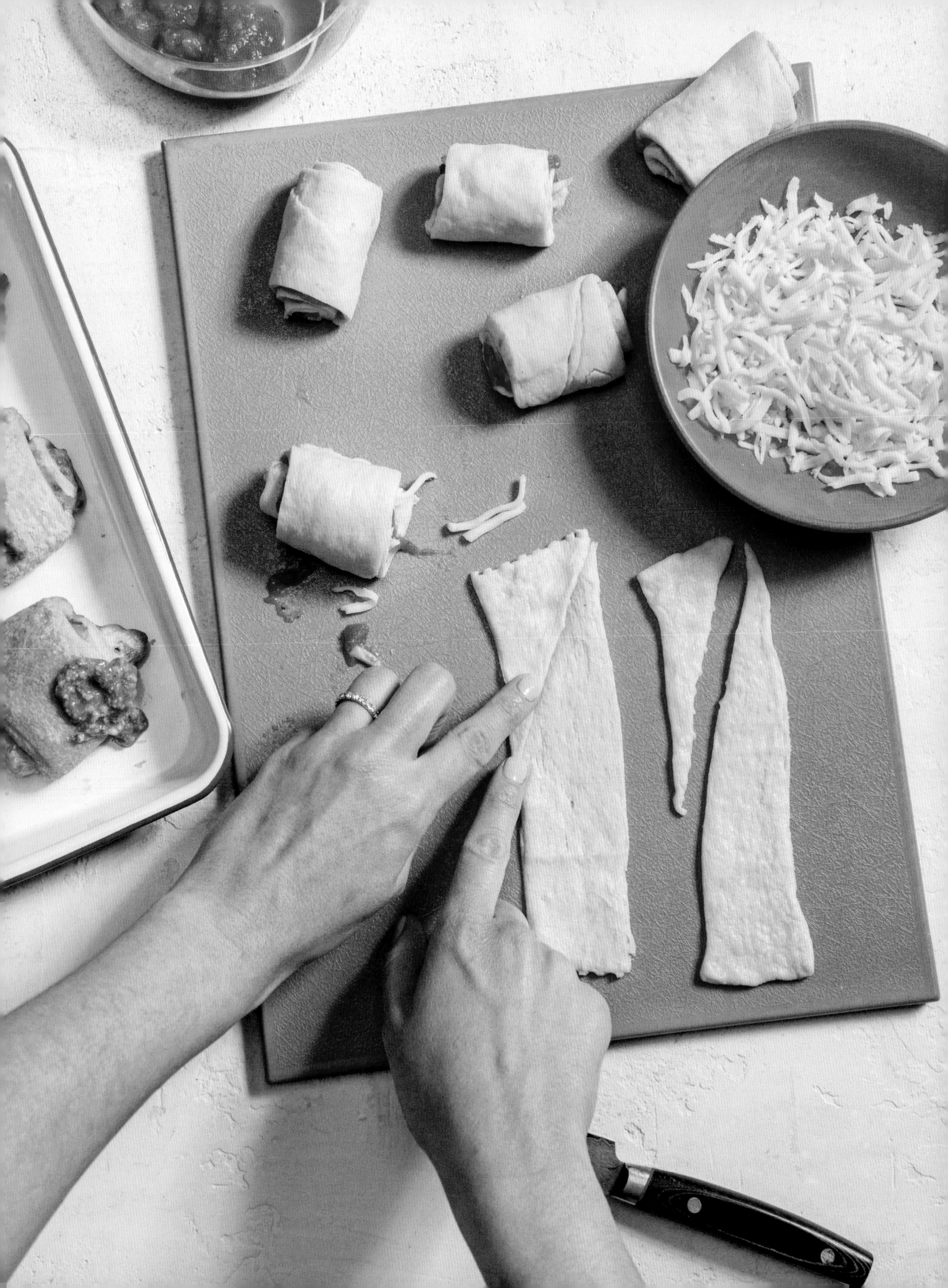

INSPIRALIZED TIP

Instead of drizzling the pesto on top of the pizza rolls, put it directly into the roll itself! Add the pesto after sprinkling on the mozzarella cheese, then roll the dough so the pesto is baked inside.

FEEDING LITTLES TIP

Serve the pesto as a dip. You can also use leftover marinara as a dip, too, especially if your child is more familiar with tomato sauce. Remember—when they see a familiar dip, they're more likely to try the less familiar food.

PREP AHEAD

You can prep these ahead of time, but for best quality, they should be made fresh. The pesto can be prepared in advance and lasts up to 5 days in the refrigerator.

roasted vegetable pasta with pesto

time to prep: 15 minutes / time to cook: 35 minutes / serves: 4

This recipe was almost titled "Fridge Cleanout Pesto Pasta," because that's how I typically make it for my family. Almost every Sunday night, I open the fridge, take out all the vegetables I have left from the past week, chop them up, drizzle with olive oil, salt, and pepper, and roast them until tender. String beans, broccoli, peppers, zucchini, corn, onions, bagged carrots, mushrooms—I roast it all! Then, I toss the roasted veggies with a box of pasta, some pesto, and we chow down. It's an easy, delicious way to reduce food waste and cram in a ton of vegetables to start the new week. Roasting veggies brings out their best flavors, and this dish is made with my usual weekly suspects: broccoli, carrots, onions, and bell peppers. You can use what you have on hand in your fridge right now, and know that this recipe is always here for you when you're all out of fresh ideas.

3 cups broccoli florets

4 carrots, peeled and sliced diagonally into 1-inch pieces

1 medium red onion, chopped into ½-inch pieces

1 red bell pepper, seeded and chopped into 1-inch pieces

Extra-virgin olive oil, to drizzle

⅓ teaspoon garlic powder

Salt and pepper

1 box (8 ounces) casarecce pasta

⅓ cup pesto sauce (try the pesto on page 95)

Preheat the oven to 400°F. Line a large baking sheet with parchment paper. On the baking sheet, toss the broccoli, carrots, onion, and pepper with olive oil. Season with the garlic powder and salt and pepper, and toss again. Roast for 35 minutes or until all vegetables are fork-tender, tossing every 10 minutes. Once roasted, roughly chop the broccoli, carrots, and pepper.

Ten minutes into cooking the vegetables, bring a pot filled halfway full with water to a boil. Add the pasta, stir, and let it cook according to the package instructions.

Drain the pasta into a colander and place it back in the pot, along with the roasted vegetables and pesto. Toss thoroughly to combine.

INSPIRALIZED TIP

Casarecce is my preferred noodle for pesto (but use whatever pasta you'd like—rigatoni, fusilli, ziti, and orecchiette work well here, too). It's also a great shape for a baby to hold.

FEEDING LITTLES TIP

To add more protein, use a bean-based pasta, top with cheese, stir in small feta cubes, or add precooked chicken sausage.

PREP AHEAD

Roast the vegetables ahead of time so that when you get into the kitchen, all you need to do is boil water and cook the pasta.

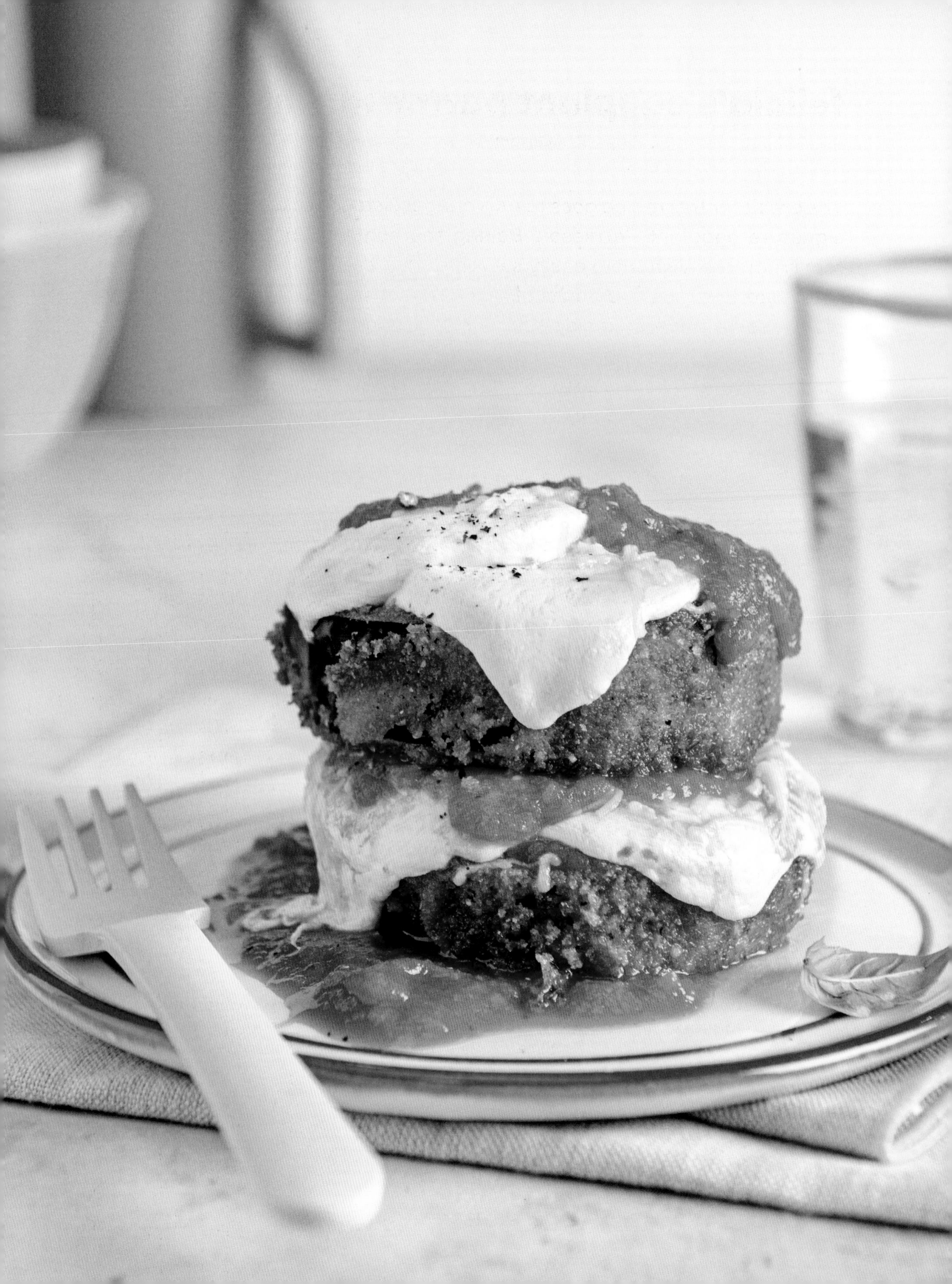

felicia's eggplant parmesan in stacks

time to prep: 25 minutes / time to cook: 45 minutes / serves: 6

The credit for this recipe goes to my younger sister, Felicia, who made us her signature eggplant Parmesan. Baking the eggplant in layers makes her family-famous dish more easily servable. Plus, there's sauce and cheese in every bite, and kids and adults alike love the crispiness of the air-fried eggplant. I serve this with a side salad or pasta and make it into a full Italian dinner. If you're making it in the summertime, take your little ones to the farmers market to show them some of the ingredients that go into it (eggplant, basil, cheese, and eggs). Thanks to Felicia for the inspiration!

½ cup almond flour

2 large eggs, whisked

1 cup seasoned Italian whole wheat breadcrumbs

1 medium eggplant, sliced crosswise into 12 (¼-inch-thick) rounds

Cooking spray, for the air fryer

1 pound fresh mozzarella cheese (a log or 2 balls will work)

¼ cup fresh basil leaves, for garnish

1 jar (24 ounces) marinara sauce

¾ cup grated Parmesan cheese

Preheat an air fryer to 400°F.

Prepare your dredging stations. Place the almond flour in a shallow plate or dish. Next to the almond flour dish, place the eggs mixed with 3 teaspoons of water in a shallow plate or dish. Next to the eggs, place the breadcrumbs in a shallow plate or dish. Line a baking sheet with parchment paper.

Dip an eggplant slice into the almond flour, dredging both sides. Next, dip both sides in the egg wash. Then, dip both sides in the breadcrumbs. Set on the baking sheet. Repeat until all the eggplant is used.

Place as many eggplant slices into the air-fryer basket as you can, spritz with cooking spray, and cook for 7 to 10 minutes, or until browned. Place the eggplant slices back on the baking sheet and continue with the remaining uncooked eggplant until all the slices are air-fried, 2 or 3 batches.

While the eggplant cooks, preheat the oven to 400°F.

Slice the mozzarella into 12 thin, round slices about ⅛ inch thick. Shred the basil. Set all aside.

(recipe continues)

Once the eggplant slices are done cooking, pour 1 cup of the marinara sauce into a 9 x 13-inch baking dish and spread it out on the bottom. Top the sauce with eggplant slices in 3 rows of 2. Top each with about 1 tablespoon of sauce or enough to cover the eggplant. Sprinkle the entire dish with one-fourth of the Parmesan cheese. Top each eggplant slice with a mozzarella slice. Next, top each mozzarella slice with 1 tablespoon of marinara sauce and sprinkle the entire dish with another ¼ cup of the Parmesan cheese, then top with the remaining eggplant slices. Top those eggplant slices each with 1 tablespoon of marinara sauce and top with the remaining mozzarella cheese. Sprinkle the entire dish with the remaining ¼ cup of Parmesan cheese. Bake for 20 minutes or until the cheese is melted. Garnish with the basil and serve.

INSPIRALIZED TIP

If you'd like to serve the eggplant pieces individually (and not make them into stacks or casserole-style), place the sauce and cheese on top of each eggplant slice and put them back in the air fryer until the cheese melts, working in batches. Serve them individually. That's how Felicia does it!

FEEDING LITTLES TIP

Eggplant is such an underappreciated vegetable. It contains a decent amount of fiber and a phytonutrient (plant nutrient) called nasunin, which is a potent antioxidant. This is a tasty way to enjoy eggplant, especially if it's something you don't eat often. And kids will love that they are eating a purple food!

PREP AHEAD

I don't recommend cooking this ahead of time, because the eggplant tends to get soggy, but you can slice the eggplant and mozzarella to save yourself some prep time.

pork chops in sun-dried tomato "cream" sauce

time to prep: 15 minutes / time to cook: 40 minutes / serves: 4

You're going to want to pour this easy, two-ingredient sun-dried tomato cream sauce over everything, but first try it with these pork chops. The chops simmer in the sauce, tenderizing and soaking up the sun-dried tomato flavor, while making the sauce tastier with their juices. Cabbage is a tough vegetable to get your little ones interested in, but this is a delicious way to offer it. When I first served this to my youngest, I chopped the cabbage up in small pieces and mixed it with couscous so it wasn't an overpowering flavor, and she gobbled it up. This is such a flavorful way to expose or introduce cabbage to your family, and also a date night–appropriate recipe for those rare and precious dinners when you get some alone time.

½ cup packed sun-dried tomatoes in oil from a jar, lightly chopped

1 can (13½ ounces) lite coconut milk, shaken

4 boneless pork chops

¼ teaspoon garlic powder

Salt and pepper

2 tablespoons extra-virgin olive oil

2 garlic cloves, minced

½ onion, diced

2 cups chopped green cabbage

1 cup low-sodium chicken broth

Barley, pasta, or your grain of choice for serving with the pork chops

Place the sun-dried tomatoes and coconut milk in a blender or food processor and blend or pulse until the coconut milk is light pink and the tomatoes are finely chopped. Set aside.

Season both sides of the pork chops with the garlic powder and salt and pepper.

Heat 1 tablespoon of the oil in a large skillet over medium-high heat. Cook the pork chops about 5 minutes per side or until seared and lightly browned. Using tongs, remove from the pan and set aside. Add the remaining 1 tablespoon of oil, the garlic, and the onion to the skillet, and cook until soft, about 5 minutes. Add the cabbage and cook for 5 minutes or until it begins to soften and wilt.

Pour the prepared cream sauce and the broth over the cabbage and nestle in the pork chops, spooning the sauce over the chops. Cook, uncovered, for about 20 minutes or until the sauce is reduced by a third or to your thickness preference.

Serve the pork chops over your preferred grain.

(recipe continues)

INSPIRALIZED TIP

Chicken, salmon, or tofu steaks work just as well as the pork chops.

FEEDING LITTLES TIP

Remember, if your kiddo scoffs at a vegetable they haven't seen before (like cabbage), it's not the end of the world. It might take twenty-plus exposures to a food for them to enjoy it. Stay calm, know your role—which is *not* to make them eat it—and hope that one day they'll like it as much as you do.

miso noodles with tofu and roasted broccoli

time to prep: 10 minutes / time to cook: 30 minutes / serves: 4

After months of my son asking for spoonfuls of our miso soups when my husband and I would order sushi, I finally included him on the order. The kid loved miso broth. I thought, "What if I made a miso noodle bowl so he could enjoy it more often? Then I could pack it with nutrients and satisfying ingredients." Thus, this dish was born, with tofu and roasted broccoli. Miso has that salty umami flavor that keeps you slurping for more, and this recipe is an easy way to expose your child to soy, which is an allergenic food.

4 cups broccoli florets

1 tablespoon extra-virgin olive oil, plus more to drizzle

¼ teaspoon garlic powder

Salt and pepper

2 garlic cloves

1-inch knob ginger

1 block (14 ounces) extra-firm tofu, drained and excess moisture pressed out

4 hard-boiled eggs

4 cups low-sodium vegetable broth

1 tablespoon white miso paste

1 tablespoon low-sodium soy sauce

1 pound ramen noodles (yakisoba or soba work fine)

Preheat the oven to 425°F. Line a baking sheet with parchment paper and lay out the broccoli. Drizzle with oil and season with the garlic powder and salt and pepper. Roast for 25 to 30 minutes or until the broccoli is fork-tender, tossing every 10 minutes to make sure it doesn't burn.

Meanwhile, prepare the soup. Mince the garlic and ginger and set aside. Cube the tofu into small ½-inch cubes. Halve the hard-boiled eggs. Set aside.

Heat the oil in a large pot over medium-high heat. Once the oil is shimmering, add the garlic and ginger and cook for 1 minute or until fragrant. Add the broth and 2 cups of water and bring to a boil over high heat. Place the miso paste in a small bowl and set aside while you bring the broth to a boil. Right before the broth is boiling, ladle about a half cup of broth into the bowl with the miso paste and stir until the miso is dissolved. Pour the dissolved miso into the pot and stir. Reduce the heat to a medium simmer and add the soy sauce, tofu, and ramen noodles. Let cook for 3 minutes, stirring, or until the noodles are loosened and cooked through.

(recipe continues)

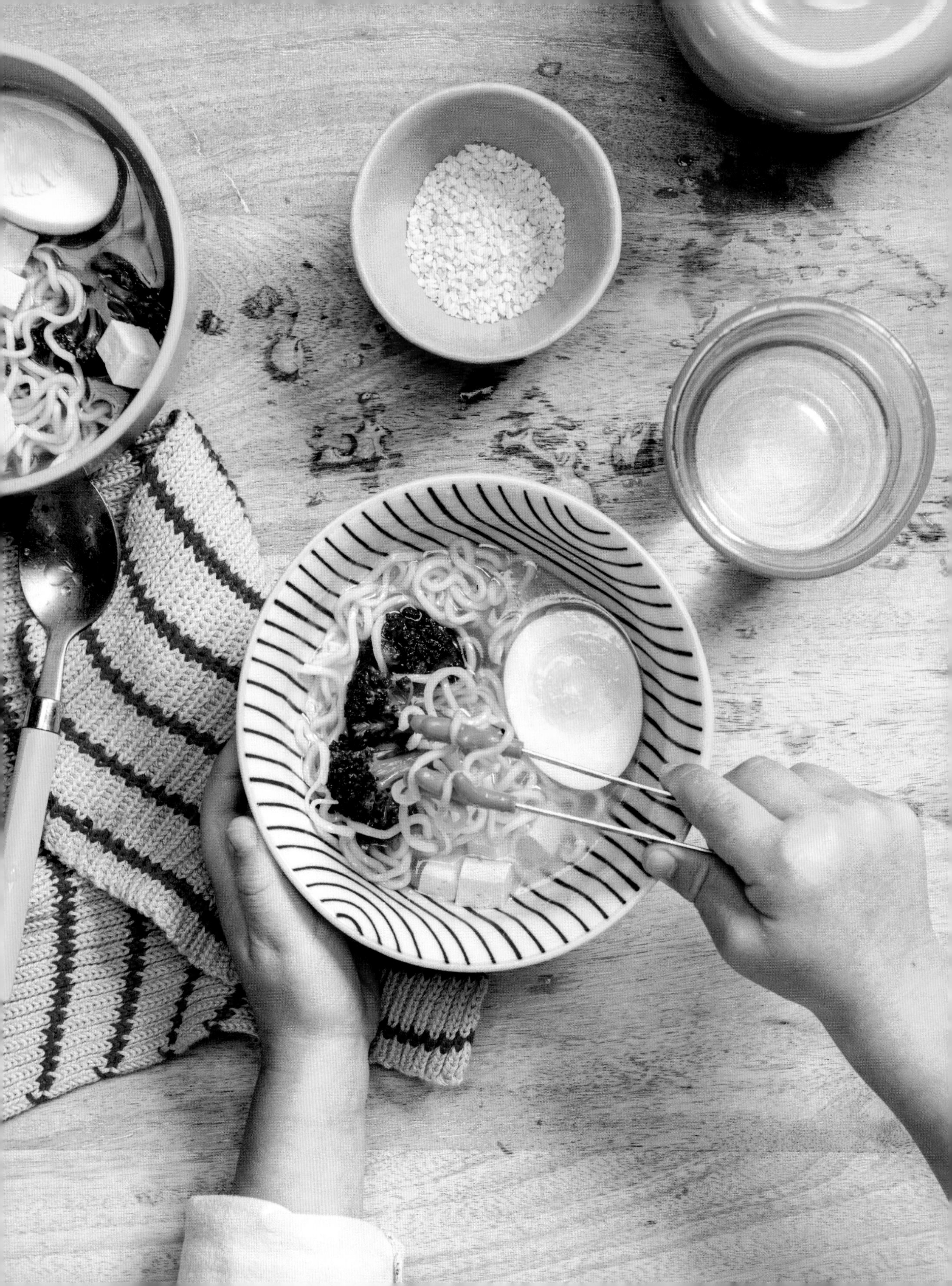

Divide the soup into bowls and top with the cooked broccoli and hard-boiled eggs.

INSPIRALIZED TIP

Omit the tofu or use a different protein, such as chicken, steak, ground meat, or shrimp.

FEEDING LITTLES TIP

The broth acts like a big dip for the broccoli. You might be surprised at how much your child enjoys broccoli this way.

I CAN'T EVEN

Buy premade hard-boiled eggs and/or steam the broccoli instead of roasting.

PREP AHEAD

Roast the broccoli ahead of time so this becomes a 15-minute meal.

dairy-free creamy potato and sausage soup

time to prep: 10 minutes / time to cook: 45 minutes / serves: 4 to 6

I've included a lot of dairy-free-but-still-creamy recipes because I know lots of families avoid dairy for allergies or intolerances but miss the flavor and texture of dairy foods. The cannellini beans are the key here. Beans are packed with protein and fiber, and they add a richness to this soup that complements the hearty flavors of the sausage. The potatoes are softened until tender and are appropriate for beginner eaters, passing the "squish test." You may be asking yourself why you ever need dairy to thicken a soup again, once you know this trick.

- 2 teaspoons extra-virgin olive oil
- 4 mild Italian sausage links
- 1 small onion, diced
- 4 garlic cloves, minced
- 2 teaspoons Italian seasoning
- 1 can (15 ounces) cannellini beans, drained and rinsed
- 1 container (32 ounces) low-sodium chicken or vegetable broth
- 4 cups cubed yellow potatoes (peeling optional)
- ½ teaspoon salt
- Pepper, to taste
- 1 cup finely chopped spinach

Heat 1 teaspoon of the oil in a large pot over medium-high heat. Once the oil is shimmering, add the sausage links, crumble, and cook until browned, about 7 minutes, stirring often. Using a slotted spoon, remove the sausage and set aside in a bowl. Immediately add the remaining teaspoon of oil, and then the onion and garlic. Cook until the vegetables soften, about 5 minutes. Add the Italian seasoning and stir well to coat the vegetables.

Add the beans and broth to the pot and stir. Using an immersion blender, blend the soup until creamy. If you don't have an immersion blender, transfer the soup mixture to a high-speed blender and blend until creamy. Return to the pot. Add the cooked sausage, potatoes, and salt and pepper, and bring the soup to a boil. Reduce the heat to a simmer, cover, and let the soup simmer for about 30 minutes or until the potatoes are tender.

Once the potatoes are tender, add the spinach to the pot. Simmer for 1 minute. Serve.

INSPIRALIZED TIP

Use a plant-based sausage here if you don't eat meat.

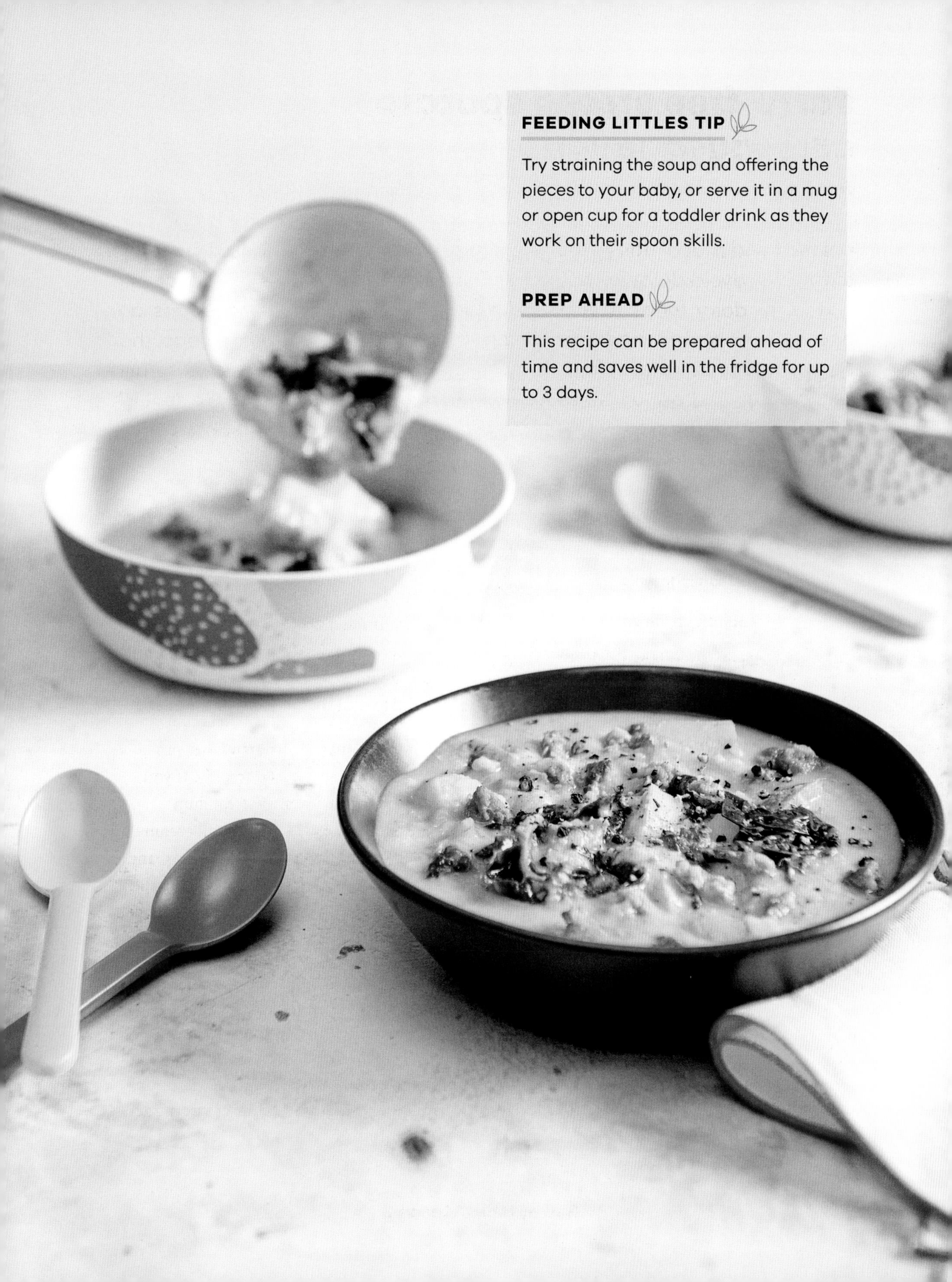

FEEDING LITTLES TIP

Try straining the soup and offering the pieces to your baby, or serve it in a mug or open cup for a toddler drink as they work on their spoon skills.

PREP AHEAD

This recipe can be prepared ahead of time and saves well in the fridge for up to 3 days.

farro minestrone soup

time to prep: 10 minutes / time to cook: 40 minutes / serves: 6

Growing up, I was always comforted by my mother's minestrone and my grandmother's pasta e fagioli. Both vegetable- and bean-based soups made me feel better emotionally or physically, and even as an adult, my mother knows when to bring me a big pot of minestrone. I'm hoping this hearty soup will be the one dish my children crave when they need some home cooking or they're not feeling their best. Unlike the soups my mother and grandmother made, this doesn't use canned tomatoes. Instead, a tablespoon of tomato paste adds enough rich, aromatic tomato flavor to bring to life the vegetables, beans, and farro. Save room for dipping a crusty bread in the leftover broth at the bottom of the bowl, savoring every last restorative drop.

2 tablespoons extra-virgin olive oil

2 garlic cloves, minced

2 celery ribs, diced

1 medium onion, diced

1 cup farro

1 tablespoon tomato paste

4 cups low-sodium vegetable broth

2 large carrots, peeled and diced

1 cup diced string beans in ¼-inch pieces

1 can (15 ounces) cannellini or Great Northern white beans, drained and rinsed

Salt and pepper

2 tablespoons thinly sliced fresh basil, for garnish

Grated or sliced Parmesan cheese, for serving (optional)

Bread, for serving

Heat the oil in a large pot or Dutch oven over medium heat. Once the oil is shimmering, add the garlic, celery, and onion. Cook until the vegetables are softened, stirring, for about 5 minutes. Add the farro and tomato paste and stir for 1 minute. Add the broth, 1 cup of water, carrots, string beans, and cannellini beans. Season with salt and pepper and bring to a boil. Reduce the heat to medium-low, cover, and simmer for 30 minutes or until the farro is cooked through. Uncover, remove from the heat, and top with the basil and Parmesan cheese, if using. Serve with bread.

INSPIRALIZED TIP

If you prefer brothier soups, add an additional cup of water when you add the broth.

FEEDING LITTLES TIP

Farro, a wheat-based whole grain that looks similar to barley, might be a new ingredient in your kitchen. It has a nutty flavor and a chewy, satisfying texture. Even though farro on its own may be too small for a baby to pick up, mixing it with the broth and other ingredients allows them to grip it better.

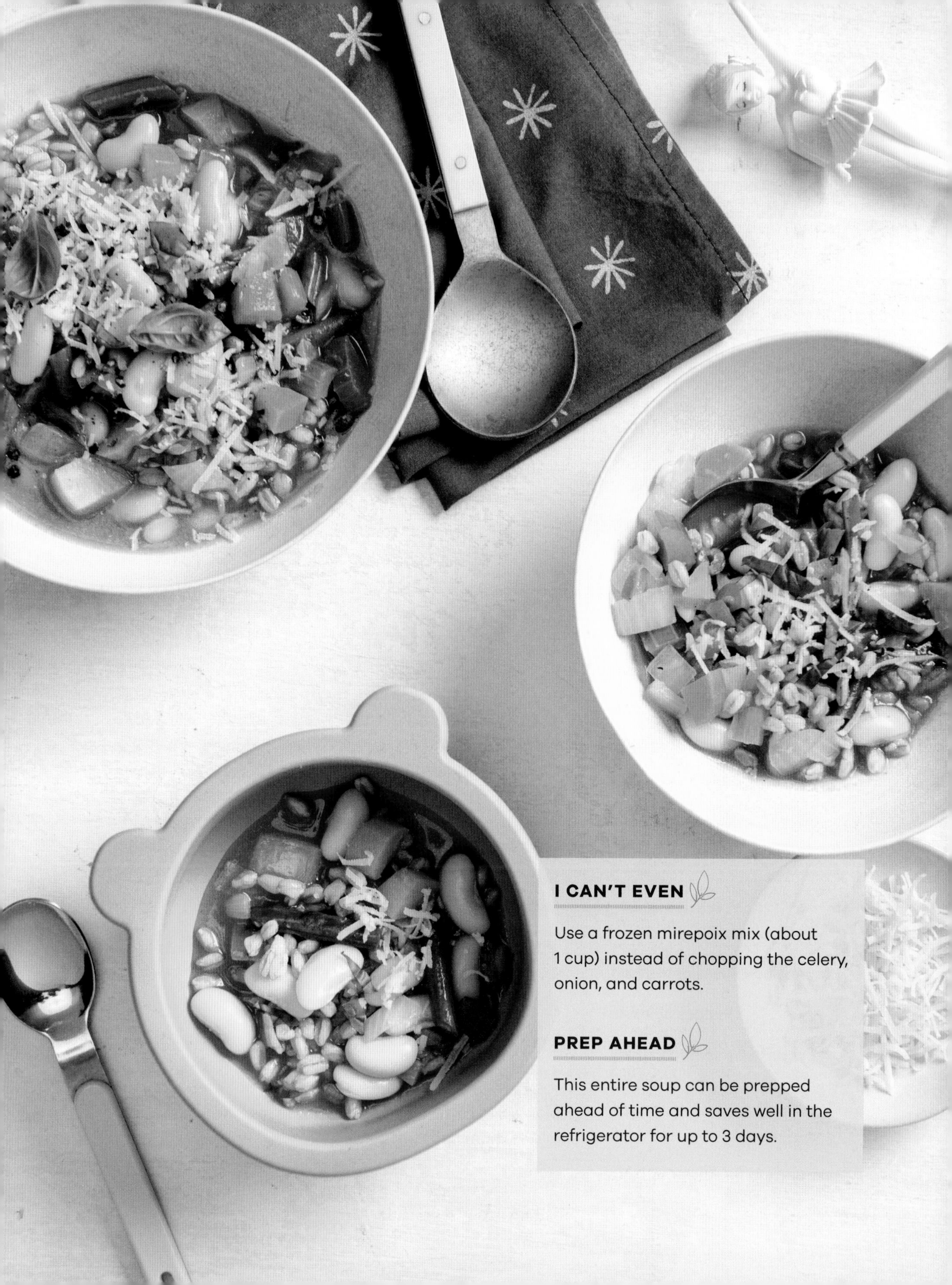

I CAN'T EVEN

Use a frozen mirepoix mix (about 1 cup) instead of chopping the celery, onion, and carrots.

PREP AHEAD

This entire soup can be prepped ahead of time and saves well in the refrigerator for up to 3 days.

spinach alfredo shells with sausage

time to prep: 10 minutes (plus 6 hours or overnight to soak cashews) / time to cook: 25 minutes / serves: 4

Attention dairy-free families: you are going to go nuts (no pun intended) for our version of this comfort food. The sauce is made with cashews, which are soaked overnight so that they can be pureed into a smooth consistency. Cashews are mild, so they're ideal to use in sauces where you don't want to add flavor, just consistency. This alfredo is lightly seasoned with cooked onion, garlic, and rosemary, and the sausage brings the flavor to a whole new level. The pasta shells are a nice shape to carry the sauce from dish to mouth.

4 Italian sausage links

1 cup raw cashews, soaked at least 6 hours (preferably overnight)

1 tablespoon extra-virgin olive oil

2 garlic cloves, sliced

½ cup diced red onion

½ teaspoon dried rosemary

½ lemon, juiced

½ teaspoon salt, plus more as needed

1 tablespoon nutritional yeast

Pepper, to taste

2 cups baby spinach, finely chopped

Preheat the oven to 425°F. Place the sausage links on a baking sheet and bake for 20 minutes or until cooked through.

Meanwhile, drain and rinse the cashews and place in a high-speed blender.

Heat the oil in a medium skillet over medium heat. Once the oil is shimmering, add the garlic and onion and cook for 5 minutes or until the vegetables are softened. Turn off the heat, stir in the rosemary, and transfer to the blender along with ¾ cup of water and the lemon juice, salt, and nutritional yeast. Season with pepper, blend until smooth, uncover, taste, and adjust with more salt if needed. Set aside.

Place the same skillet back over medium heat and add the spinach. Stir and let cook until dark green and wilted, about 3 minutes. Set aside.

Fill a large pot halfway with water and bring to a boil. Once boiling, add the shells and cook for 10 minutes until al dente or according to package instructions. Drain into a

8 ounces shells pasta

Red pepper flakes, for garnish

colander and place back into the pot along with the spinach. Slice the cooked sausage into ¼-inch-thick rounds and add to the pot. Pour over half of the alfredo sauce. Stir well to combine and add more alfredo sauce, if desired. Transfer to a serving dish and serve, garnished with red pepper flakes.

INSPIRALIZED TIP

You can skip the nutritional yeast if you don't have any handy, but the dish won't have that cheesy Parmesan taste. (It will still be yummy, though.)

FEEDING LITTLES TIP

Make sure to dice the sausage into quarters or small pieces for kids younger than four.

I CAN'T EVEN

Use a jarred dairy-free (or regular) alfredo sauce instead of making this one from scratch.

PREP AHEAD

Cook the sausage and make the sauce ahead of time, so that all you need to do at dinnertime is cook the pasta and add the spinach.

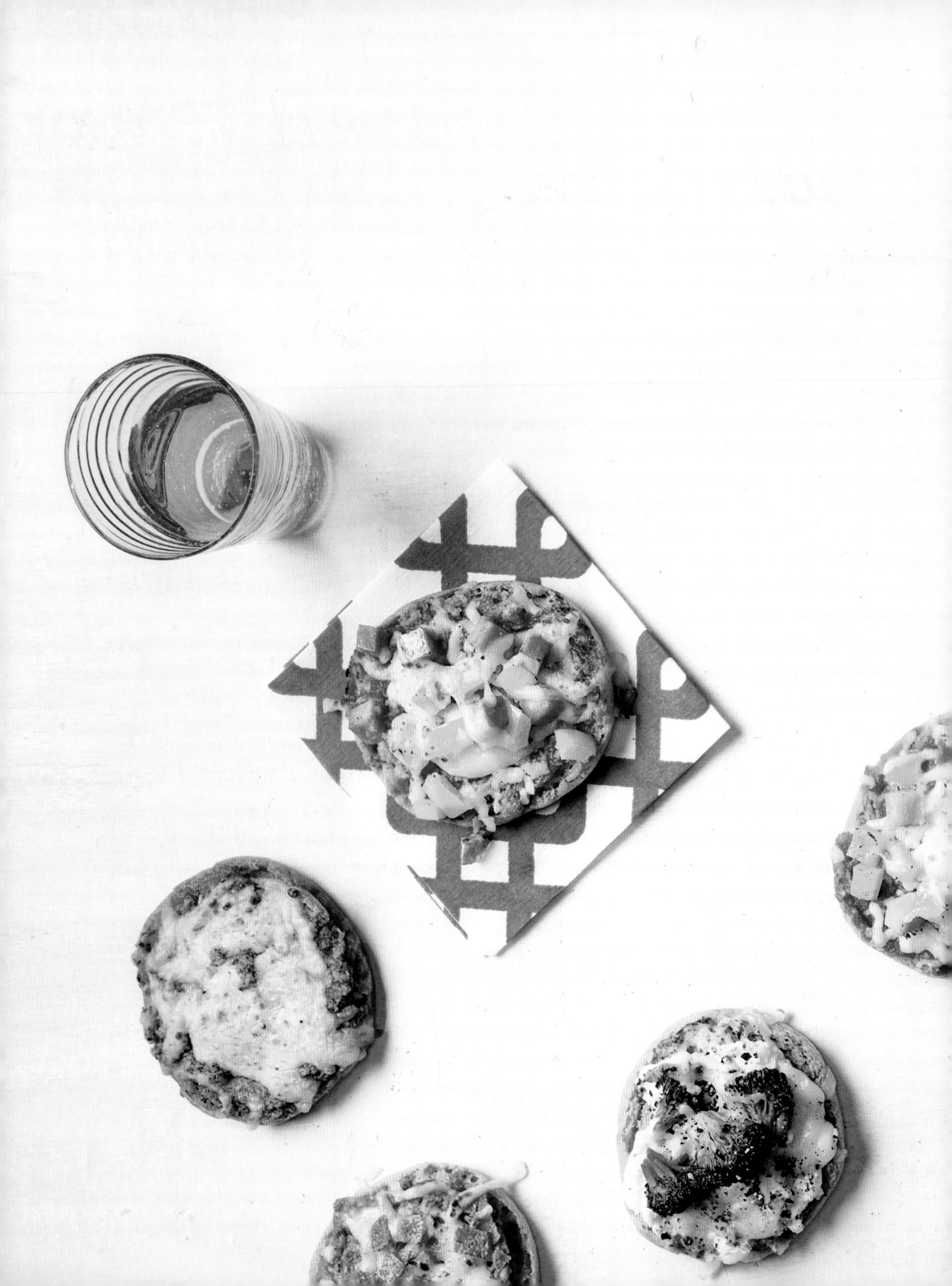

easy go-tos

Have extra time on a Sunday and want to prep the week's lunches for your kids?

Finally going on a date night and have fifteen to twenty minutes to throw a meal together before the babysitter arrives?

Going out with friends and need a simple recipe for your partner to give the kids while you get ready?

Ordering takeout and want to enjoy it after the kids go down, but still need something to feed them at dinnertime?

Nauseous from pregnancy and just want to eat crackers, but you still need to feed your family?

Need something easy and quick that you know your kid will eat?

Welcome to our easy go-tos. This chapter is full of meals that are designed for kids' palates and are quick and easy to throw together when you're cooking for the under-eighteen set. (That said, what adult wouldn't want Crunchy Oven-Baked Grilled Cheese (page 125)? It's the only way we can make grilled cheeses now, and we'll never go stovetop again.)

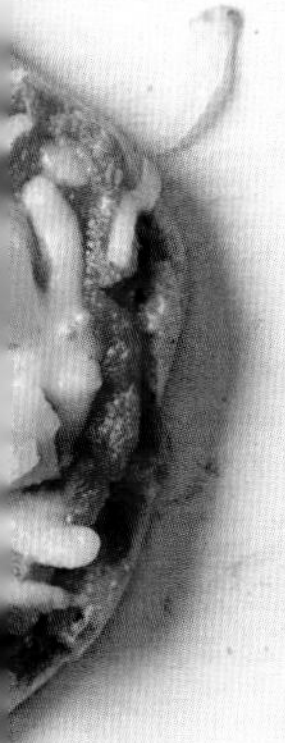

For the most part, when we are going out and need to feed our kids before the babysitter arrives, we order pizza. However, if your kid has specific nutritional needs, allergies, or you're just trying to clear out the fridge, take fifteen minutes to throw together some Penne with Chickpea Sauce and Spinach (page 131) or some Secret Salsa Black Bean Burrito Bowls (page 130). Bonus: the leftovers are easy to pack into a lunch box the next day.

While we don't encourage short-order cooking—i.e., extra work for overtaxed parents—sometimes we need another option for our kids, and these recipes make cooking something

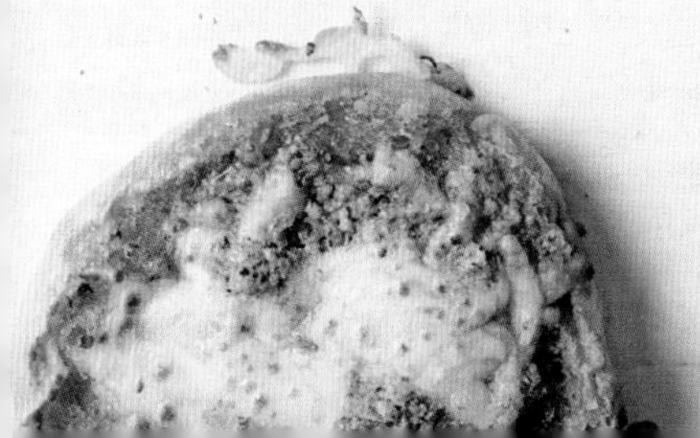

special for them a little less time-consuming. Then, the adults in the family can enjoy a quiet mealtime or much-needed night out.

But wait! Before we get into the main recipes, we've included two other types of go-to meals that take little effort and time but are still tasty and nutritious, whether we're cooking for the kids or for the whole family: Simple Staples and I Can't Even (the absolute simplest) dishes.

Simple Staples

Some of our most beloved recipes are the ones that you don't even need a recipe for—just start chopping and heating and you've got a tasty meal in minutes. Below are the staple ideas to have in your back pocket for an easy lunch or dinner.

BURRITOS OR TACOS

- Warm up corn or flour tortillas and gather fillings to serve tacos or burritos family-style. Think beans, cheese, rice, cooked vegetables, meat, salsa, sour cream, sliced avocado, or guacamole.
- Serve tortillas with the fillings in bowls on the table. Everyone gets to make their own tacos or burritos.

SIMPLE TERIYAKI STIR-FRY

- Cook a fresh or frozen protein in a neutral oil, add vegetables and cook until tender, then toss in some bottled teriyaki sauce and cook until heated through. Serve with rice or noodles.
- Combination examples: Shrimp and Broccoli, Shrimp and Snow Peas, Pork and Green Beans, Tofu with Carrots and Bell Peppers
- Note: frozen bell peppers are handy here because they are soft enough for babies once they defrost in the skillet.

ONE-PAN GROUND MEAT RICE SKILLETS

- Sauté any ground meat or ground vegetable product in a skillet, add cooked rice and vegetables and/or a can of tomatoes, seasonings, and cheese (optional). If using cheese, cover the skillet with a lid and cook until the cheese melts.
- Combination examples (just add cooked rice!):
    - Taco Beef Skillet: ground beef, garlic and onions, with corn, beans, can of tomatoes, taco seasoning, Mexican cheese blend and top with avocado
    - Italian Turkey Skillet: ground turkey, garlic and onions, can of crushed tomatoes, broccoli, Italian seasoning, mozzarella, and Parmesan cheese
    - Mediterranean Lamb Skillet: ground lamb, garlic and onions, can of diced tomatoes, chopped green bell peppers, cumin, oregano, and top with feta and parsley

PASTA NIGHT

- Pasta + Protein + Sauce + Veggies = Pasta Night
- Combination examples:
    - Sausage, Parmesan Sauce, and Broccoli: To make a Parmesan sauce, reserve ½ cup of pasta water. Then, place your pasta, sausage, and broccoli back into the pot, add shredded or grated cheese, and stir while you drizzle in the pasta water. Stop adding water when your pasta is saucy to your liking. Add Italian seasoning or garlic powder for flavor.
    - Ground Turkey, Marinara Sauce, and Mushrooms
    - Chopped Chicken, Alfredo Sauce, and Spinach
    - Shrimp, Pesto, and Peas

POUR AND COOK CHICKEN MEAL IDEAS

Pour and cook meals are ones where you place protein and vegetables in a slow cooker, pressure cooker, or oven, top with a premade sauce, and let the device do the cooking for you. We like using this method best for boneless chicken breasts or thighs. If you are vegetarian, we've included an option with tofu. Serve these proteins with sides, if needed, and over pasta, noodles, or grains.

While you may have to wait for the food to cook, the effort and cleanup are a breeze.

Here are some examples of sauces to use: salsa, marinara, cream of mushroom soup, BBQ sauce, low-sodium lentil soup, alfredo, bruschetta sauce, Indian simmer sauce, marsala sauce.

Boneless, Skinless Chicken Breasts or Skinless Thighs (use 1 cup of sauce per 1 pound of meat)

COOKING DEVICE	COOK TIME
Oven	400°F for 22 to 25 minutes
Pressure cooker	High pressure for 8 minutes
Slow cooker	Low on 3 to 4 hours or until internal temperature of 165°F is reached

Meal combination examples:

- Salsa Chicken Rice Bowl with Avocado
- Marsala Chicken with Penne and Steamed Broccoli

Cubed Extra-Firm Tofu (use 1 cup of sauce per 14 ounces of cubed tofu)

COOKING DEVICE	COOK TIME
Oven	400°F for 30 to 40 minutes
Pressure cooker	High pressure for 2 minutes
Slow cooker	Low for 4 to 6 hours or high for 2 to 3 hours

Meal combination examples:

- Tofu "Tikka" Masala and Peas with Brown Rice
- Barbecue Tofu and Sweet Potatoes with Quinoa and Avocado

I Can't Even

I Can't Even is the name we give the mood when you just don't have it in you to cook, but you still need to feed your family. It's not like you need an excuse; sometimes, you just don't want to. Perhaps you had a long day at work or with the kids. Maybe you're having family issues and you're just emotionally broken down. Or maybe this is your first time feeding your little one and you're feeling overwhelmed. We all have those days, and that's when the "I Can't Even" meals pull through. We make them when we just don't have the energy to turn on the oven. We still need to put food on the table, but we don't want to spend more than ten or fifteen minutes in the kitchen and certainly don't want a lot of cleanup.

If you have the time to wait for delivery, awesome. We support that. But if you have hangry little hands tugging at your legs and need to make something quickly, here are some ideas to get you over the hump.

And please know that anything you feed your family is served with love, and that's what matters. Whether it's a PB&J, a grilled cheese, a bowl of cereal, or cookies, it's all food. You're doing great.

BREAKFAST FOR DINNER

- Eggs (or omelets) + Toast + Fruit
- Toaster waffles + Fruit
- Yogurt with granola + Fruit + Nut (or sun) butter
- Bagel and cream cheese + Fruit
- Oatmeal with nut butter + Fruit
- Cereal + Fruit + Milk

THE FREEZER IS YOUR FRIEND

Pick a frozen protein and serve with frozen vegetables and an additional side. Consider frozen sweet potato fries, frozen or boxed rice, or frozen premade gnocchi. Cook according to package directions.

Frozen protein ideas: veggie or meat burgers, fish sticks, chicken nuggets, edamame, pizza, sausages, meatballs. Follow package instructions.

STUFFED BAKED POTATOES

Heat up a can of premade chili and pour it over baked potatoes. Top with sour cream or Greek yogurt. To make quick baked potatoes, place a trivet in the bottom of a pressure cooker and add 1 cup of water. Wash medium russet potatoes and pierce them all over with a fork. Place the potatoes on top of the trivet, cover with the lid, and set the valve to the sealing position. Cook on High pressure for 15 minutes. Let the pressure release naturally (if you're in a rush, you can do this manually, but the potatoes won't be as tender). Test for doneness by piercing the potatoes with a knife, and if it goes in smoothly, the potatoes are done.

MAC AND CHEESE

Cook pasta per box instructions. During the last minute of cooking, add frozen peas so they heat through. Drain pasta and peas. Stir in cheese packet and butter as instructed. If you want to add more protein and a creamy texture, sub unsweetened Greek yogurt for milk in equal quantities.

For other combos, stir in black beans, leftover cooked butternut squash cubes, or leftover ground meat.

ADDITIONAL FAVORITES:

- Heated leftover entrée + Cut-up bell peppers or fruit
- Snack tray (see page 135)
- Peanut butter and jelly + Heated veggies from frozen + Blueberries
- Avocado toast + Hard-boiled egg
- Frozen pizza + Bagged Caesar salad or fruit
- Grilled cheese + Tomato or vegetable soup
- Egg, tuna, bean, or chicken salad + Crackers + Cut-up veggies

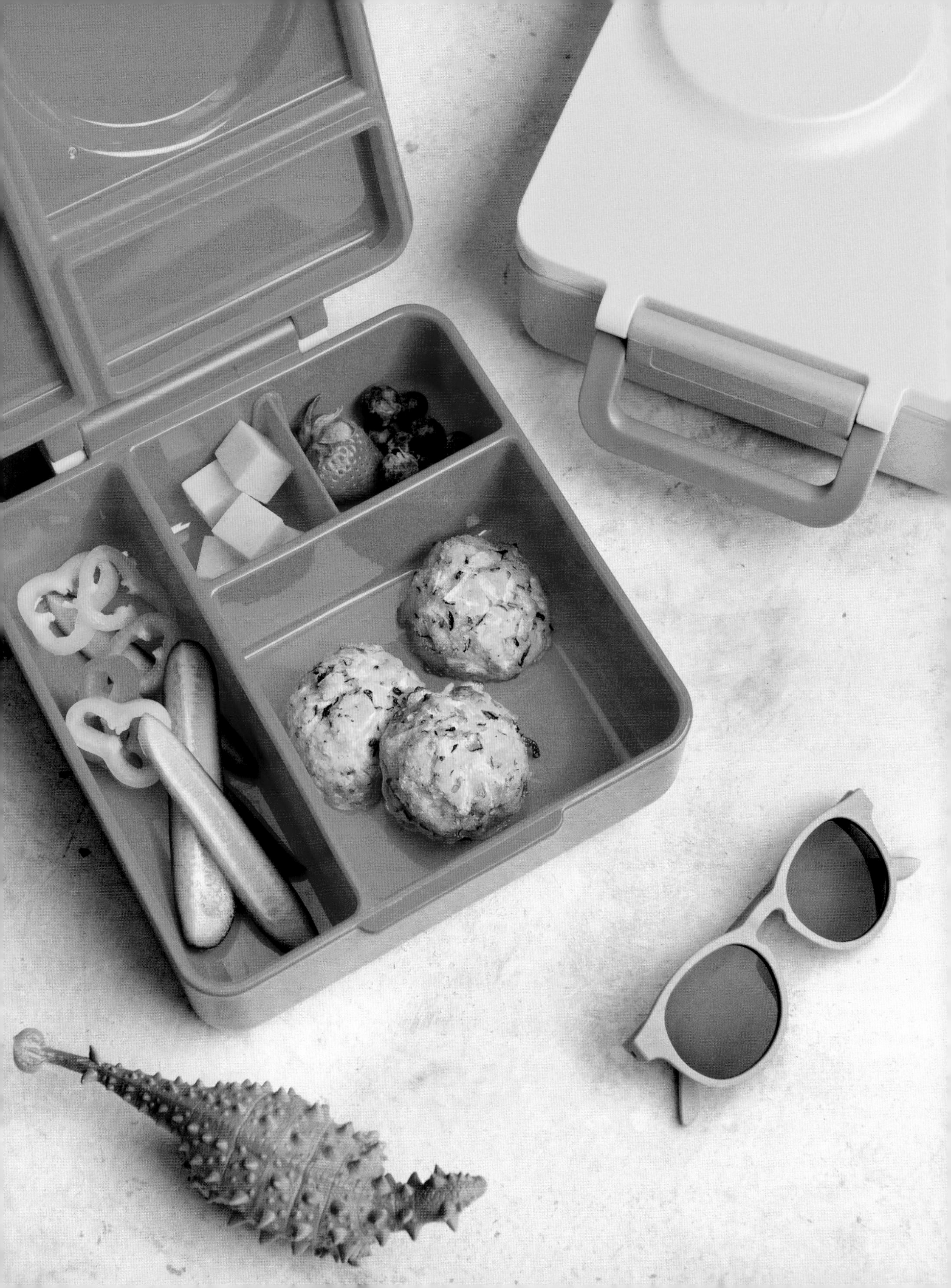

veggie bites two ways

time to prep: 15 minutes / time to cook: 20 minutes / makes: about 6 bites

Snackable, portable, hearty, flavorful, and fun, these veggie bites are the ultimate kids' food. After making the base recipe for years, I decided to switch it up for a nostalgic pizza flavor, and my kids asked for me to make a second batch. Made with pantry and fridge ingredients, this is the kind of recipe you'll default to when you want to put something nutritious on your kid's plate, but you don't have the energy to come up with something new. We always have a batch in the freezer, because they heat up well, and I pack them whenever we're on the go. I can't wait to see what flavor combination you come up with—but don't skip the pizza one.

The Base Recipe

⅓ cup almond flour (whole wheat or oat flour work well, too)

1 cup shredded or grated vegetable (carrot, sweet potato, and zucchini work best)

⅓ cup grated Parmesan cheese

1 large egg

¼ teaspoon garlic powder

1 teaspoon dried oregano

Salt and pepper, to taste

Pizza Veggie Bites

⅓ cup almond flour (whole wheat or oat flour work well, too)

(ingredients continue)

Preheat the oven to 375°F. Line a baking sheet with parchment paper.

Mix together the ingredients for either of the veggie bites in a medium bowl. Mold the mixture into ball-shaped pieces and place on the parchment paper, making 6 or 7 bites. Bake for 15 minutes, turn the heat up to 400°F, and bake for another 5 minutes or until golden brown on the edges.

Let cool slightly before serving.

(recipe continues)

1 cup shredded or grated vegetable (carrot, sweet potato, and zucchini work best)

⅓ cup shredded mozzarella cheese

1 large egg

2 tablespoons marinara sauce

¼ teaspoon garlic powder

¼ teaspoon dried oregano

¼ teaspoon dried rosemary

¼ teaspoon dried basil

Salt and pepper, to taste

INSPIRALIZED TIP

Mold these into whatever shape you like. They work well as little rectangles or squares or even rounded ovals. If you have a special mold your little ones like, try that out as well.

FEEDING LITTLES TIP

These veggie bites are appropriate for babies since they're soft and easy to hold. They're also an awesome way to use up vegetables that are about to go bad in your fridge.

PREP AHEAD

These bites can be entirely prepped ahead and stored in the freezer for up to 3 months.

crunchy oven-baked grilled cheese with broccoli

time to prep: 10 minutes / time to cook: 10 minutes / makes: 2 sandwiches

When I asked Megan to send me her go-to family recipes, she said, "Well, I don't know if this counts, but I make my grilled cheese sandwich in the toaster oven and it gets nice and crispy." Um, genius. I'm the official recipe developer here, so how have I never thought to put a grilled cheese sandwich in the toaster oven?! I tested it immediately and, long story short, I will never make grilled cheese any other way again. Neither will you!

1 cup frozen broccoli florets

⅔ cup low-sodium chicken or vegetable broth (or water)

1 tablespoon unsalted butter

4 slices multigrain bread

4 slices cheddar cheese

Preheat the oven (or toaster oven on the Bake setting) to 350°F.

Combine the broccoli and broth (or water) in a small pot and bring to a boil. Boil until the broccoli is cooked through, about 3 minutes. Transfer the broccoli to a cutting board and slice the stems off the florets and finely chop the florets. Set aside.

Lightly spread ¼ tablespoon of butter on 4 slices of bread. Place 2 pieces of bread butter side down on a baking sheet. Add a slice of cheese on the left side of each slice of bread. Sprinkle the broccoli on top. Top the right side of the bread with the remaining cheese. Top with the remaining slices of bread, butter side up. Place in the oven and bake for 5 to 7 minutes or until the cheese is melted and the bread is crispy, pressing down with a spatula to compress each sandwich every 2 to 3 minutes. Remove from the oven and let the sandwiches cool for 5 minutes before slicing to serve.

FEEDING LITTLES TIP

Serve the cooked broccoli on the side of the grilled cheese if your tot is hesitant to try the assembled sandwich.

INSPIRALIZED TIP

To elevate this grilled cheese for an adult, use sautéed Brussels sprouts instead of broccoli, and a Gruyère or Swiss cheese instead of cheddar. Your kids might like it, too.

sweet potato, ham, and cheese cups

time to prep: 15 minutes / time to cook: 15 minutes / makes: 12 cups

Ham and cheese is a classic combo for a reason. I've made ham and cheese frittatas, ham and grilled cheese sandwiches, and ham and cheese roll-up snacks. Here, we're making ham and cheese cups with sweet potatoes, which add a hint of sweetness (and a nutritional boost). Pack them in a lunch box or serve them as an easy meal with fruit and a dipping sauce on the side.

Olive oil spray, for greasing the muffin pan

4 cups grated sweet potato

1 teaspoon garlic powder

Salt and pepper, to taste

2 large eggs

3 slices deli ham, cubed

½ cup shredded cheddar cheese

Preheat the oven to 400°F. Grease a 12-cup muffin pan with olive oil spray.

Stir together the sweet potato, garlic powder, salt, pepper, eggs, ham, and cheese in a large mixing bowl, and toss to combine. Pack the muffin cups two-thirds of the way full, using about ⅓ cup of mixture in each cup. Bake for 15 minutes or until the eggs set and the cups are firm. If you want, trim off any of the burnt parts on top of the muffins—or keep them for a nice crunch.

INSPIRALIZED TIP

If you have leftover hot dogs from a barbecue, substitute diced dogs for the ham for a different flavor.

FEEDING LITTLES TIP

Look for deli meat with no added nitrates/nitrites when possible.

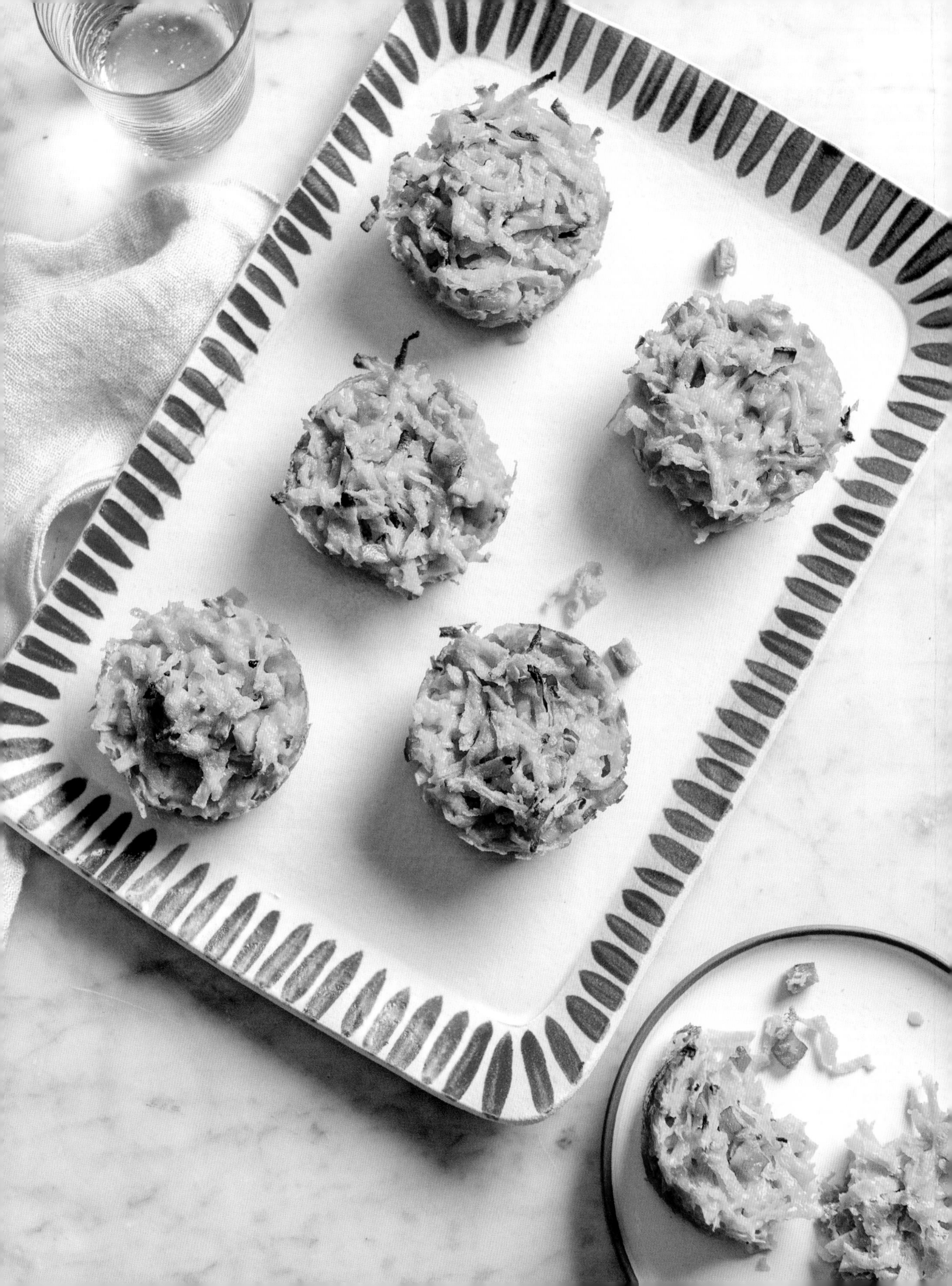

strawberry chia jam and cream cheese squares

time to prep: 25 minutes / makes: 2 sandwiches

Cream cheese and jelly was my ultimate after-school snack. Somewhere along the way to adulthood, though, I forgot about it—until I had children of my own. We use a strawberry chia jam that's super easy to make, and it's handy to keep in mind if you're out of jelly but have a carton of berries in the fridge.

1 cup strawberries, stems trimmed

1 tablespoon chia seeds

Cream cheese

4 slices bread

Place the strawberries in a food processor and pulse until jamlike. Pour the mixture into a small bowl, stir in the chia seeds, and set in the refrigerator, covered, for 20 minutes to let the chia seeds gel up with the strawberries.

Once the jam is ready, spread cream cheese onto 2 slices of bread. On the other slices of bread, spread out the jam. Close the sandwiches and slice. Triangles or fun shapes with cookie cutters can make these even more interesting to your tot.

INSPIRALIZED TIP

If you use a different fruit, like a raspberry, you need to be cautious of tartness. Strawberries strike the perfect balance between tart and sweet, so no added sugars are needed, but if you want to use another berry, add a teaspoon of maple syrup, sugar, or honey to sweeten.

FEEDING LITTLES TIP

Mix this jam into plain yogurt for babies, toddlers, and older kids alike. If adding additional sweeteners, avoid honey for kids younger than one year.

hawaiian fried rice with veggies

time to prep: 10 minutes / time to cook: 10 minutes / serves: 2

This is a tasty, quick version of fried rice that's extra kid-friendly, thanks to sweet pineapple and familiar ham. The ham can be substituted for your little one's protein of choice, like chicken, salmon, edamame, or tofu. It's a great way to introduce flavors such as sesame and soy sauce; before you know it, you'll be serving Sesame Ginger Steak, Pepper, and String Bean Stir-Fry (page 86). If you're making it for yourself, elevate it with chopped onion, fresh veggies and scallions, ground pork or pork loin instead of ham, and extra seasonings.

1 tablespoon sesame oil

1 garlic clove, minced

1 cup frozen veggies of choice (I use a combination of string beans, carrots, corn, and peas)

½ cup frozen pineapple chunks

1½ cups cooked brown rice

2 slices deli ham, diced

Pepper, to taste

1 large egg

1 tablespoon low-sodium soy sauce

Heat the sesame oil in a large skillet over medium-high heat. Once the oil is shimmering, add the garlic, frozen vegetables, and pineapple, and cook for 5 minutes or until heated through and fork-tender.

Add the rice and ham, and season with pepper. Stir well. Create a hole in the center of the mixture and add in the egg. Stir until scrambled and then break up well with a spatula, and stir with the rice mixture to combine. Add the soy sauce and stir well. Divide the mixture into bowls, and if there are any large chunks of pineapple, halve them with a knife.

PREP AHEAD

Similar to takeout, leftover fried rice tastes even better the next day. I recommend adding a splash of broth or water into a pan along with the fried rice to add a bit of moisture back in.

INSPIRALIZED TIP

If you're ordering takeout but your kid isn't interested, serve this dish in a takeout container and they'll feel included, too.

FEEDING LITTLES TIP

Fruit is a gateway food for many kids—they see it on their plate and suddenly they want to dig into the rest of the meal. Pineapple is the gateway food here. However, if you don't enjoy pineapple mixed with savory foods, serve it on the side.

secret salsa black bean burrito bowls

time to prep: 5 minutes / time to cook: 5 minutes / serves: 2 large bowls or 4 small bowls

The secret ingredient in this recipe is—you guessed it—salsa. No, we're not trying to sneak it onto our kid's plate. But salsa can serve as a ready-to-add sauce that you might not have considered. This is a pared-down version of a burrito bowl, using mostly canned and frozen foods, and the salsa flavors the rice, so there's no need to add seasonings. I keep these ingredients in my pantry and freezer, so it's one of those meals that gets made over and over again, when I haven't grocery shopped for the week or don't feel like making a mess in the kitchen but still want to cook something filling, nourishing, and tasty.

1 tablespoon neutral cooking oil, such as avocado oil or other vegetable oil

1½ cups cooked brown rice

⅔ cup canned black beans, drained and rinsed

½ cup frozen corn

¼ cup mild salsa

Salt and pepper

½ cup guacamole or mashed avocado, for serving

2 tablespoons full-fat plain Greek yogurt, for serving

Heat the oil in a large skillet over medium heat. Once the oil is shimmering, add the rice, black beans, corn, and salsa. Season with salt and pepper, stir, and cook for about 5 minutes or until warmed through. Divide the rice mixture into bowls and serve with the guacamole and yogurt.

INSPIRALIZED TIP

You can switch this up by using a salsa verde instead of red salsa.

FEEDING LITTLES TIP

Some kids love spicy foods—others hate them. Even mild salsa has a little kick, and for some kids it can be too much. Learning to love spicy foods is all about patience and gradual exposure. If your child can't handle the salsa, try subbing it out for chopped tomato, or add more chopped tomato to the salsa to lighten the kick.

I CAN'T EVEN

Use microwavable rice.

penne with chickpea sauce and spinach

time to prep: 5 minutes / time to cook: 20 minutes / serves: 2

You know the kids who are so obsessed with ketchup that you could literally serve anything as long as it's slathered in the stuff and they'd try it? Well, I have a friend whose child feels the same way about hummus, so she adds hummus to everything—eggs, meat, cheese, soups; the list is endless. She even serves her pasta with hummus as a dip. I live by the mantra "don't fix it unless it's broken," but when she told me she wished that her child would try pasta with a sauce, I came up with this easy in-between option: hummus and pasta water, with nutritional yeast for an inviting and familiar cheesy flavor. Try it with kids who love mild flavors or hummus in particular.

4 ounces favorite pasta (I like tagliatelle, penne, or bowties here)

½ cup hummus

2 cups baby spinach, well chopped

1 teaspoon nutritional yeast

Salt and pepper

2 teaspoons seasoned Italian whole wheat breadcrumbs (you can also use gluten-free breadcrumbs)

Bring a pot filled halfway with water to a boil. Once boiling, add the pasta and cook according to the package directions. Reserve ½ cup of pasta water and drain the pasta into a colander. Place the pasta back into the pot and add the hummus, reserved pasta water, spinach, and nutritional yeast. Season with salt and pepper, and stir well to coat the pasta in the sauce. Stir until the spinach is wilted, about 5 minutes. Divide the pasta into bowls and top with the breadcrumbs.

INSPIRALIZED TIP

Experiment with hummus varieties, like roasted red pepper, garlic, or one with a hint of lemon.

FEEDING LITTLES TIP

Sometimes calling new food by a silly name helps your child feel less overwhelmed. If you use bowtie pasta in this dish, consider calling it "butterfly pasta." Penne noodles make clever "witch fingers." Spinach can be "monster leaves." Of course, calling food by its real name is important, too, but letting your kid use their imagination can help them have fun—and feel more adventurous—at the table.

english muffin mini pizzas

time to prep: 5 minutes / time to cook: 10 minutes / makes: 4 pizzas

English muffins make perfectly kid-sized meals, whether you're serving a burger, grilled cheese sandwich, egg salad sandwich, tuna melt, peanut butter and jelly sandwich, or pizza. When I make a pizza for the kids (or the whole family), I always try to add a vegetable, whether that's as a topping or pureed and stirred into the sauce like it is here. When your little one takes a bite, they'll taste a little of the peas and more of the salty pepperoni and gooey cheese, which will keep them reaching for more. Seeing veggies in their whole form is important, but adding them to sauces in this way adds a nutritional kick that's an approachable way to learn to love them. Remember, every exposure to an ingredient helps in the long run. If the flavor is too much for your kids, serve the peas on the side instead.

¼ cup peas, thawed if frozen

¼ cup marinara sauce or tomato basil sauce

2 whole-grain English muffins

½ cup shredded mozzarella cheese

8 slices turkey pepperoni, chopped (or regular pepperoni)

Preheat the oven to 400°F.

Place the peas with 1 tablespoon of water in a small food processor and pulse until creamy, adding tablespoons of water as needed until it looks like a puree. Alternately, you can mash the peas completely and then stir in the water until it is pureed. Place the puree in a small bowl along with the marinara sauce and stir to combine.

Spread the marinara sauce out on the muffins. Top with mozzarella cheese and then pepperoni. Place in the oven for 10 minutes or until the cheese melts.

INSPIRALIZED TIP

Other purees work well here, such as carrot (which blends in better with the sauce).

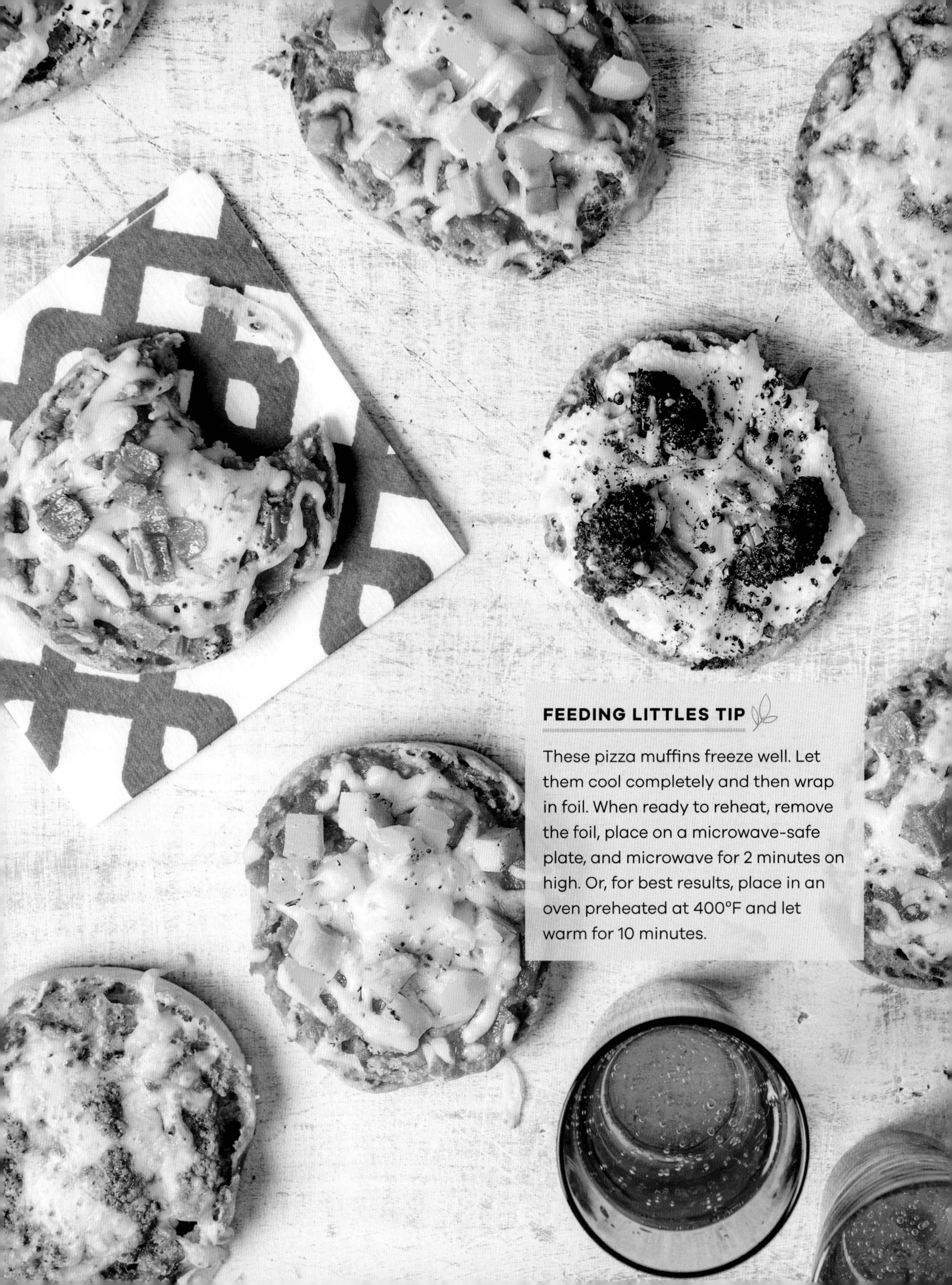

FEEDING LITTLES TIP

These pizza muffins freeze well. Let them cool completely and then wrap in foil. When ready to reheat, remove the foil, place on a microwave-safe plate, and microwave for 2 minutes on high. Or, for best results, place in an oven preheated at 400°F and let warm for 10 minutes.

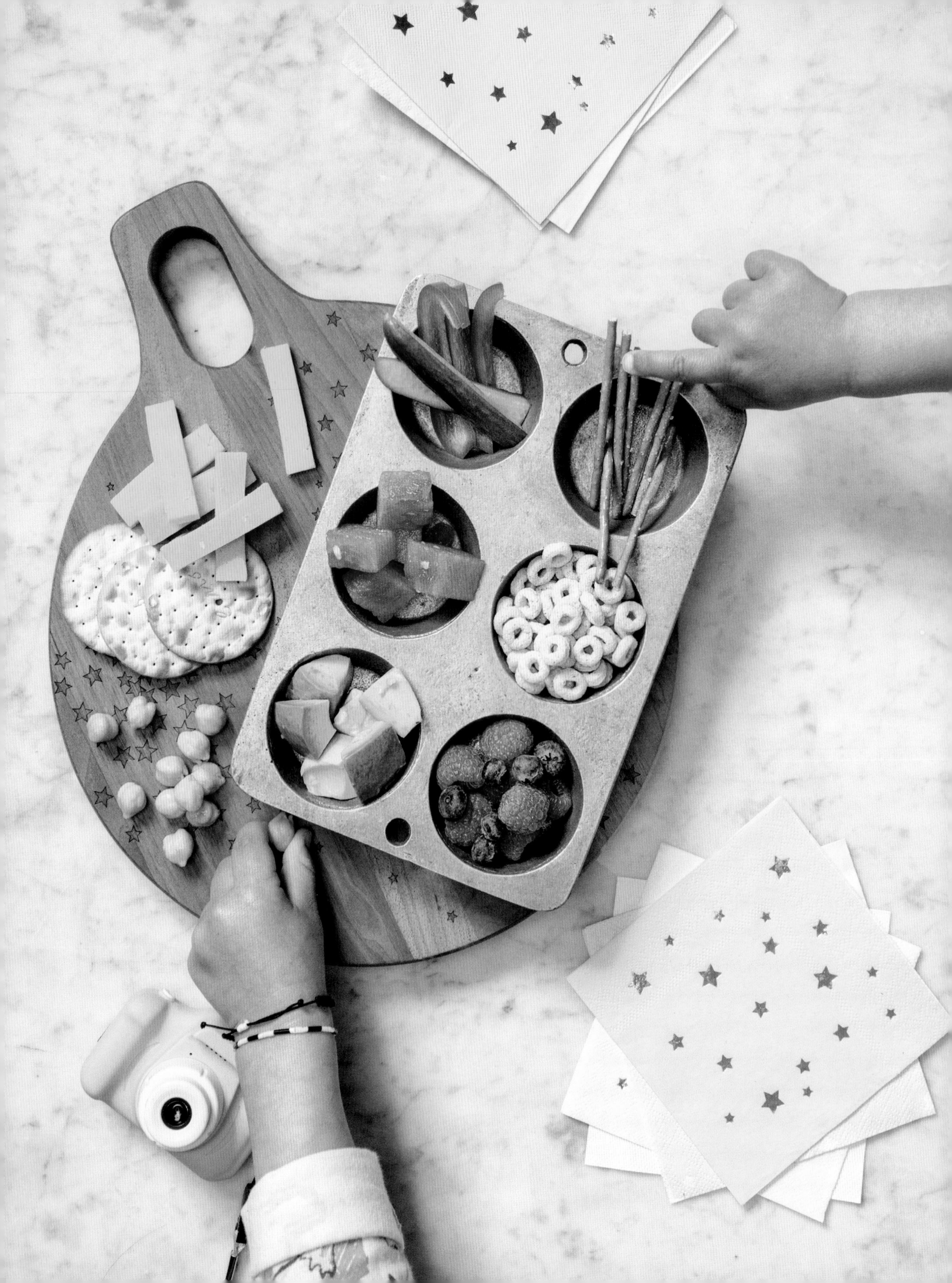

snack tray dinner

serves: 2 children

Sometimes, you don't feel like cooking dinner or, frankly, you just miss the old days when you could make a bowl of popcorn or a plate of cheese and crackers and call it dinner. Lean into that nostalgia with a Snack Tray Dinner.

Take out a muffin pan, ice cube mold, or container that has spaces big enough to fill with small, snackable foods. Silicone muffin cups or individual mini ramekins also work. Fill each space with your child's favorite snacks as well as some not-so-loved vegetables or foods. Not only is this meal easy and quick for parents, but it's exciting and novel enough for kids that they may just end up eating some foods they normally don't.

Some Ideas for Your Snack Tray Dinner

- Crackers, rice cakes, pretzels, and chips
- Steamed vegetables (like peas, broccoli, green beans) or any leftover cooked veggies you have on hand
- Raw vegetables (age-appropriate—bell peppers, cucumbers, jicama, quartered cherry tomatoes, broccoli, cauliflower; if using carrots/celery for kids younger than age four, slice very thin)
- Fruit (berries work especially well)
- Legumes and beans (like edamame, black beans, pinto beans, and chickpeas)
- Avocados
- Cooked corn
- Tomatoes
- Nuts (age four and older for whole nuts)
- Sliced or rolled-up deli meats
- Cheese
- Cheerios or similar cereal
- Raisins
- Celery sticks with almond butter or cream cheese (age four and older for whole celery sticks)

(continued)

The Snack Tray Can Also Be Themed for a Specific Occasion:

- Make a toddler charcuterie board with fruit, cheese, crackers, and meats.
- Call it "breakfast for dinner" and fill it with toasted and sliced freezer waffles, fruit, yogurt (with a spoon on the side), cereal, cubed granola bars, and sliced hard-boiled eggs.
- Make it extra special for a holiday, like on Valentine's Day with a heart-shaped cookie cutter to make veggie, fruit, bread, and even pepperoni hearts. And, of course, include a chocolate candy for dessert.
- However you choose to build your Snack Tray Dinner, it'll take the pressure off mealtime and it may just become your new go-to weeknight dinner. Remember to make yourself your own version to enjoy alongside your littles.

megan's amped-up boxed mac and cheese

For a truly elevated mac and cheese, Megan has the secret sauce . . . and it's Greek yogurt. I would have never thought to do this, but by stirring Greek yogurt into your cheese sauce, the mac and cheese is creamier, thicker, and has a little tang that makes all the difference. Plus, it adds a satisfying source of fat and protein. Amp up the meal even more by incorporating different vegetables and toppings. To get you started, here are some of our favorite ways to jazz up boxed mac and cheese—no shame in that box game!

Base Recipe with Greek Yogurt

Cook the pasta according to the box directions. When making the cheese sauce, add ¼ cup plain, full-fat Greek yogurt to the pan instead of the milk and butter as instructed. Add in the cheese packet, stir, and then add back in the cooked pasta.

Suggested Fillings and Toppings to Upgrade Boxed Mac and Cheese

- Simple additions: frozen peas, beans, or cubed chicken
- Bacon + Chopped tomatoes + Avocado + Shredded romaine
- Sausage + Chopped spinach
- Shredded chicken + Drizzle of barbecue sauce
- Buffalo sauce + Blue cheese
- Canned tuna + Frozen peas + Chopped crackers or panko breadcrumbs
- Ground turkey + Finely chopped kale
- Cooked and finely chopped broccoli + Chopped ham
- Ground beef + Taco seasoning + Avocado
- Note: if adding frozen peas, chopped broccoli, or kale, add it to the boiling water during the last minute of cooking the pasta so it cooks through.
- Play with these ideas until you find your family's favorite mac and cheese.

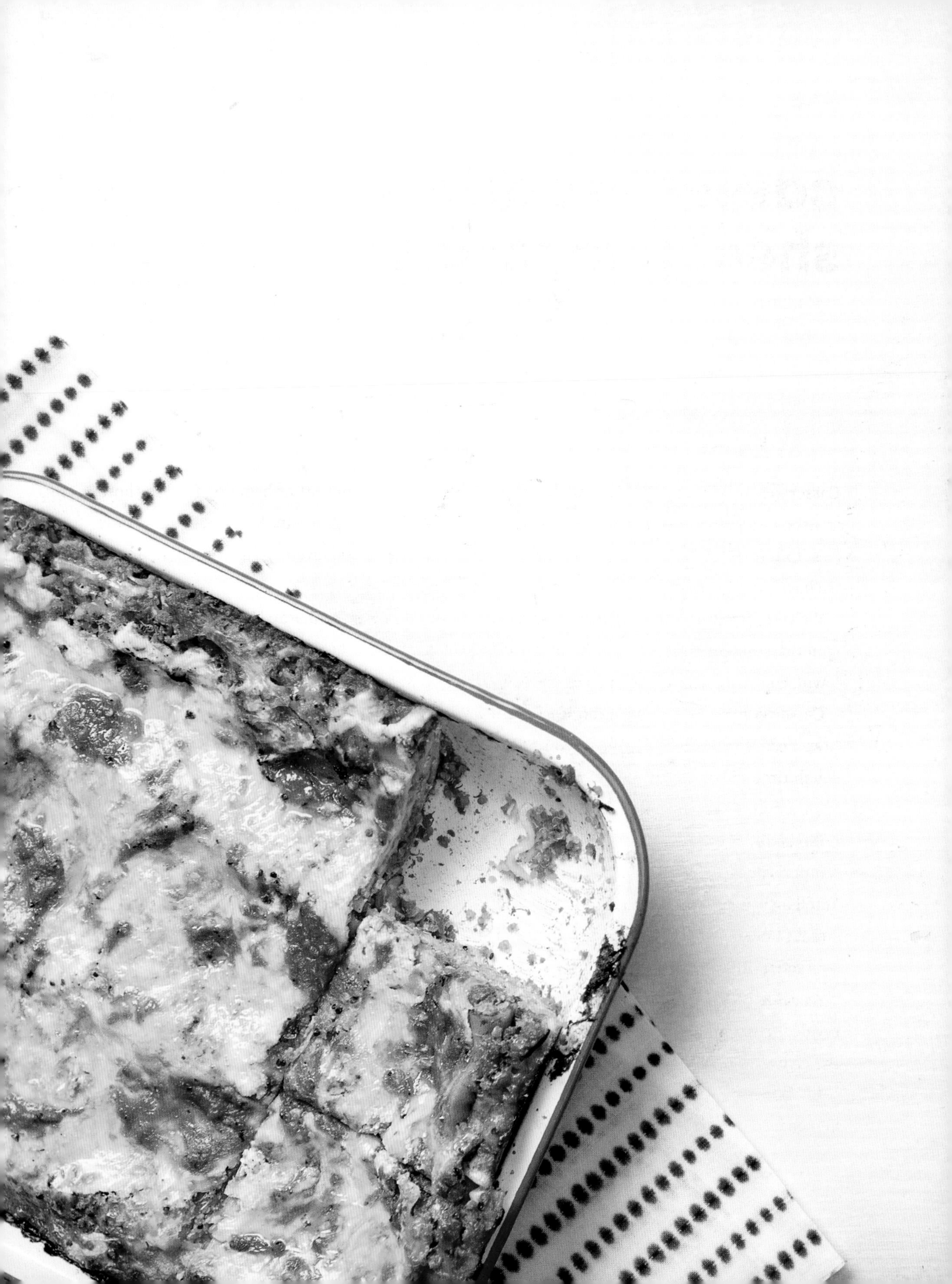

casseroles and sheet pan meals

Casseroles and sheet pan meals are ideal when we're craving comfort or bringing food to those in need of comfort. They're also handy when we're feeding a large group, or we don't have time to stand over the stovetop and just want to pop something in the oven. Whatever your reason, we have plenty of flavorful and nutritious options for you.

We've reimagined some of the classics (like the Cauliflower Parmesan Bake, our vegetarian spin on a classic meat Parmesan, page 143) while elevating others by using vegetables to add flavor, color, and nutrients (such as our Pumpkin and Kale Lasagna Roll-Ups, page 165).

Casseroles can be saved for leftovers for a week of easy meals and they're ideal for pre-baby prep because they freeze well. If you have a friend or family member who's going through a rough time or has a little one on the way, nothing says "I'm here for you" like bringing over food such as our vegetarian Zucchini and Quinoa Lasagna (page 149). We've included dairy-free options, for folks with dairy allergies, those who eat vegan, or for those perhaps who have to temporarily abstain from dairy (perhaps you're breastfeeding and have a baby with a sensitivity). You'll love our Sweet Potato Spaghetti with Chicken Meatballs (page 150), which uses spiralized sweet potatoes as "spaghetti" ("swaghetti," if you will), a familiar food in a familiar shape to encourage more vegetable eating!

As casseroles are considered a "combined food," we've also included recipes that can be easily divided to make the dish more palatable and approachable for a selective eater. For example, all the elements in the Baked Beef Stew with Parsnips (page 159) can be separated on a plate.

In short, these casseroles and sheet pan recipes are the set-it-and-forget-it meals that we all need.

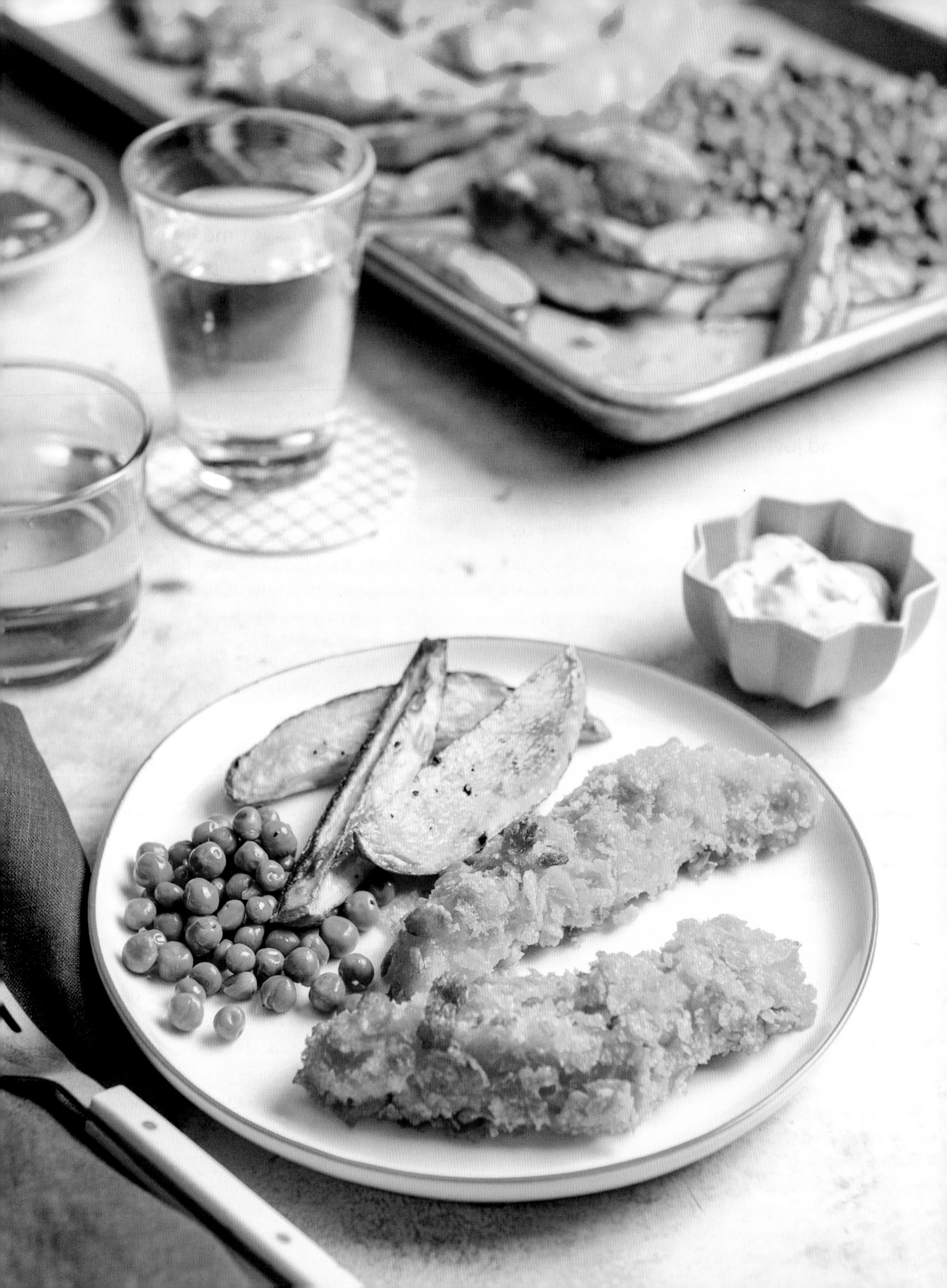

sheet pan corn flake fish and chips

time to prep: 20 minutes / time to cook: 30 minutes / serves: 4

I love recipes that have you baking half the meal while preparing the remaining part—by the time you're done prepping, the cook time is almost done. Preparing a dredge and then dredging proteins one by one can make it feel like you'll never make it to mealtime. Here, you pop the potatoes in the oven and then get to coating the fish. Once the fish is in the oven alongside the veggies, you can spend the next fifteen minutes out of the kitchen while dinner finishes up. Instead of a traditional panko breading, these corn flakes create a lighter crust that can be easier on beginner eaters and nostalgic and joyful for adults.

2 pounds russet potatoes, sliced into wedges

Extra-virgin olive oil, to drizzle

Salt and pepper

3 cups corn flakes

½ cup vegan mayonnaise

⅓ cup Dijon mustard

4 pieces (4 ounces each) skinless and boneless cod

1½ cups green peas (if using frozen, take them out when you start the recipe to let them start to defrost)

Cooking spray, for the peas

Tartar sauce or ketchup, for serving

Preheat the oven to 425°F. Line two sheet pans with parchment paper. On one end of a sheet pan, spread out the potatoes. Drizzle with olive oil, toss to coat, and season generously with salt. Season with pepper and bake for 15 minutes.

Meanwhile, pour the corn flakes into a large zip-tight bag and lay out on a flat surface. Smash the corn flakes into little pieces and pour into a baking dish or large rimmed plate or bowl. Set aside. Place the mayonnaise and mustard in the bottom of a large bowl and whisk together. Set aside.

Cut the cod pieces crosswise into 1-inch-thick pieces and pat dry. Place the fish in the bowl with the mayonnaise mixture. Toss gently to coat the fish pieces. Then, one by one, dip the fish pieces in the corn flakes and gently roll to coat. Set aside on the other prepared sheet pan. Repeat until all the fish are coated.

When the potatoes have baked for 15 minutes, remove the pan from the oven and on the other side of the pan, add the peas and spritz generously with cooking spray. Place the pan back into the oven, along with the pan with the fish. Bake the potatoes, peas, and fish for 12 to 15 minutes or until the fish flakes easily with a fork.

(recipe continues)

Serve the fish, potatoes, and peas with your favorite tartar sauce or ketchup.

INSPIRALIZED TIP

Make sure you smash the corn flakes enough so they adhere to the fish. If the pieces are too large, they won't stick easily. Since there's no flour or egg here, the breading will have a gentler stick than a traditional coating. Handle the fish carefully when serving so the corn flakes don't fall off.

FEEDING LITTLES TIP

Serve with a familiar dip. Maybe you don't think fish and hummus or ketchup go well together, but your kid will appreciate the familiarity of their favorite dip.

PREP AHEAD

The potatoes can be cooked ahead of time and will save for up to 3 days in the refrigerator, but the fish should be prepared fresh.

cauliflower parmesan bake

time to prep: 20 minutes / time to cook: 50 minutes / serves: 4

If your child has never eaten cauliflower before, make this dish and let me know if that changes. It has all the satisfying texture and flavor of a hearty bake, but it's completely vegetarian. The cauliflower transforms, softening as it absorbs the sauce while crisping up thanks to the Parmesan breading. Now, if you're looking at the total time to make this dish and you're thinking it seems long, know that most of that time is in the oven, so it's pretty hands-off. And yes, the juice is worth the squeeze.

2½- to 3-pound cauliflower head, outer leaves removed and stem intact, rinsed and patted dry

1 large egg, whisked

⅓ cup finely grated Parmesan cheese, plus more for dusting

⅔ cup panko breadcrumbs

1¼ tablespoons Italian seasoning

1 pound baby red potatoes

Extra-virgin olive oil, to drizzle

½ teaspoon garlic powder

Salt and pepper

1 jar (24 ounces) marinara or tomato basil sauce

1 to 1½ cups shredded mozzarella cheese

Sliced fresh basil, for garnish

Preheat the oven to 425°F. Line two baking sheets with parchment paper.

Slice the cauliflower lengthwise from the center into 1-inch-thick slabs (depending on the size of your cauliflower, this should yield 2 or 3 slabs). If any florets fall off, that's OK. Keep them—you'll use them all.

Whisk together the egg and ½ tablespoon of water in a shallow dish. Combine the Parmesan, breadcrumbs, and Italian seasoning in another shallow dish. Carefully dip a cauliflower slab into the egg wash, then place in the breadcrumb mixture and coat completely. Set on one of the prepared baking sheets. Repeat until all of the cauliflower slabs and florets are used.

Place the baking sheet with the cauliflower in the oven and bake for 20 minutes. Flip the cauliflower and bake for another 15 to 20 minutes or until fork-tender and golden brown.

Once you flip the cauliflower after 20 minutes of baking, place the potatoes on the other prepared baking sheet and drizzle with olive oil. Sprinkle with the garlic powder, season with salt and pepper, and toss to coat. Bake until fork-tender, 15 to 20 minutes. Smash each potato with the

(recipe continues)

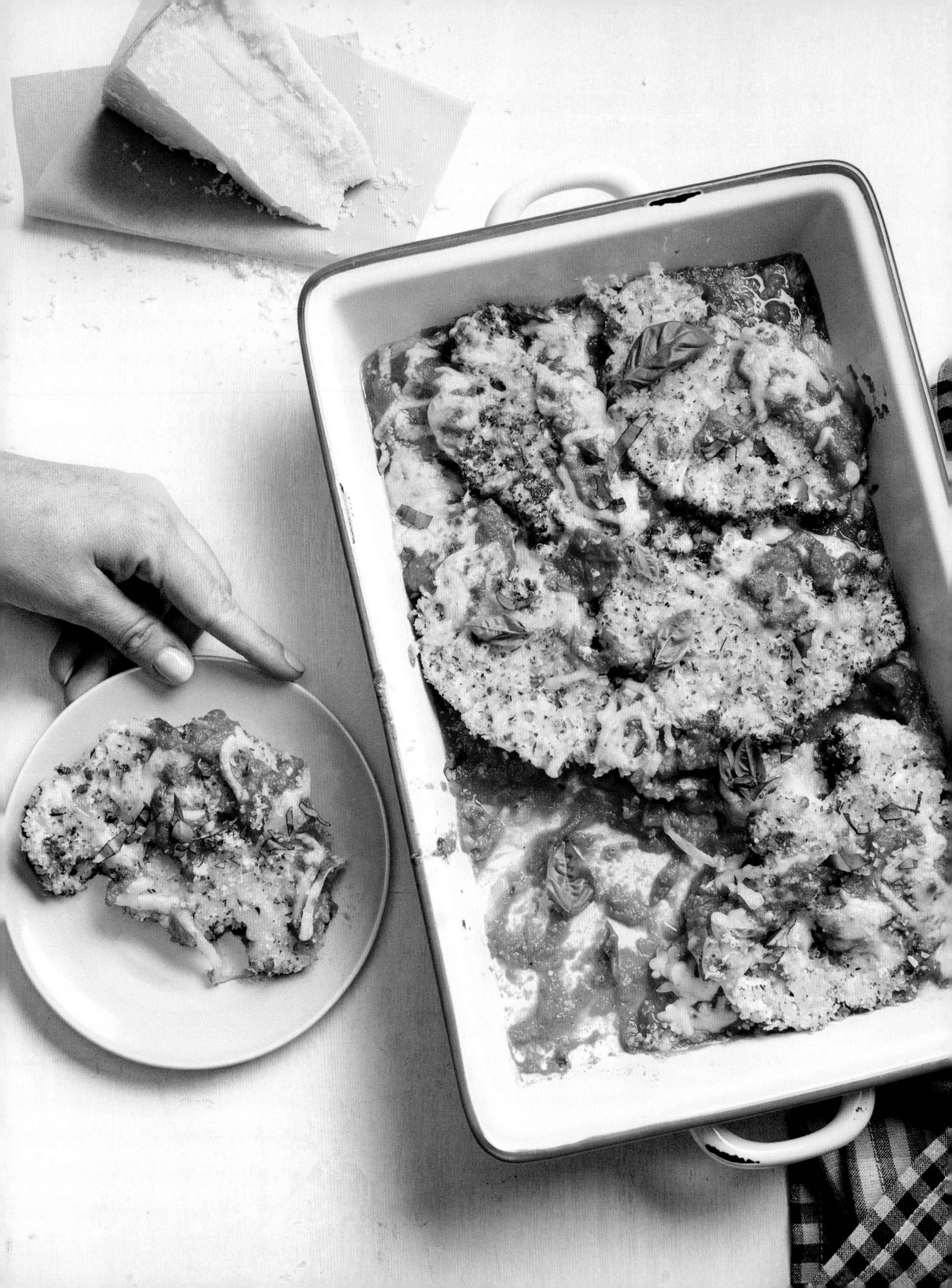

back of a fork until the potato is almost flat, dust lightly with grated Parmesan cheese, and set aside.

While the cauliflower and potatoes bake, pour half the jar of sauce into the bottom of a large 9 x 13-inch baking dish. Once the cauliflower is done baking, transfer the slabs and florets into an even layer on top of the sauce. Spoon more sauce over the cauliflower, just slightly covering the cauliflower (you won't use all of the remaining sauce). Sprinkle the mozzarella cheese over the top, and bake for 7 to 10 minutes or until the cheese melts. Immediately garnish with extra Parmesan cheese and basil. Serve with the potatoes.

INSPIRALIZED TIP

For a more traditional presentation, serve the cauliflower with buttered pasta or crusty bread.

FEEDING LITTLES TIP

To add color to your child's meal, serve with some fresh blueberries and blackberries. Fruit can be your child's "gateway food" that helps them want to try more on their plate.

PREP AHEAD

This entire dish can be made in advance and reheated in the oven at 400°F for 20 minutes.

sheet pan chicken and veggie quesadillas

time to prep: 5 minutes / time to cook: about 30 minutes / serves: 4

Quesadillas are one of the easiest foods to make when you're in a pinch—just sprinkle with cheese and fillings and let melt. However, when your family grows and your time shrinks, making quesadillas for everyone can take up more time than you want. That's where this sheet pan version comes in. *Everything* is easier in a sheet pan. Tortillas are laid down, topped with fillings and more tortillas, and baked with another sheet pan on top to seal the quesadillas—no need to stand over a stovetop. My kids love shredded carrot here, but bell pepper or even mushrooms would work well, too. Serve with your preferred quesadilla dips, such as salsa, sour cream, and guacamole.

Cooking spray, for greasing the sheet pan

1 tablespoon extra-virgin olive oil

1 pound boneless, skinless chicken breasts, butterflied (or buy chicken cutlets)

1 teaspoon taco seasoning

Salt and pepper

8 (8-inch) tortillas, warmed

⅓ cup shredded carrot, diced bell pepper, diced onion, or diced mushroom (or another preferred veggie)

2 cups shredded Mexican cheese blend

Preheat the oven to 425°F. Grease a sheet pan with cooking spray and set aside.

Heat the oil in a large skillet over medium-high heat. Once the oil is shimmering, add the chicken, sprinkle with the taco seasoning, and season with salt and pepper. Cook the chicken for 3 minutes, flip, and cook another 4 to 5 minutes or until the chicken is white and its juices run clear. Transfer the chicken to a cutting board and, using two forks, shred the chicken. Set aside.

On the prepared sheet pan, lay out 4 tortillas, not touching. Top with half of the shredded vegetable and half of the cheese, then the cooked chicken, and then the remaining veggie and cheese.

Place a tortilla on top of each filled tortilla to close the quesadilla. Place another sheet pan on top to keep the quesadillas from opening. Bake for 15 minutes, remove from the oven and spritz with cooking spray, and cook for another 5 minutes or until the tops are crispy. Slice into triangles and serve.

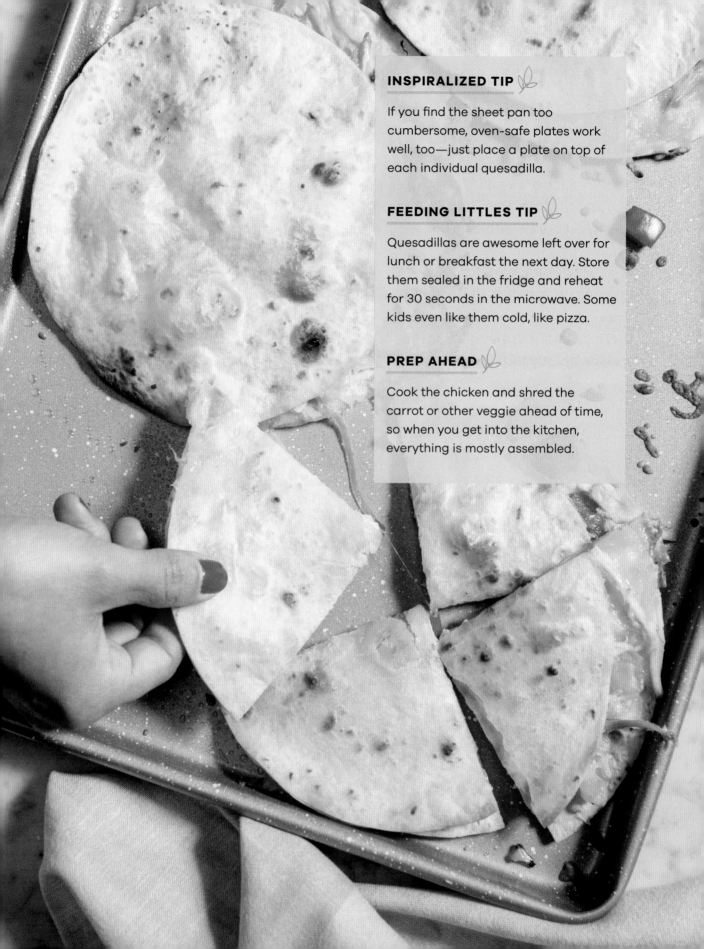

INSPIRALIZED TIP

If you find the sheet pan too cumbersome, oven-safe plates work well, too—just place a plate on top of each individual quesadilla.

FEEDING LITTLES TIP

Quesadillas are awesome left over for lunch or breakfast the next day. Store them sealed in the fridge and reheat for 30 seconds in the microwave. Some kids even like them cold, like pizza.

PREP AHEAD

Cook the chicken and shred the carrot or other veggie ahead of time, so when you get into the kitchen, everything is mostly assembled.

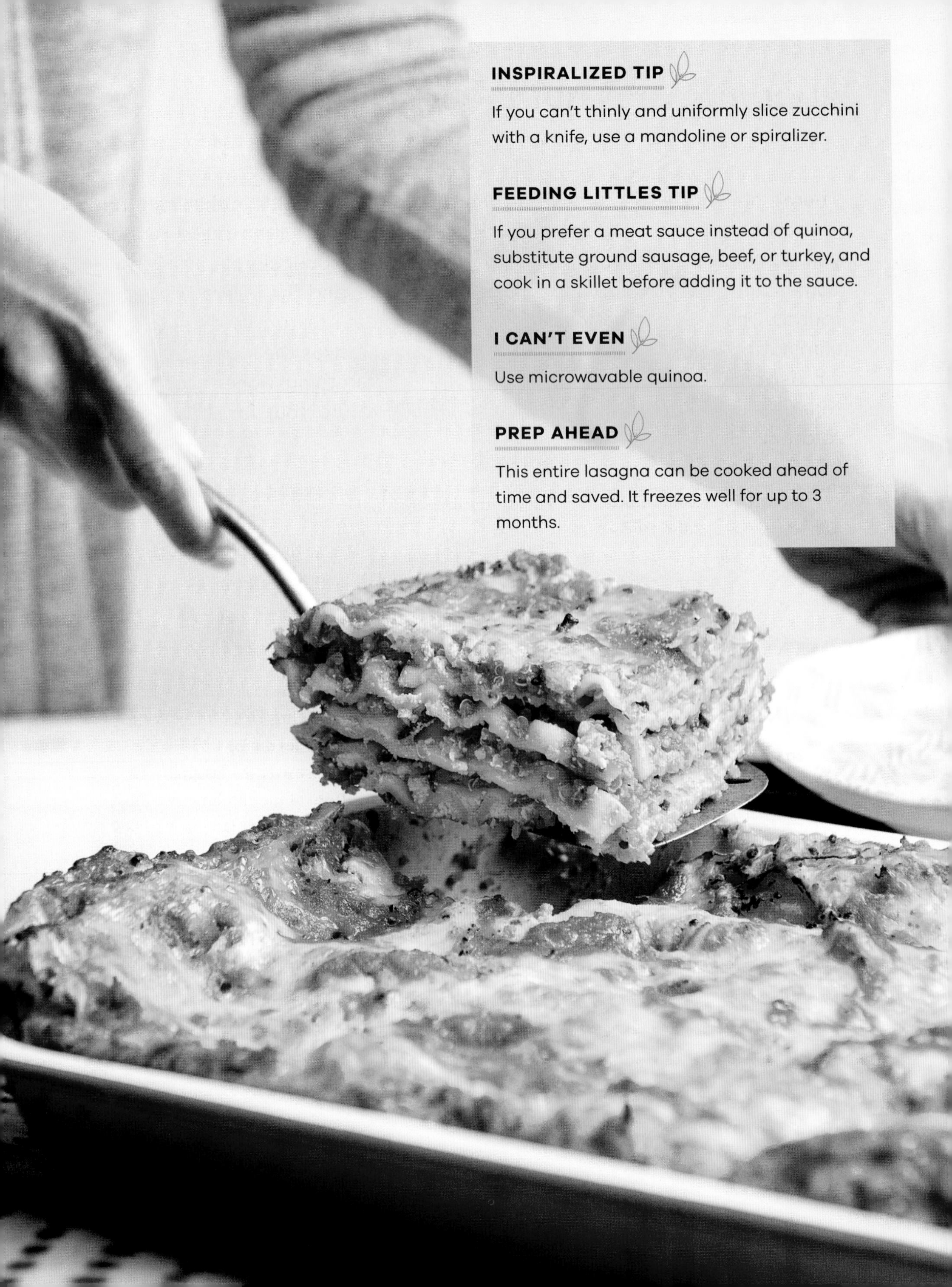

INSPIRALIZED TIP

If you can't thinly and uniformly slice zucchini with a knife, use a mandoline or spiralizer.

FEEDING LITTLES TIP

If you prefer a meat sauce instead of quinoa, substitute ground sausage, beef, or turkey, and cook in a skillet before adding it to the sauce.

I CAN'T EVEN

Use microwavable quinoa.

PREP AHEAD

This entire lasagna can be cooked ahead of time and saved. It freezes well for up to 3 months.

zucchini and quinoa lasagna

time to prep: 30 minutes / time to cook: about 45 minutes / serves: 6 to 8 adults

There's only one way my children will eat zucchini, and it's in this lasagna. There's something magical about this dish. Not only is it no-boil (I repeat: you don't need to precook these noodles), but it's super simple. The magic comes both from the quinoa and sauce mixture and the layered zucchini rounds. The zucchini softens to the same al dente texture of the lasagna, eliminating any off-putting texture. The quinoa makes the lasagna creamier, as it thickens and fluffs up the sauce. Everything works seamlessly together to yield a dish that will soon make it into your family's regular rotation.

1 jar (24 ounces) tomato basil sauce

2 cups cooked quinoa

1½ cups ricotta cheese

⅓ cup grated Parmesan cheese

1 large egg

Salt and pepper, to taste

12 no-boil lasagna noodles

1 large or 2 medium zucchini, sliced into ⅛-inch-thick rounds

1 cup shredded mozzarella cheese

Shredded fresh basil, for garnish (optional)

Preheat the oven to 400°F.

Place the tomato basil sauce and the quinoa in a large bowl and stir together to combine well. Set aside.

In a medium bowl, whisk together the ricotta, Parmesan cheese, egg, and salt and pepper. Set aside.

In the bottom of a 9 x 13-inch baking dish, spread out enough of the sauce mixture to lightly cover the bottom, about 1 cup. Place 3 lasagna noodles on top to cover the sauce. Spread ½ cup of the cheese over the lasagna noodles, then top with one-third of the zucchini rounds, then about ⅓ cup sauce. Top with 3 more lasagna noodles and repeat with more cheese, zucchini, and sauce. Repeat again with the lasagna noodles, cheese, zucchini, and sauce. Top with lasagna noodles and repeat with the remaining cheese and sauce, and then sprinkle with mozzarella cheese. Cover with foil and bake for 40 to 45 minutes or until the lasagna noodles are cooked through.

Uncover, garnish with basil, if using, and let cool slightly. Slice and serve.

sweet potato spaghetti with chicken meatballs

time to prep: 40 minutes / time to cook: about 45 minutes / serves: 4

Have you ever made spaghetti and meatballs in the oven? The trick is to swap regular spaghetti for spiralized vegetables, which cook alongside the meatballs for an al dente spaghetti-like texture. The cleanup is minimal, and it's an inventive way to incorporate more vegetables into your meals. In this recipe, chia seeds bind the meatballs together and add fiber, protein, and omega-3 fatty acids. With adult supervision, the spiralizing can be done by your toddler for an interactive meal; kids are always amazed when a vegetable turns into noodles. Switching up your usual spaghetti is a novel way to serve dinner that you may become obsessed with (as I surely am).

1 pound ground chicken breast

3 garlic cloves, grated or finely minced

1 tablespoon Italian seasoning

2 tablespoons chia seeds

Salt and pepper

2 medium sweet potatoes, peeled and spiralized into spaghetti-shaped noodles

Extra-virgin olive oil, to drizzle

1 jar (24 ounces) tomato basil sauce

Grated Parmesan cheese, for garnish

Shredded fresh basil, for garnish

Preheat the oven to 400°F. Line two baking sheets with parchment paper and set aside.

In a medium bowl, combine the chicken, garlic, Italian seasoning, and chia seeds, and season with salt and pepper. Using your hands, mix all of the ingredients together. Cover and refrigerate the meatball mixture for 30 minutes, to bind the meat together.

While the meatballs gel, lay out the sweet potato noodles on one of the prepared baking sheets. Drizzle with olive oil and season with salt and pepper. Bake for 25 to 30 minutes or until the noodles are al dente or soft enough for your family's preferences. Set aside, covering with plastic wrap or foil to keep warm.

Once the meatball mixture is ready, dampen your hands and roll heaping tablespoons into balls. Arrange them on the second prepared baking sheet, with at least ½ inch of space between each meatball, making about 18 meatballs total.

Place the meatballs in the oven and bake for 10 minutes. Using tongs, carefully turn the meatballs over and bake for another 10 minutes, until lightly browned and cooked through.

(recipe continues)

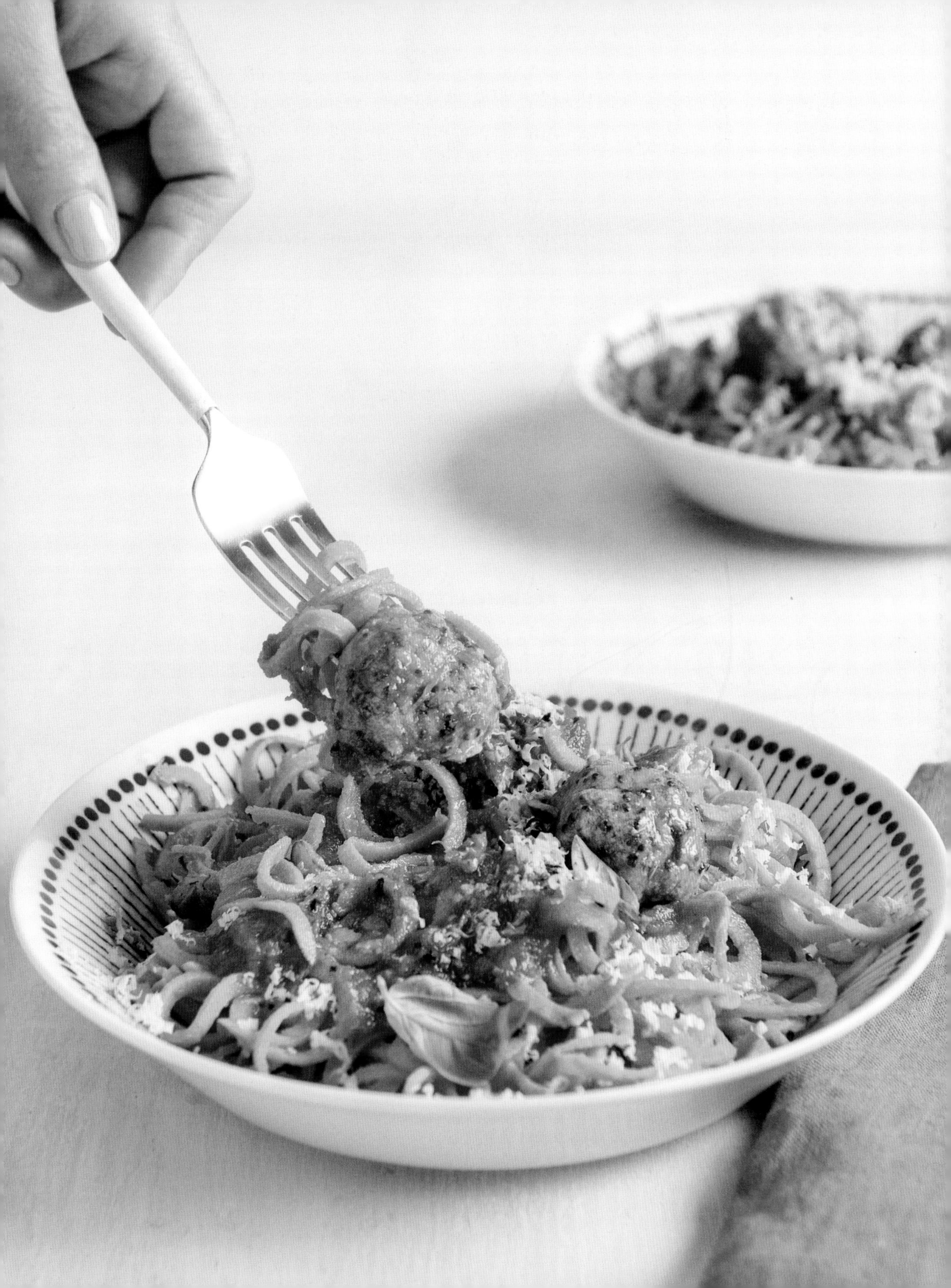

Meanwhile, pour the tomato sauce into a large skillet. Once the meatballs are 5 minutes from being fully baked, heat the pan to medium-high and bring the sauce to a simmer. Once the meatballs are ready to come out of the oven, place them into the sauce and turn the meatballs to coat them in the sauce. Let the tomato sauce and meatballs simmer together for 5 minutes. Transfer to a serving dish and garnish with cheese and basil.

Serve the sweet potato noodles topped with the meatballs, or separately, family-style.

INSPIRALIZED TIP

If you don't have a spiralizer, buy pre-spiralized sweet potatoes, or carefully use a mandoline or julienne peeler to slice the sweet potatoes into strands. You can also use regular cooked spaghetti noodles and boil them in water per the package instructions.

FEEDING LITTLES TIP

Young kids can be finicky with meat because if it's dry, it's hard to chew. That's why meatballs or breaded chicken are often a better bet, as they retain moisture. If you'd like, double the meatball ingredients to keep extras in the freezer.

PREP AHEAD

This entire meal can be prepped ahead and stored for up to 3 days in the refrigerator. The meatballs can last up to 3 months in the freezer, but I don't recommend freezing the sweet potato noodles.

butternut squash sage baked ziti

time to prep: 10 minutes / time to cook: 50 minutes / serves: 6 to 8

Toasted sage gives a gourmet touch to this one-pan baked ziti, infusing flavor into the oil that cooks the rest of the ingredients. Simple ingredients and a little bit of pouring, stirring, and baking adds up to a sumptuous pasta dish that's easy to clean up, saves well for reheating, and is a cozy way to welcome the fall and winter seasons (but since we're using canned vegetables, it can be made all year long). Ziti is a solid, easy-to-hold shape for beginner eaters that absorbs the broth and pureed butternut squash.

1 tablespoon extra-virgin olive oil

4 fresh sage leaves

2 garlic cloves, minced

½ cup diced red onion

2 tablespoons tomato paste

1 can (15 ounces) butternut squash puree (or pumpkin or sweet potato)

3½ cups low-sodium chicken or vegetable broth

½ teaspoon salt

Pepper, to taste

1 box (16 ounces) ziti pasta (penne also works well)

¾ cup ricotta cheese

1 to 2 cups shredded mozzarella cheese

Preheat the oven to 400°F.

Heat 1 teaspoon of the oil in a large, wide oven-safe skillet or Dutch oven over medium-high heat. Add the sage and let it fry for 1 minute, flip, and fry for another 1 to 2 minutes or until crispy. Set aside on a paper towel.

Immediately add the remaining 2 teaspoons of oil and the garlic and onion and cook for 3 minutes or until the vegetables soften. Turn off the heat. Add the tomato paste and stir well to coat the vegetables. Add the butternut squash and stir to combine. Then, add the broth, salt, and pepper, and stir well to combine. Add the uncooked ziti and stir to combine. Add tablespoon dollops of the ricotta throughout the pasta, pushing the ricotta into the pasta.

Sprinkle the pasta mixture with the mozzarella. Cover with aluminum foil or a tight-fitting lid and bake for 40 minutes or until the ziti is cooked through and al dente. If you don't like crispy pasta edges, make sure all of the noodles are submerged in the liquid (add more liquid, if needed).

Uncover and top with the sage, crumbling to sprinkle. Serve.

(recipe continues)

INSPIRALIZED TIP

If any of the pieces of pasta are poking through the top of the mixture, (i.e., not submerged in liquid) they will end up a bit crunchier. I love the crunchy texture, but if you're worried about your little eaters, take those pieces out before serving it to them (and save for your plate) or make sure you submerge all noodles prior to oven baking.

FEEDING LITTLES TIP

For extra protein and minerals, use low-sodium chicken bone broth instead of regular broth.

I CAN'T EVEN

Skip the sage, which is mostly aromatic and doesn't impart much flavor.

PREP AHEAD

This meal can be prepped entirely ahead of time.

no-boil tomato, pea, and sausage rigatoni

time to prep: 10 minutes / time to cook: about 50 minutes / serves: 4

For a classic pasta bake, this tomato rigatoni with sausage and peas can't be beat. The peas are negotiable, too. I like adding them for a pop of color, I usually have them in my freezer, and they add only the mildest flavor. The sauce is creamy, thanks to the Parmesan cheese, which adds a salty, nutty flavor to every bite. Rigatoni is the pasta shape that has the most surface area for sauce and ingredients to cling to, making this flavor-packed from the first bite.

1 teaspoon extra-virgin olive oil

4 Italian sausage links, decased

1 jar (24 ounces) tomato basil sauce

1 cup frozen peas

⅓ cup grated Parmesan cheese

1 cup low-sodium vegetable or chicken broth, plus more as needed

1 box (8 ounces) rigatoni pasta

1 cup shredded mozzarella cheese

PREP AHEAD

This meal can be entirely prepped ahead of time.

Preheat the oven to 400°F. Heat the oil in a large, oven-safe skillet. Once the oil is shimmering, add the sausage, crumble, and cook until no longer pink, about 7 minutes. Turn off the heat and add the tomato basil sauce, peas, Parmesan cheese, broth, and rigatoni. Stir well to combine evenly, and if any large pieces of pasta are not submerged, add more broth. Sprinkle the top with the mozzarella cheese. Cover the skillet with aluminum foil, and bake for 35 to 40 minutes or until the rigatoni is al dente.

Uncover and serve.

INSPIRALIZED TIP

This recipe works well with plant-based sausages, too. If your family is vegetarian, you can also omit the meat.

FEEDING LITTLES TIP

This dish pairs well with crusty garlic bread or soft breadsticks. Since many kids love bread and other "beige" foods, it's a surefire way to encourage them to come to the table. Show them how to dip the bread in the sauce.

chicken fajita casserole

time to prep: 15 minutes / time to cook: 15 minutes / serves: 4

In our house, fajita night is a family tradition. But as easy as they are to make, there's lots of stovetop time involved, and on a busy weeknight, I'm looking for a pour-and-bake meal, which is where this casserole version comes in.

If you've ever made fajitas, you know that it takes a while to cook peppers down so they're soft enough for beginner eaters. That's why it's key to slice the peppers very thin so they bake through. If you're not serving this to little eaters (under fourteen to sixteen months), then don't worry either way.

Serve with toasted tortillas or a side of fluffy brown rice. I hope fajita night becomes your family's tradition, too.

Cooking spray, for the baking dish

1 teaspoon ground cumin

2 teaspoons chili powder (or less, if you don't like spice)

1 teaspoon dried oregano

1 teaspoon garlic powder

¼ teaspoon onion powder

2 teaspoons paprika

¼ teaspoon salt

1 pound skinless, boneless chicken breasts (if your package comes with 2 breasts, split lengthwise to yield 4 pieces, otherwise use 1 pound chicken cutlets), sliced into strips

2 bell peppers, seeded and sliced thinly into ⅛-inch-thick strips

Preheat the oven to 400°F. Lightly grease a large (about 9 x 13-inch) baking dish. In a small bowl, stir together the cumin, chili powder, oregano, garlic powder, onion powder, paprika, and salt.

Place the chicken in the baking dish. Sprinkle with half of the spice mixture and toss to coat. Top with the peppers and onion, sprinkle with the remaining spice mixture, toss to coat the vegetables, and top with the cheese. Bake for 15 minutes or until the chicken is cooked through and no longer pink on the inside, or the internal temperature reaches 165°F. Garnish with the cilantro.

Serve with tortillas, lime wedges, avocado, and lettuce.

1 large red onion, sliced thinly

1 cup shredded Mexican cheese blend

1 tablespoon chopped cilantro, for garnish

Tortillas, lime wedges, sliced avocado, shredded romaine lettuce, for serving

INSPIRALIZED TIP

To make these fajitas vegetarian, swap the chicken breasts for a can of black beans, letting the beans and vegetables bake together until the peppers are soft.

FEEDING LITTLES TIP

Boneless, skinless chicken thighs also work here. They have a little more fat so can be more tender for new eaters. Ensure that the meat is fork-tender when you serve it.

I CAN'T EVEN

Use taco seasoning (1½ to 2 tablespoons) instead of the homemade seasoning.

PREP AHEAD

This entire meal can be prepped ahead.

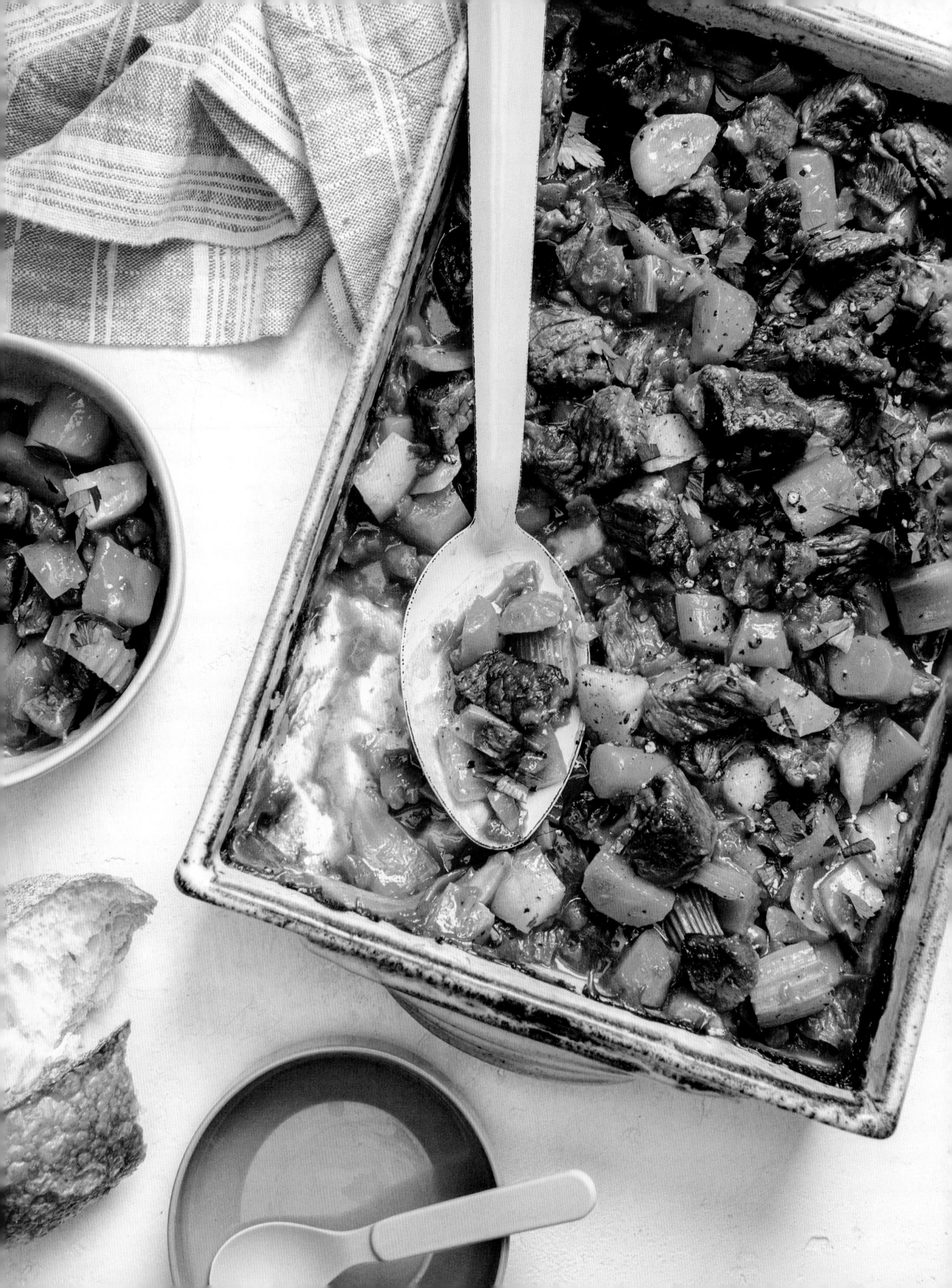

baked beef stew with parsnips

time to prep: 15 minutes / time to cook: 2 hours / serves: 8

There's nothing like a cozy, inviting stew simmering on the stovetop. Actually, you know what's better? Those same smells filling your kitchen and wrapping around you like a warm hug, but coming from the oven, where you don't have to worry about something bubbling over. I'm all about finding shortcuts or easier methods of cooking my family's favorite meals, and this beef stew is just as hearty, and the meat's just as tender, as in the traditional version. It'll also make you a fan of parsnips (if you're not already), which have a fantastic nutty flavor but can be overwhelming if underprepared. They're foolproof here, as the stew juices soften and embolden the parsnips. With some warmed crusty sourdough for dipping, this is the meal you'll serve to guests on a cold night. When you tell them it was made in a baking dish, they'll beg you for the recipe.

1 can (15 ounces) diced tomatoes, no salt added

1 cup low-sodium beef broth

3 tablespoons arrowroot powder (or all-purpose flour)

1 teaspoon salt, plus more as needed

Pepper, to taste

2 pounds beef stew meat, cut into 1-inch cubes

6 carrots, peeled and cut into 1-inch chunks

2 large parsnips, peeled and cut into ½-inch chunks

(ingredients continue)

Preheat the oven to 375°F.

Combine the tomatoes, broth, arrowroot powder, salt, and pepper in a large bowl.

Place the beef, carrots, parsnips, celery, onion, and bay leaf in a 9 x 13-inch baking dish. Pour the broth mixture on top. Cover with aluminum foil and bake for 2 hours or until the meat and vegetables are tender. Remove the bay leaf, taste, and if the beef stew needs more salt, season with more salt and give a big stir.

Right before serving, place the sourdough in the oven alongside the stew for 5 to 10 minutes, to warm. Garnish the stew with parsley, and serve the bread alongside.

INSPIRALIZED TIP

If you can't find parsnips, substitute potatoes, rutabaga, or turnips.

(recipe continues)

2 celery ribs, cut into 1-inch pieces

1 medium onion, cut into 1-inch pieces

1 bay leaf

1 loaf sourdough bread, for serving

Chopped fresh parsley, for garnish

FEEDING LITTLES TIP

This meal is easy to deconstruct if your child is overwhelmed by the combination. Try putting the liquid in a cup for them to drink with a straw once it has cooled. If serving the broth this way, offer the meat and vegetables on a plate.

PREP AHEAD

This entire meal can be made ahead, but the meat won't be as tender as it is on the first day.

southwestern salsa rice bake with chipotle sauce

time to prep: 20 minutes + overnight for soaking the cashews / time to cook: 60 minutes / serves: 4 to 6

Since a jar of salsa usually contains aromatic seasonings like cilantro, garlic, and lime juice, there's no need for additional flavoring. We're big chips and salsa fans in our house, and this meal brings in those same Southwestern flavors, no muss or fuss. The sauce is one of my all-time go-tos that goes well with almost everything—as a dip, on tacos, drizzled over roasted veggies, or on a burger. Here it gives the rice a creamy garnish, making it easier to serve to beginner eaters on a preloaded spoon. Make extras and keep it in a jar in the fridge for up to 4 days or freeze it in cubes and store in the freezer for up to 3 months. I guarantee you'll find your own unique ways to use it!

3 cups low-sodium vegetable broth

1 cup chunky mild salsa

2 bell peppers, seeded and diced

2 cans (15 ounces each) black beans, drained and rinsed

1½ cups frozen or fresh corn

1 cup dry white basmati rice

1 cup cilantro leaves

2 avocados, peeled, pitted, and diced

(ingredients continue)

Preheat the oven to 400°F.

Stir together the broth and salsa in a medium pot and bring it to a boil over high heat. Once boiling, reduce the heat to a medium simmer.

While the broth mixture comes to a boil, in a 9 x 13-inch baking dish, place the peppers, black beans, corn, and top with the rice. Shake the pan so the ingredients are in an even layer. Pour the boiling broth mixture evenly over the top. Cover the baking dish with aluminum foil and bake for 60 minutes.

While the casserole bakes, prepare the sauce. Drain the cashews and place them in a high-speed blender with ¾ cup water, the garlic, adobo sauce and pepper, lime juice, paprika, and salt and pepper. Blend until smooth and set aside.

Top the finished rice bake with the cilantro and avocados, and drizzle with chipotle sauce.

(recipe continues)

For the chipotle sauce

1 cup cashews, soaked for at least 6 hours (or overnight)

1 garlic clove, minced

1½ tablespoons sauce from a can of chipotle peppers in adobo, plus 1 pepper

½ ripe lime, juiced

⅛ teaspoon smoked paprika

Salt and pepper, to taste

INSPIRALIZED TIP

If you're a nut-free household, substitute ½ cup mayonnaise or ½ cup full-fat coconut milk for the cashews in the cream sauce.

FEEDING LITTLES TIP

If serving this to a baby, mix the peppers, beans, corn, rice, and avocados with the sauce to give it more grip for them to pick up with their hands or eat off a loaded utensil. This is a gateway recipe for introducing a little—but not too much—spiciness.

I CAN'T EVEN

Skip the cashew cream sauce and use a chipotle mayo or similar condiment.

PREP AHEAD

This entire dish can be made ahead, but rice doesn't save very well in the refrigerator, so I recommend making it fresh.

judy's shepherd's pie

time to prep: 15 minutes / time to cook: about 65 minutes / serves: 6

Judy here! My husband, Louie, loves to cook. When our kids were little, Louie made this recipe at least a few times a month during the winter. We lived in Wisconsin, Utah, and Colorado, so we needed recipes that would warm our tummies when it was cold outside. Our son, Prescott, loved to stick a baby carrot into the mashed potatoes, so it looked like a single candle in a birthday cake. As silly as it sounds, it's something I remember so fondly about meals when our kids were little. I hope this recipe helps you make fond memories, too.

1½ pounds potatoes, peeled and cubed

½ cup milk

3 tablespoons butter

Salt and pepper

2 tablespoons extra-virgin olive oil

1 medium onion, diced

1 carrot, diced

1 celery stalk, diced

1 pound ground lamb (can use ground beef or other ground protein)

1 tablespoon all-purpose flour

¾ cup low-sodium beef stock

(ingredients continue)

Fill a large pot two-thirds of the way with water and bring to a boil. Add the potatoes and boil for 10 minutes or until completely tender. Using a slotted spoon, transfer the potatoes to a large bowl and mash the potatoes with a fork or potato masher. Add the milk, 1 tablespoon of the butter, and season with salt and pepper.

Preheat the oven to 400°F.

Heat the oil in a large skillet. Once the oil is shimmering, add the onion, carrot, and celery and cook until softened, about 7 minutes. Push the vegetables to the side and add the lamb, crumbling and cooking for 10 minutes or until cooked through and browned. Spoon off any fat and discard. Combine the meat with the vegetables. Add the flour, stir, and cook for another 2 to 3 minutes. Add the stock, thyme, rosemary, and nutmeg. Season with salt and pepper and stir.

Bring the mixture to a boil and once boiling, reduce the heat to a simmer and stir occasionally until thickened, about 5 minutes. Transfer the mixture into a 9-inch pie pan or baking dish. Spread the mashed potatoes over the top, making irregular peaks with the tines of a fork. Chop the remaining 2 tablespoons of butter and sprinkle over the top.

(recipe continues)

1 tablespoon chopped fresh thyme, or 1 teaspoon dried

1 tablespoon chopped fresh rosemary, or 1 teaspoon dried

Pinch of ground nutmeg

Bake the casserole until the potatoes are browned and the dish is heated all of the way through, 30 to 35 minutes. Let cool slightly and serve.

INSPIRALIZED TIP

For a fun way to add more vegetables, replace ½ pound of the potatoes with 1 cup cauliflower florets and boil them with the potatoes.

FEEDING LITTLES TIP

If you stick a carrot out of the top as described above, your kids can pretend to blow out the "birthday candle" when the dish is done. This is a fun, simple way to bring them into the kitchen and learn to love cooking.

I CAN'T EVEN

Even though the mashed potatoes are the best part of any recipe, they're also the most time-intensive. If you want to make this but don't have the capacity to whip them up, try microwavable mashed potatoes. Target's Good & Gather brand has a Yukon Gold version that's tasty and made with wholesome ingredients.

PREP AHEAD

This entire meal can be prepped ahead of time.

pumpkin and kale lasagna roll-ups

time to prep: 20 minutes / time to cook: about 45 minutes / serves: 4 to 6 (makes 12 roll-ups)

I'm not sure which I love more: lasagna or lasagna roll-ups. Lasagna roll-ups are simply cooked lasagna noodles that are spread with a cheese sauce, sprinkled with a stuffing, rolled up, and baked. The main pro of roll-ups is that they are easier to serve. The main con of roll-ups is that they take longer to prepare, because you have to cook the lasagna first and then prepare each roll-up. But when you feel like mixing up your pasta game, try this combination of pumpkin, cheese, and egg for a fluffy filling that's absolutely drool-worthy—and a tasty way to incorporate pumpkin into your family's diet. So, who is Team Roll-Ups and who is Team Original?

12 lasagna noodles (two-thirds of a 16-ounce box)

1 tablespoon extra-virgin olive oil

½ large onion, chopped

3 garlic cloves, minced

Kosher salt and freshly ground black pepper

½ teaspoon red pepper flakes

2 cups finely chopped curly kale

½ teaspoon lemon zest

1 container (15 ounces) ricotta cheese

1 large egg

1 cup freshly grated Parmesan

1 can (15 ounces) pumpkin puree

1 cup shredded mozzarella

Preheat the oven to 350°F. Bring a large pot of water to a boil and cook the lasagna noodles according to the package directions until al dente. Drain.

Heat the oil in a large skillet over medium heat. Add the onion and garlic and season with salt, pepper, and the red pepper flakes. Cook until the onion is soft, about 5 minutes. Add the kale and cook until wilted. Stir in the lemon zest and remove the skillet from the heat.

Stir the ricotta, egg, and ½ cup of the Parmesan in a large bowl until combined. Add the pumpkin, stir to combine, and season with salt and pepper.

In a large 9 x 13-inch baking dish, spoon a layer of the ricotta and pumpkin mixture on the bottom of the dish, about 1 cup. Set aside.

Spread the ricotta and pumpkin mixture onto one side of each lasagna noodle. Top with the kale mixture, then roll up tightly. As they are finished, add to the baking dish seam side down to create 3 rows of 4 roll-ups in a single layer.

Sprinkle the mozzarella and remaining Parmesan over the assembled roll-ups. Bake until bubbly and melted, about 20 minutes. Serve.

(recipe continues)

INSPIRALIZED TIP

If you can't find canned pumpkin (this happens to me all the time in those seasonal baking months like November and December), you can use four 4-ounce pouches of pumpkin puree instead. Just be sure to pick a variety that isn't overly sweetened with fruit.

FEEDING LITTLES TIP

Kale is a polarizing veggie—people either love it or they avoid it. In this recipe, the strong flavor of the kale pairs well with the richness of the pumpkin and cheese, but if it's not your family's thing you can omit it or substitute with chopped spinach instead.

PREP AHEAD

This entire meal can be made ahead of time. Save in the refrigerator for 3 days or in the freezer for 3 months.

sheet pan sesame tofu and broccoli trees

time to prep: 10 minutes / time to cook: 30 minutes / serves: 3

When I was vegan, tofu and broccoli over rice was my jam. I made this combo all the time and it was always the dish I made for friends when they would ask, "What do you *eat*?!" (Plant-based diets weren't as mainstream as they are now.) It's still the dish that I fall back on when I want to eat more plants with a comforting basic. After having children, I realized my quick-cooking method of sautéing the broccoli and tofu in a wok didn't soften the vegetables or firm up the tofu enough for them to enjoy. Here, everything is baked to ensure the broccoli is fork-tender and suitable for the littlest of eaters. And I find it even more flavorful than my old-school original. Plus, this sauce is a major upgrade from the bottled one I used to use and it's one-size-fits-all for pretty much any dish you can image: drizzle it on proteins and veggies for stir-fries and other East Asian–inspired meals.

1 package (14 ounces) extra-firm tofu, drained

2 tablespoons extra-virgin olive oil

5 tablespoons soy sauce

1 large head of broccoli (about 1½ pounds)

Cooking spray, for the broccoli

Salt and pepper

1 tablespoon sesame oil

1 garlic clove, grated

½-inch piece ginger, peeled and grated

(ingredients continue)

Preheat the oven to 400°F. Line a large sheet pan with parchment paper and set aside.

Place the tofu on two paper towels or a thin kitchen towel and top with more towels. Press firmly down on the tofu to remove excess moisture. Repeat with new paper towels or kitchen towels until the moisture is mostly drained. Slice the tofu into 1-inch cubes.

Whisk together the olive oil and 2 tablespoons of the soy sauce in a large mixing bowl. Add the tofu and toss well to coat. Set aside to marinate while you prepare the rest of the recipe.

Slice the broccoli off the stem, leaving 1 to 2 inches of the stem intact, to make tree-like broccoli florets. Discard the unused stems. Place the broccoli on one end of the prepared sheet pan and spritz generously with cooking spray or brush with olive oil. Season with salt and pepper.

(recipe continues)

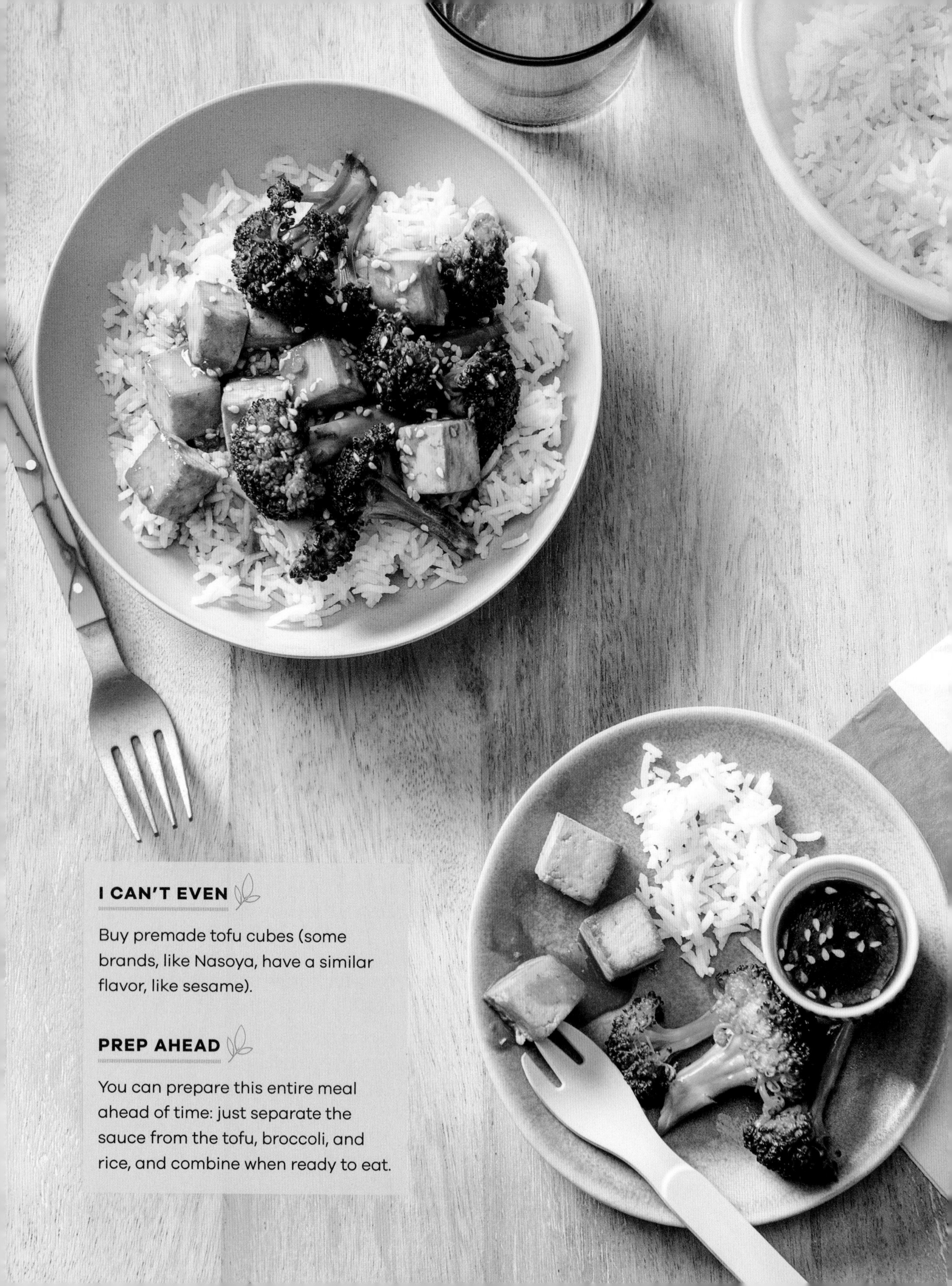

I CAN'T EVEN

Buy premade tofu cubes (some brands, like Nasoya, have a similar flavor, like sesame).

PREP AHEAD

You can prepare this entire meal ahead of time: just separate the sauce from the tofu, broccoli, and rice, and combine when ready to eat.

1 tablespoon rice vinegar (white vinegar also works)

½ tablespoon chili garlic sauce, sriracha, or hot sauce (whatever you have on hand)

1 teaspoon arrowroot powder (can also use cornstarch)

2 teaspoons sesame seeds, for garnish

Noodles or cooked rice, for serving

Place the tofu at the other end of the sheet pan. Put the sheet pan in the oven and roast for 30 minutes or until the broccoli is fork-tender and the tofu is firm.

While the tofu and broccoli bake, prepare the sauce. Whisk together the sesame oil, garlic, ginger, rice vinegar, the remaining 3 tablespoons of soy sauce, and the chili garlic sauce (or other hot sauce) in a small pot and set aside. Whisk together the arrowroot powder with 2 teaspoons of water in a small bowl. Pour that slurry mixture into the pot with the sauce mixture and stir. Place the pot over medium-low heat and stir until thickened, about 3 minutes. Turn the heat off.

Divide the broccoli and tofu into bowls and pour the sauce over the top evenly. You can also pour the sauce over the broccoli and tofu on the sheet pan and toss to coat that way. Sprinkle with the sesame seeds. Serve with noodles or rice.

INSPIRALIZED TIP

If tofu's not your thing, use chicken, pork, beef strips, salmon, or shrimp instead.

FEEDING LITTLES TIP

Get inspired and pretend the broccoli florets are little trees. Ask your child to have the trees swim in the "pool" (sauce) or line them up in a forest. Every time kids interact with a food, they're one step closer to wanting to try it.

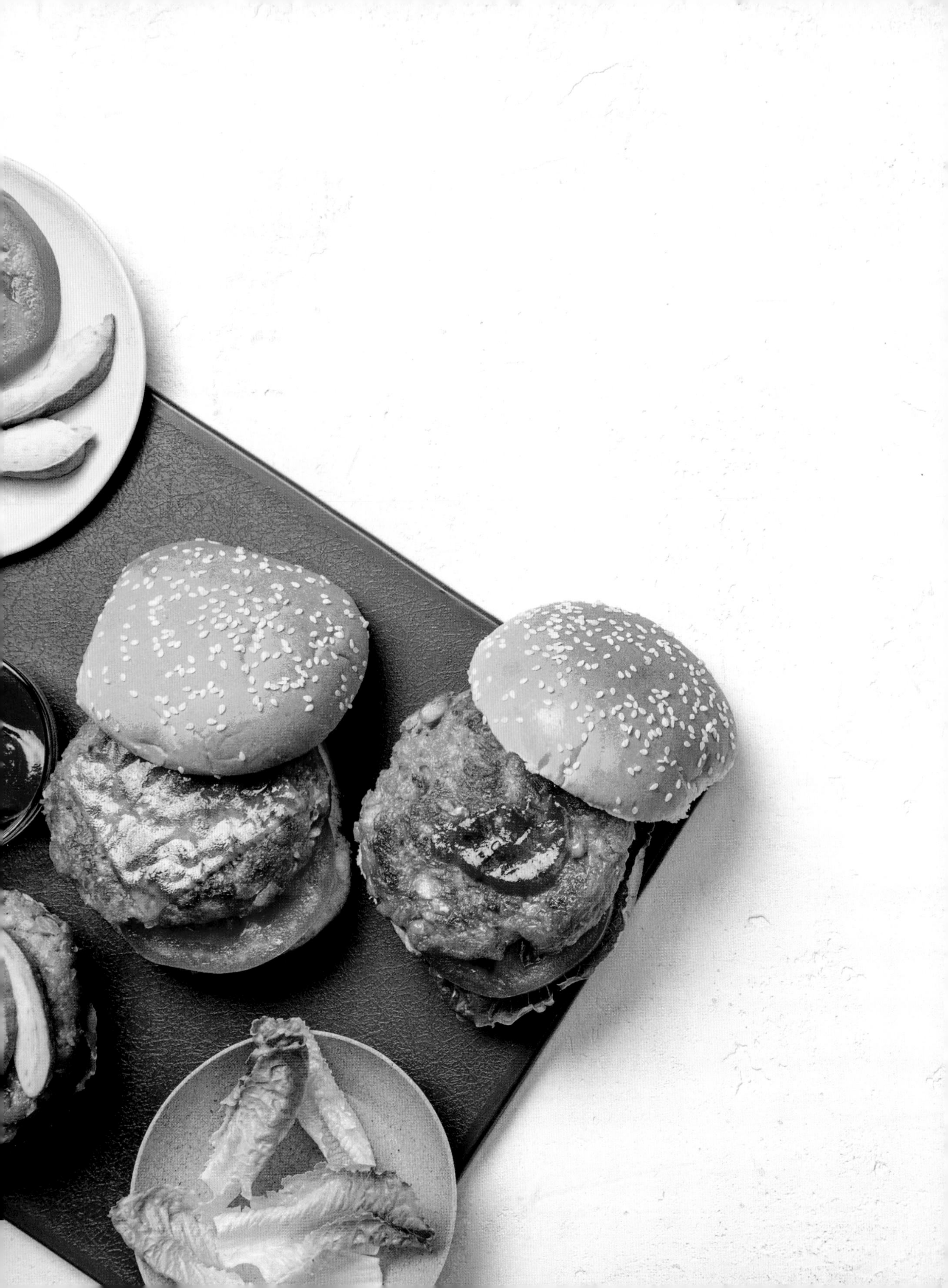

enjoy your veggies

As you surely know, vegetables are packed with vitamins, minerals, and plant nutrients that help us feel our best. However, kids don't always love vegetables, and it can be a point of stress for many parents. Rest assured, friends: kids can—and do—thrive even if they're more interested in eating fruit at the moment, but we've also worked our hardest to create recipes that make veggies inviting, approachable, and absolutely tasty. Our goal is for your family to truly enjoy vegetables, if you don't already. To do this, we're getting inventive with our preparation, cooking, and presentation to show that they can be delicious and exciting but also approachable and even nostalgia-inducing (hello, French fry–shaped veggies). While steamed or roasted veggies have their time and place, step up your veggie game with these inspired ways to eat these nutritional powerhouses.

Now, it's important to note that our goal is never to "hide" or "sneak" vegetables into our meals. Sneaking anything into your child's diet will likely backfire since it can erode their trust, but regularly cooking with them—and having your kiddo help so they see what's going in their food—will allow them to learn that they can enjoy the flavor and texture of vegetables in many different ways.

When cooked properly and paired with the right seasonings and accompaniments, vegetables can truly be the main event. You will love our hearty Sweet Potato Fajita Quinoa Bowls (page 175), thanks to the fork-tender, meaty, thick-cut sweet potato slices. With our Indian Butter Tempeh with Cauliflower Rice (page 181), the cauliflower acts as a rice-like "grain" and is topped with an aromatic and creamy Indian butter sauce. Or integrate red peppers into a pasta dish with our Shrimp and Asparagus in Red Pepper Sauce with Penne (page 172). No more boring vegetables; it's time to level up.

shrimp and asparagus in red pepper sauce with penne

time to prep: 15 minutes / time to cook: 20 minutes / serves: 6

I'll be completely honest, I've made roasted red pepper sauce from scratch by roasting my own peppers, and I couldn't tell a difference. I'm all about scratch cooking if you're into it, but sometimes it's not necessary. And by using jarred peppers, this meal goes from taking 1 hour to make to 30 minutes. This sauce is light but flavorful enough to work well with pasta, while not overpowering the shrimp flavor. Asparagus is fun for little hands, too, especially those who haven't nailed the pincer grasp yet.

For the red pepper sauce

1 tablespoon extra-virgin olive oil

3 garlic cloves, minced

1 shallot, minced

1 jar (16 ounces) roasted red peppers, drained

½ cup full-fat coconut milk or half-and-half (or use ⅓ cup low-sodium chicken or vegetable broth for a less creamy version)

1 tablespoon freshly squeezed lemon juice

2 tablespoons chopped fresh basil

Salt and pepper, to taste

Heat the oil in a large and wide skillet over medium heat. Once the oil is shimmering, add the garlic and shallot and cook for 1 minute or until fragrant. In a high-speed blender, combine the cooked vegetables, peppers, coconut milk, lemon juice, basil, and salt and pepper. Puree until creamy.

Bring a large pot filled halfway with water to a boil. Add the pasta and cook according to the package instructions. Drain the pasta and transfer to a large serving bowl.

Meanwhile, heat 1 tablespoon of the oil in a large skillet over medium heat. Once the oil is shimmering, add the asparagus and season with the garlic powder and salt and pepper. Combine well and let cook for 5 minutes. Add ¼ cup of water and cook 5 minutes more or until fork-tender.

Once the asparagus is cooked, set aside in a bowl. Immediately place the skillet back over medium heat and add in the remaining 1 tablespoon of olive oil and the shrimp. Season the shrimp with salt and pepper and cook for 3 minutes, flip, and cook for another 2 minutes or until the shrimp is opaque and C-shaped. Set the shrimp aside

For the shrimp and pasta

1 box (12 ounces) penne pasta

2 tablespoons extra-virgin olive oil

1 pound asparagus, trimmed and chopped into 1-inch pieces

½ teaspoon garlic powder

Salt and pepper

1½ pounds medium shrimp, peeled and deveined

1 tablespoon shredded fresh basil, for garnish

in the bowl with the asparagus. Pour the red pepper sauce into the skillet, back over medium heat. Bring the sauce to a simmer and then add the shrimp and asparagus to the skillet.

Pour the sauce, shrimp, and asparagus over the pasta, toss to combine, and serve garnished with the basil.

INSPIRALIZED TIP

Revive this recipe over and over again by switching up the protein, vegetable, and pasta.

FEEDING LITTLES TIP

Roasted red pepper sauce can be used as a dip, so if you want to serve this deconstructed, let your kids dip the asparagus, pasta, and shrimp in the sauce.

PREP AHEAD

Prep the sauce ahead of time—it saves well for up to 3 days in the refrigerator.

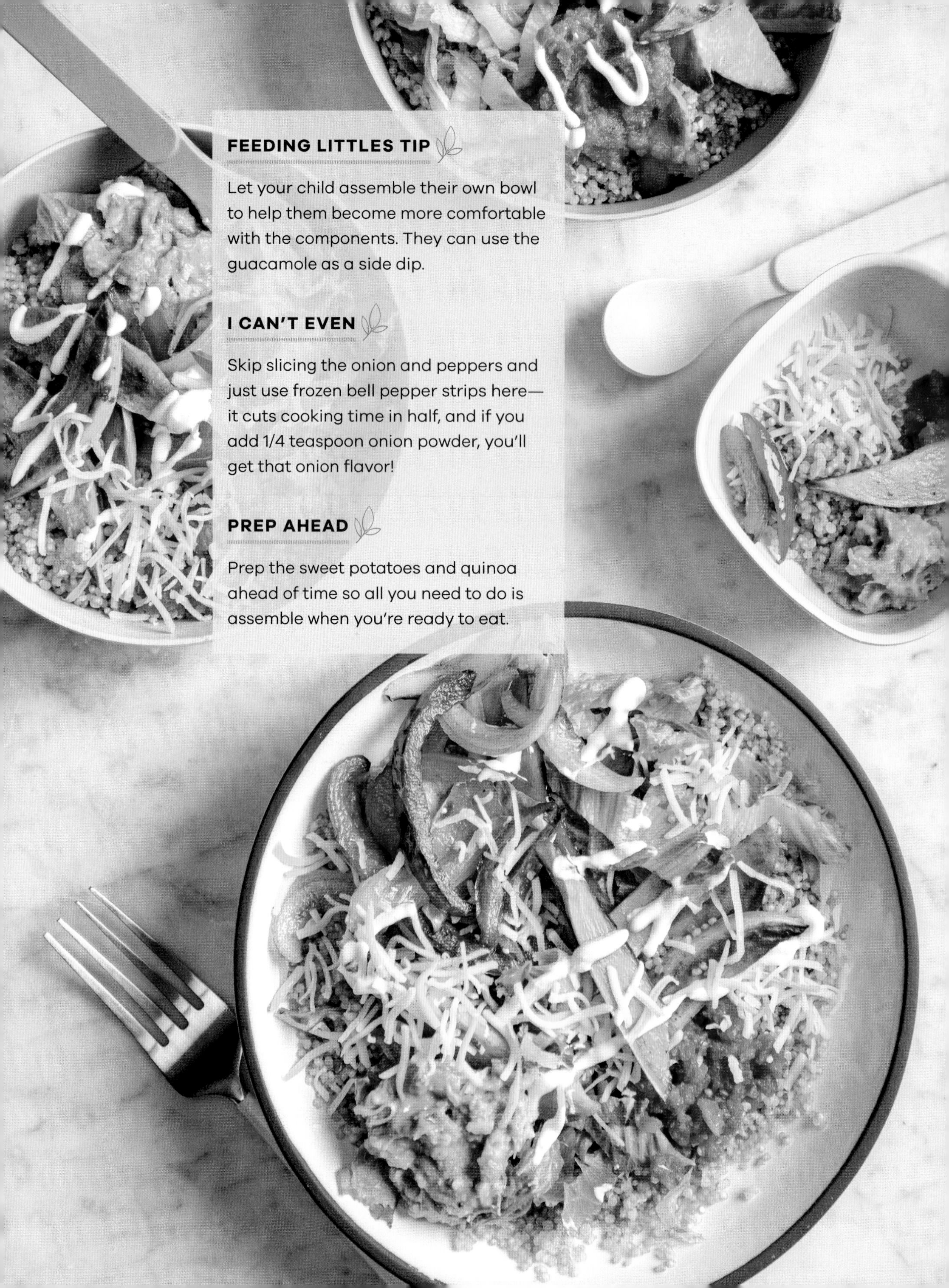

FEEDING LITTLES TIP

Let your child assemble their own bowl to help them become more comfortable with the components. They can use the guacamole as a side dip.

I CAN'T EVEN

Skip slicing the onion and peppers and just use frozen bell pepper strips here—it cuts cooking time in half, and if you add 1/4 teaspoon onion powder, you'll get that onion flavor!

PREP AHEAD

Prep the sweet potatoes and quinoa ahead of time so all you need to do is assemble when you're ready to eat.

sweet potato fajita quinoa bowls

time to prep: 10 minutes / time to cook: about 25 minutes / serves: 4

In 2016, *The Wall Street Journal* reported that the "bowl trend" was catching fire on Instagram (it's a pretty presentation, so I get it). Regardless of whether the craze sticks around, it's a handy way to build a meal. Bowls are for those times when you are craving a lot of different textures and flavors and don't want to commit to just one. Here, we're making a quinoa-based version of a can't-miss meal: sweet potato fajitas. The sweet potatoes are hearty and meaty and the quinoa adds a complete protein; tortillas optional.

1 cup dry quinoa

1 large sweet potato (or 2 medium), sliced into wedges

2 tablespoons extra-virgin olive oil

½ teaspoon chili powder

Salt and pepper

3 bell peppers, seeded and sliced

1 small onion, thinly sliced

1 teaspoon taco seasoning

½ cup salsa

1 cup chunky guacamole

1 cup shredded Mexican cheese blend

1 (packed) cup shredded romaine lettuce

Sour cream, for garnish (optional)

Preheat the oven to 425°F.

Combine the quinoa and 2 cups of water in a small pot and bring to a boil. Reduce the heat to low, cover, and cook for about 15 minutes or until the quinoa is fluffy. Set aside and cover to keep warm.

Meanwhile, set the potato out on a baking sheet, brush with 1 tablespoon of the oil, season with the chili powder and salt and pepper, and bake for 20 minutes or until fork-tender.

While the potato is baking, heat the remaining 1 tablespoon of oil in a large skillet over medium heat. Once the oil is shimmering, add the bell peppers and onion, sprinkle with taco seasoning, and cook until the vegetables are fork-tender, about 10 minutes. Set aside.

Assemble the bowls. Divide the quinoa into 4 bowls. Top with the peppers and onion, salsa, guacamole, cheese, romaine, and sweet potatoes. Serve, drizzled with sour cream, if using.

INSPIRALIZED TIP

If your family likes steak, shrimp, or chicken fajitas, add the cooked protein to the bowl before serving.

carrot crescent roll puffs

time to prep: 20 minutes / time to cook: 20 minutes / makes: 16 puffs

Kids dig food that comes in small bites. Think of these puffs as children-friendly hors d'oeuvres that are easy to hold and dip, and as a fun way to enjoy carrots, dressed up like pigs in a blanket. With buttery, sumptuous crescent rolls and plenty of smoky flavor, these are both scrumptious and adorable.

6 large carrots

1 cup low-sodium soy sauce

2 tablespoons maple syrup

1 teaspoon liquid smoke

1 teaspoon paprika

1 teaspoon smoked paprika

1 teaspoon garlic powder

1 container (8 ounces) crescent rolls

¼ cup melted unsalted butter

Salt and pepper

Mustard and ketchup, for serving

Peel the carrots, chop into 2-inch pieces, and round the edges of each piece using a vegetable peeler.

In the pot of a pressure cooker, stir together the soy sauce, 1 cup water, maple syrup, liquid smoke, paprikas, and garlic powder. Add the carrots. Set the pressure cooker to High pressure and cook for 4 minutes, then manually release the pressure. Once the carrots are done cooking, if desired, place them on a grill pan or grill over medium-high heat to get grill marks.

While the carrots cook, preheat the oven to 375°F. Lay out a large piece of parchment paper on the countertop, unroll the crescent sheets, and tear where perforated. Cut each triangle in half to yield two triangles. If you want to use less crescent roll, cut each triangle into thirds.

Place a carrot piece on the thick side of each triangle and roll to the thinner side. Transfer to a parchment paper–lined baking sheet, brush with butter, and sprinkle with salt and pepper. Bake for 12 to 15 minutes or until golden brown.

Serve the puffs with mustard, ketchup, or your favorite dip.

INSPIRALIZED TIP

Once you've assembled your puffs and they're ready for the oven, brush with a little melted butter and sprinkle with everything bagel seasoning for something extra!

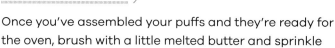

FEEDING LITTLES TIP

These make a hearty snack or can be the star of a meal when paired with protein, like a side of beans or hummus.

PREP AHEAD

To save time, prep the carrots ahead of time and reheat in a microwave or on the stovetop until heated through. Then wrap in the dough and bake.

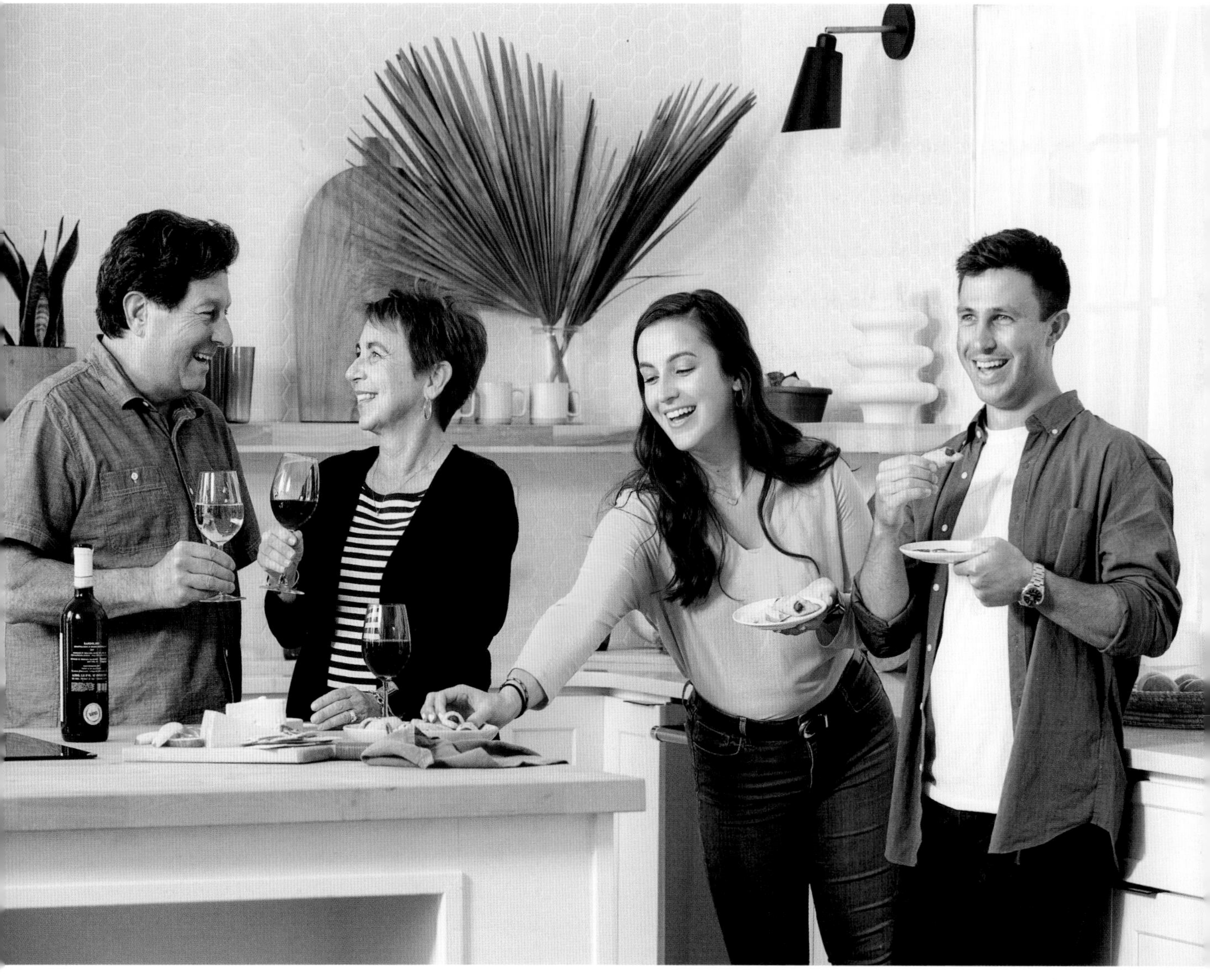

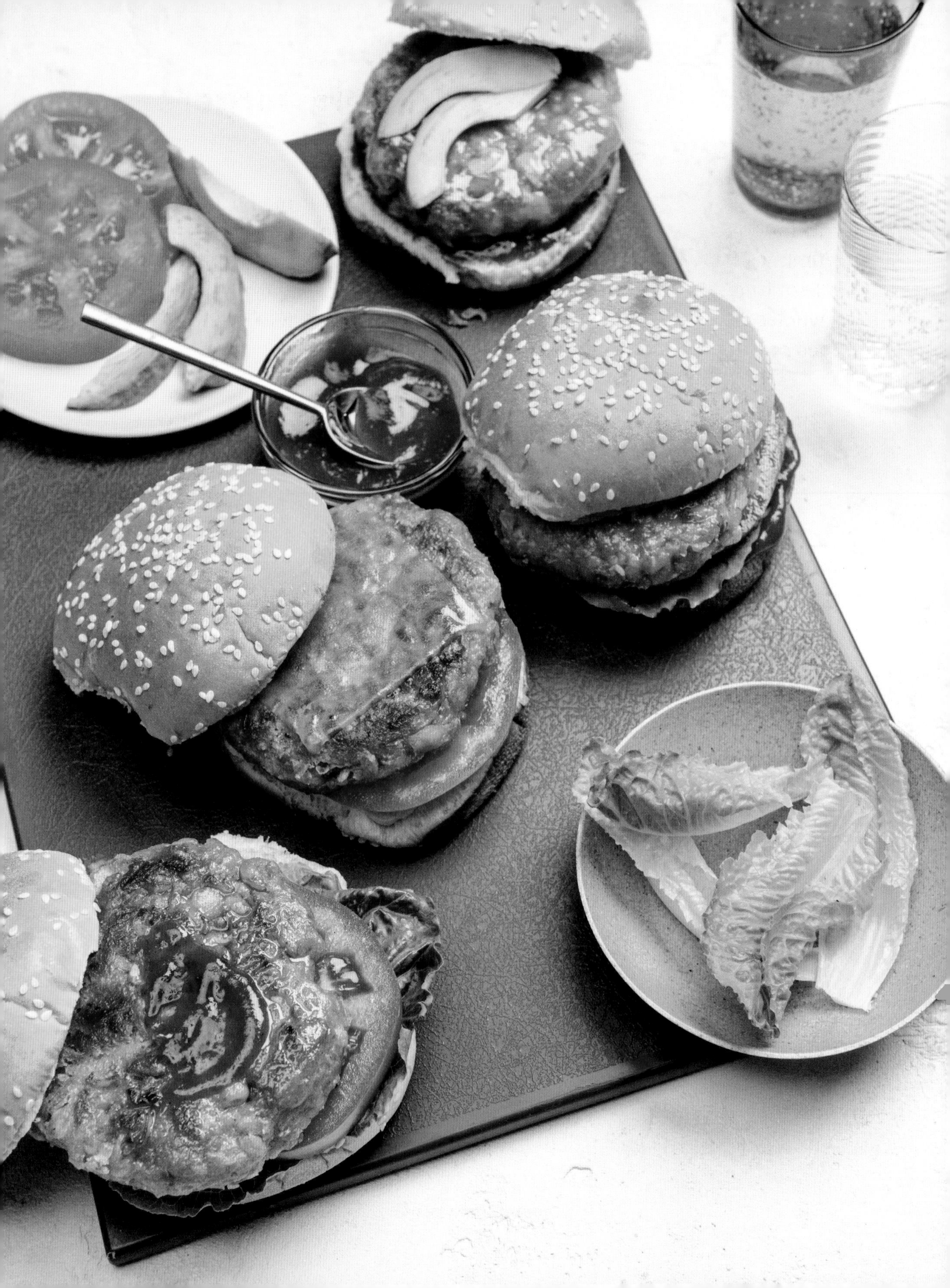

barbecue white bean veggie burgers

time to prep: 15 minutes / time to cook: 20 minutes / makes: 6 to 8 patties

For years, I experimented with my own veggie burger recipe. Everything I had found in cookbooks and online were too bean-y, too grain-y, or too crumbly. Finally, I developed a winner. Every time I make them (with an ample side of fries), my family scarfs them down, and it makes me happy to serve a wholesome meal that everyone enjoys. It's simple, it's veggie-packed, it does not crumble, and it freezes well for last-minute meals.

2 tablespoons extra-virgin olive oil

1 garlic clove, minced

½ cup diced onion

½ cup grated carrot, sweet potato, or golden beet

1 can (15 ounces) cannellini beans, drained and rinsed

1 cup cooked farro (or cooked brown rice)

½ cup oat flour (if you have oats, just pulse in a food processor until flour-like) or whole wheat or all-purpose flour

1 tablespoon ground cumin

2 tablespoons mayonnaise

2 tablespoons barbecue sauce, plus more for serving

Sliced cheese, for serving (optional)

(ingredients continue)

Heat 1 tablespoon of the oil in a medium skillet over medium heat. Once the oil is shimmering, add the garlic and onion and cook for 30 seconds or until fragrant. Add the carrot and cook until softened, about 3 minutes. Remove from the heat and set aside.

In a large mixing bowl, add the cannellini beans and mash with the back of a fork until mostly mashed. Add the cooked farro, cooked onion mixture, oat flour, cumin, mayonnaise, and barbecue sauce.

Line a sheet pan with parchment paper. Form the burgers into patties (about ½ cup per burger) and place on the sheet pan.

Heat the remaining 1 tablespoon of oil in a large skillet. Once the oil is shimmering, add the veggie burgers and cook for 5 minutes per side, pressing down with the back of a spatula to keep firm. Once you flip the burgers, top with slices of cheese, if using.

Serve the burgers on the buns with desired toppings and drizzle with more barbecue sauce, if desired.

(recipe continues)

6 hamburger buns, for serving

Burger toppings, for serving (e.g., sliced avocado, romaine lettuce, tomatoes)

INSPIRALIZED TIP

Let's chat about substitutions. While you can substitute vegan mayo here, the burger won't quite bind as well as it will with traditional mayo. If you have a gluten allergy, use gluten-free oats and substitute short-grain brown rice for the farro. If you can't have tomatoes, omit the barbecue sauce.

FEEDING LITTLES TIP

If your toddler can't hold a big assembled burger, cut it into little wedges.

I CAN'T EVEN

Substitute microwavable brown rice for the farro.

PREP AHEAD

These burgers can be completely prepped ahead, or you can at least cook the farro ahead of time.

indian butter tempeh with cauliflower rice

time to prep: 15 minutes / time to cook: about 30 minutes / serves: 4

If this is your first time seeing the word "tempeh," or you've heard of it but have never cooked with it, let me explain. Tempeh is a fermented soybean product that's formed into a rectangular cake, often combined with whole grains for extra nutrients and consistency. Now, I know that doesn't sound all that tempting, but trust me, tempeh rocks. I use it in stir-fries, in stuffed peppers, crumbled in the place of sausage in lasagnas, and sliced into strips like bacon. It's a tasty, fulfilling way to introduce soy to your little ones and it absorbs whatever flavors you cook it in, so it's versatile and adaptable. Here, it's the ideal conduit for the butter sauce, and every forkful is nourishing, packed with veggies and protein. Are you convinced?

2 packages (8 ounces each) tempeh

1 tablespoon extra-virgin olive oil

6 cups riced cauliflower or florets from 1 large head cauliflower, riced

Salt and pepper

1 tablespoon coconut oil

1 small onion, sliced

3 large garlic cloves, minced

1 tablespoon peeled and freshly grated ginger

1 tablespoon garam masala

1 teaspoon chili powder

(ingredients continue)

Boil ½ inch of water in a medium pot. Add the tempeh and cook for 10 minutes or until the moisture evaporates. Cube into 1-inch pieces.

While the tempeh cooks, heat the olive oil in a wide, deep skillet. Once the oil is hot, add the riced cauliflower and season with salt and pepper. Cook until softened, about 5 minutes, stirring often. Divide the cauliflower rice into plates or bowls and cover with foil or something similar to keep warm.

Prepare the sauce: Carefully wipe down the skillet used to cook the cauliflower rice, add the coconut oil, and set the skillet over medium heat. Once the oil is shimmering, add the onion, garlic, and ginger, and cook for 5 minutes or until the vegetables soften. Add the garam masala and chili powder and cook for 1 minute, stirring occasionally. Add the tomato paste, stir to coat, and then add the coconut milk. Stir and bring to a boil. Once boiling, reduce to a medium simmer and cook for 10 minutes or until slightly thickened. Add the tempeh cubes and cook for

(recipe continues)

1 can (6 ounces) tomato paste

2 cups canned unsweetened full-fat coconut milk

¼ cup cilantro leaves (about a handful), for garnish

Warmed naan, for serving (optional)

another 5 minutes, stirring occasionally.

Divide the tempeh over the cauliflower rice and garnish with the cilantro. Serve with naan, if using.

INSPIRALIZED TIP

If you're nervous to try tempeh but want to make this flavorful Indian-inspired dish, substitute the tempeh with chicken for a more traditional pairing.

FEEDING LITTLES TIP

If this dish is overwhelming to your kiddo, deconstruct it. Separate the tempeh and sauce from the cauliflower rice. If you want to serve the cilantro to your baby, finely chop it and mix into the sauce.

I CAN'T EVEN

Buy pre-riced cauliflower in the freezer or refrigerator section to speed up this recipe. You can also purchase premade Indian butter sauce, if you need to save time.

PREP AHEAD

The sauce can easily be prepped ahead of time. When you're ready to prepare the meal, cook the tempeh and transfer to the skillet along with the premade sauce, letting it simmer for 5 to 10 minutes before serving over the riced cauliflower.

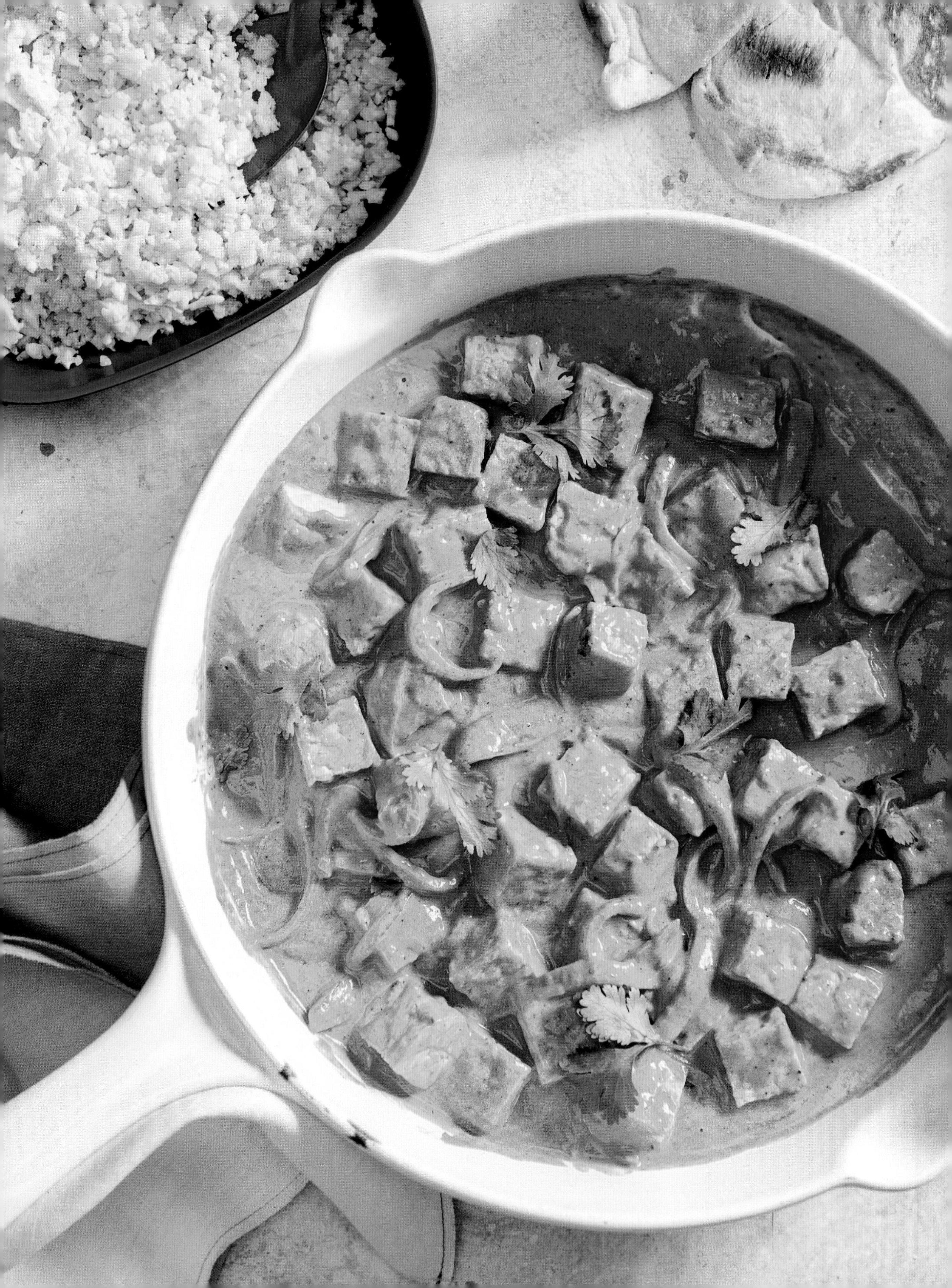

weeknight beef tacos with edamame avocado mash

time to prep: 20 minutes / time to cook: 15 minutes / serves: 4 (2 tacos per person)

When I was a kid, taco night was the highlight of any week. My mother would put all the taco fillings in bowls alongside crunchy shells and let us dive in. I loved having the independence to build my own meal. It's untraditional, but you can put a twist on taco night with this guacamole-inspired dip, which has a similar flavor, with the slightest crunch. By using edamame, we bring more protein into the whole meal and an allergen exposure (soy).

½ cup frozen shelled edamame, thawed

2 garlic cloves, roughly chopped

2 ripe avocados, peeled and pitted

¼ cup finely diced red onion

1 small jalapeño, finely diced

¼ cup minced cilantro

1 ripe lime, juiced

Salt and pepper

1 pound ground beef

2 teaspoons taco seasoning

8 tortillas (hard or soft, your preference), for serving

Shredded Mexican cheese blend, shredded romaine lettuce, chopped tomatoes, for serving

Put the edamame in a food processor and pulse until creamy with some chunks. Place the edamame in a medium mixing bowl and add the garlic, avocados, onion, jalapeño, cilantro, and lime juice. Season generously with salt and some pepper. Mix until the avocado mash is made to your preferred consistency. Set aside.

Heat a large skillet over medium heat. Once the pan is hot, add the beef and crumble with a spatula or wooden spoon. Add the taco seasoning, season with salt and pepper, and stir to coat. Let the beef cook, stirring occasionally, until it is cooked through.

While the beef cooks, warm your tortillas over a burner, in a skillet, or in the oven.

Place all of your toppings (cheese, lettuce, tomatoes) in separate bowls to serve family style along with the avocado mash, beef, and warmed tortillas.

INSPIRALIZED TIP

If you have a soy allergy in your family, omit the edamame or substitute with peas.

FEEDING LITTLES TIP

Add variety to this recipe by changing up the meat—ground chicken, turkey, or pork can also work well. Vegetarian? Substitute with black beans.

PREP AHEAD

The taco meat can be prepared ahead of time, but it's best to make the avocado mash right before serving, to avoid browning from the oxidization of the avocados.

spinach falafel with carrots and hummus

time to prep: 15 minutes / time to cook: 40 minutes / serves: 5 (4 falafels per person)

Spinach is a tough one to make palatable or servable for babies and toddlers. Like meatballs, falafel are an appealing size and shape for little eaters and a tasty way to introduce flavors like cumin. This version is served with large carrots, too, which are fun for them to eat. Serve it with hummus and you have a yummy deconstructed pita sandwich.

10 carrots, peeled and trimmed

Extra-virgin olive oil, to drizzle

½ teaspoon garlic powder

Salt and pepper

For the falafel

1 small onion, diced

2 garlic cloves, minced

½ cup fresh flat-leaf parsley, chopped

½ cup cilantro leaves, chopped

1 cup packed baby spinach

1 tablespoon ground cumin

Salt and pepper

2 cans (15½ ounces each) chickpeas, drained and rinsed

Preheat the oven to 400°F. Line a large baking sheet with parchment paper.

Place the carrots on the baking sheet and drizzle with olive oil. Season the carrots with the garlic powder and salt and pepper. Toss to coat. Bake for 40 minutes or until fork-tender.

While the carrots roast, make the falafel. In a large food processor, place the onion, garlic, parsley, cilantro, spinach, and cumin. Season with salt and pepper. Process for 30 seconds, then add the chickpeas and flour, and process until coarse.

If using an air fryer for the falafel, preheat it to 400°F.

Form the mixture into 2-inch balls and set aside, or if baking the falafel in the oven, place on the baking sheet alongside the carrots. Bake for 15 to 25 minutes, or until firm and golden brown.

If using an air fryer, set the balls inside the preheated air-fryer basket and spritz with cooking spray. Cook for about 15 minutes or until golden brown, shaking the air-fryer basket every 5 minutes and cooking in batches if necessary.

While the falafel and carrots cook, warm the pitas in the oven, directly on the rack, for about 10 minutes. Remove and cut each pita into 8 slices.

2 tablespoons all-purpose, whole wheat, chickpea, or oat flour

Cooking spray, for the air fryer

2 whole wheat pitas

Hummus, for serving

Once the carrots and falafel are done cooking, divide the hummus onto 5 plates, add the pita slices, and add the falafel and carrots.

INSPIRALIZED TIP

Do not prep any of the ingredients for the falafel until you place the carrots in the oven to roast.

FEEDING LITTLES TIP

See if your kids want to pretend that they're a bunny rabbit as they eat their big carrot.

PREP AHEAD

This entire meal can be prepared ahead of time. To serve, microwave or oven-bake the falafel and carrots at 400°F until warmed through, 10 to 15 minutes.

stovetop butternut squash mac and "cheese"

time to prep: 10 minutes / time to cook: 30 minutes / serves: 6 to 8

As far as comfort food goes, it doesn't get better than mac and cheese. If you're avoiding dairy for any reason, you need an equally satisfying version in your repertoire. While the boxed variety will always have a place in my family's pantry (and heart), this dairy-free, veggie-packed recipe is so simple and delicious, I find myself making it even more often. Plus, it has a more sophisticated flavor that adults enjoy, too. The creamy sauce coats every forkful of macaroni, and with its golden-brown crunchy crust, this mac and cheese has it all (except the cheese). It's important to let kids see foods in their whole form, so we have some options for veggies you can mix in as well.

1 cup peeled and cubed butternut squash

1 box (16 ounces) elbow macaroni

Peas, spinach, broccoli (optional, if you'd like to add whole vegetables to this meal)

1 tablespoon extra-virgin olive oil

2 garlic cloves, minced

½ medium red onion, diced

1 cup canned unsweetened full-fat coconut milk

1 tablespoon nutritional yeast

½ teaspoon paprika

½ teaspoon dried thyme

Place a medium skillet over high heat, add the butternut squash, and cover with water. Bring to a boil, reduce the heat to medium to simmer, and cook until the squash is fork-tender, about 10 minutes. Drain the squash and pat dry. Set aside.

Meanwhile, fill a large pot halfway with water, place it over high heat, and bring to a boil. Once boiling, add the pasta (and any raw vegetables, if using) and cook according to the package directions. Drain the pasta into a colander, rinse, and pour the pasta back into the pot.

Heat the oil in a large skillet over medium heat. Once the oil is shimmering, add the garlic and onion and let cook until the vegetable mixture is translucent, about 5 minutes. Transfer to a blender along with the squash, coconut milk, nutritional yeast, paprika, thyme, the ¼ teaspoon of salt, and pepper. Blend, taste, and adjust with more salt, as needed.

Pour the prepared sauce over the pasta, stir well to coat, and transfer to a serving bowl. Season with more pepper, top with the crackers, and serve.

¼ teaspoon salt, plus more as needed

Pepper, to taste

½ cup well-chopped crackers

INSPIRALIZED TIP

Get intentional with your crust and buy flavored crackers, such as barbecue or rosemary, or use a true cheddar cracker for extra cheesy deliciousness.

FEEDING LITTLES TIP

Toppings are made for mac and cheese. Try diced precooked chicken sausage, scallions (omit for babies), chopped tomatoes, or avocado.

I CAN'T EVEN

Buy frozen butternut squash, so you don't have to peel and chop your own.

PREP AHEAD

The sauce can be prepped ahead of time, and leftovers save well in the fridge for up to 3 days.

loaded baked potato and zucchini soup

time to prep: 25 minutes / time to cook: 20 minutes / serves: 6

This soup is perfect as an appetizer or a light meal when served with crusty, warm bread and a satiating salad. It's also a creative way to squeeze in vegetables with all the deliciousness of a baked potato. If you'd rather skip the shredded cheese topping, the soup will be completely dairy-free and still have that cheesy taste, thanks to nutritional yeast.

- 1 tablespoon extra-virgin olive oil
- ½ red onion, diced
- 2 garlic cloves, minced
- ½ cup small-cubed zucchini
- 1½ cups small-cubed potatoes
- ½ cup raw cashews
- 1 teaspoon nutritional yeast
- 2 cups low-sodium chicken broth
- ½ teaspoon salt, plus more to taste
- Pepper, to taste
- 1 tablespoon freshly squeezed lemon juice
- 6 strips bacon, cooked and crumbled, for serving
- 1½ cups shredded cheddar cheese, for serving
- ¼ cup sliced scallions or chives, for serving

Heat the oil in a large skillet over medium-high heat. Once the oil is shimmering, add the onion and garlic. Cook until fragrant, about 1 minute, and then add in the zucchini and potatoes. Add the cashews, nutritional yeast, broth, 2 cups of water, the ½ teaspoon of salt, and pepper. Bring to a boil, then reduce the heat, cover, and simmer for 20 minutes or until the potatoes are fork-tender.

Transfer the vegetable mixture to a blender along with the lemon juice and blend until smooth. Alternately, you could use an immersion blender and blend the soup right in the pot. Taste and adjust with more salt, if needed.

Pour the soup into bowls and top with bacon, cheese, scallions or chives, and anything else you like on top of your baked potato. Serve.

INSPIRALIZED TIP

For a creamier, dairy soup, drizzle generously with heavy cream, or add a dollop of sour cream.

FEEDING LITTLES TIP

Try serving this in a cup with a wide reusable straw if your child struggles to use a spoon. You can also serve it with toast strips for dipping in the soup.

chicken and broccoli rice casserole

time to prep: 15 minutes / time to cook: about 45 minutes / serves: 4

Chicken and broccoli is the king of comforting combos, and this dairy-free casserole version is so tasty and creamy, you'll never miss the dairy. If you find that your younger eaters are intimidated by casseroles, you can deconstruct this by boiling the broccoli separately from the rice and more simply serving this casserole as a chicken, broccoli, rice, and dip meal. Then, the next time you make this dish, try combining a couple of the components until your child builds up the confidence to dive right into this casserole.

1 medium sweet potato, peeled and cubed

2 boneless, skinless chicken breasts, chopped into ½-inch cubes

¼ teaspoon garlic powder

¼ teaspoon salt, plus more as needed

Pepper

3 tablespoons extra-virgin olive oil

2½ cups low-sodium chicken broth, plus more as needed

1¼ cups dry white long-grain rice

3 cups broccoli florets

2 garlic cloves, minced

½ medium red onion, diced

1 cup canned unsweetened full-fat coconut milk

½ teaspoon paprika

½ teaspoon dried thyme

Place a medium skillet over high heat, add the sweet potato, and cover with water. Bring to a boil, reduce the heat to medium to simmer, and cook until the sweet potato is fork-tender, about 10 minutes. Drain and pat dry. Set aside.

Season the chicken with the garlic powder and salt and pepper.

Heat 1 tablespoon of the oil in a large pot or wide, deep large skillet over medium-high heat. Once the oil is shimmering, add the chicken and cook until browned and no longer pink on the inside, about 10 minutes. Transfer to a plate and set aside.

Add the broth, 1 tablespoon of the oil, and the rice to the pot and bring to a boil. Once boiling, reduce the heat to a simmer, cover, and cook for 10 minutes. Uncover the pot, add the broccoli and extra broth (another cup) if it has already evaporated, cover the pot again, and cook for 10 more minutes. Turn off the heat and let the rice stand for 10 more minutes, covered. Uncover the pot, smash the broccoli with the back of a fork, and stir to combine.

Meanwhile, heat the remaining 1 tablespoon of oil in a medium skillet over medium heat. Once the oil is shimmering, add the garlic and onion and let cook until translucent, about 5 minutes. Transfer the vegetable

(recipe continues)

mixture to a blender along with the sweet potato, coconut milk, paprika, thyme, the ¼ teaspoon of salt, and pepper to taste. Taste and adjust with more salt, as needed. Set aside.

Add the cooked chicken to the broccoli and rice, and pour the sauce mixture over the top. Stir well to combine. Taste and adjust with salt as needed. Transfer to a dish and serve.

INSPIRALIZED TIP

Make this completely plant-based by replacing the chicken with chickpeas or roasted extra-firm tofu. If you're not dairy-free, you can add 1 cup of shredded cheddar cheese into the sauce mixture and stir until melted.

FEEDING LITTLES TIP

Sometimes selective eaters pick out one or two components of a casserole and just eat that. Don't get discouraged. It's a good sign that they're interacting with the food, even if they're not ready to try the whole thing just yet. Remember, exposure is how they get there.

I CAN'T EVEN

Use 4 cups of microwavable rice, and boil the broccoli on its own.

PREP AHEAD

This entire meal can be prepped ahead of time, but for optimal freshness and consistency, cook the rice the same day.

salmon cakes and fries with avocado dill aioli

time to prep: 15 minutes / time to cook: 30 minutes / serves: 4 (1 large cake or 2 small cakes per person)

From burgers to meatballs to macaroni salad to fried rice, canned salmon is an accessible and affordable way to enjoy this heart-healthy, versatile fish. Whenever I make salmon cakes, I'm pleasantly surprised and think, "Why don't I make these more often?" What makes these cakes particularly delectable is the balance of zesty dill, lemon, and Dijon mustard. Each bite is bright and satisfying and melds with a simple but exquisite aioli, made with dill, avocado, lemon, and mayonnaise. With plenty of familiar textures *and* opportunities for flavor introductions, this meal hits all the notes.

Note: Canned salmon might contain small bones. Oftentimes they are very soft and edible, but if they are hard make sure to remove them.

2 pounds Japanese sweet potatoes, sliced into sticks or "fries"

1 tablespoon extra-virgin olive oil, plus more to drizzle

¼ teaspoon salt, plus more as needed

Pepper

1 can (14¾ ounces) salmon, drained (or 3 5-ounce cans work, too)

1 large egg

¼ cup mayonnaise

½ cup breadcrumbs (seasoned or plain)

1 garlic clove, grated or finely minced

(ingredients continue)

Preheat the oven to 425°F. Line a baking sheet with parchment paper. Lay out the sweet potatoes, drizzle with olive oil, and toss to coat. Season with the ¼ teaspoon of salt and pepper to taste. Roast for 25 to 30 minutes, flipping halfway through, or until the potatoes are fork-tender and starting to crisp up and deeply brown on the edges.

Combine the salmon with the egg, mayonnaise, breadcrumbs, garlic, dill, mustard, and scallions in a large bowl. Season with salt and pepper and stir until combined, then form into 4 patties or 8 smaller patties.

Heat the 1 tablespoon of oil in a large skillet over medium-high heat. Once the oil is shimmering, add the patties and cook until browned and firm, 5 to 7 minutes per side.

(recipe continues)

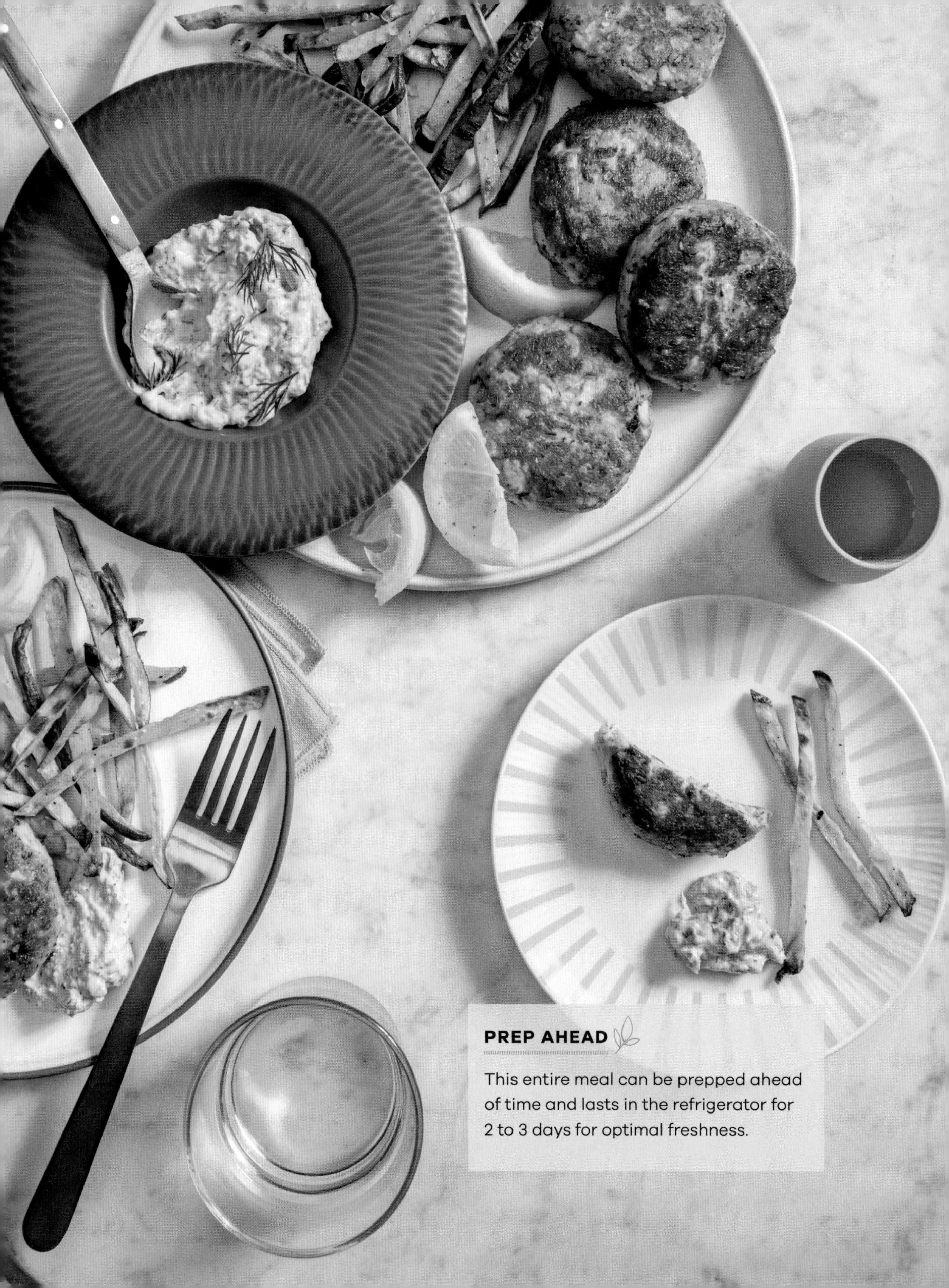

PREP AHEAD

This entire meal can be prepped ahead of time and lasts in the refrigerator for 2 to 3 days for optimal freshness.

2 tablespoons chopped fresh dill

1 tablespoon Dijon mustard

¼ cup finely chopped scallions

For the avocado dill aioli

1 large avocado, peeled, pitted, and mashed

⅓ cup mayonnaise

1 lemon, juiced

1 tablespoon chopped fresh dill

Salt and pepper

While the salmon cooks, prepare the aioli. In a medium bowl, place the avocado, mayonnaise, lemon juice, and dill, season with salt and pepper, and whisk together until combined. You can also do this in a small food processor for a smoother consistency.

Serve the patties with the sweet potatoes and aioli.

INSPIRALIZED TIP

Sweet potatoes come in many different shapes, sizes, and colors: Japanese sweet potatoes have a lovely nutty texture and are much heartier than the orange-fleshed ones you might be familiar with. When peeled, they resemble traditional Russets, since they're white on the inside.

FEEDING LITTLES TIP

These salmon cakes are an especially great way for babies to try salmon, since they can be easily cut into strips and are pretty soft.

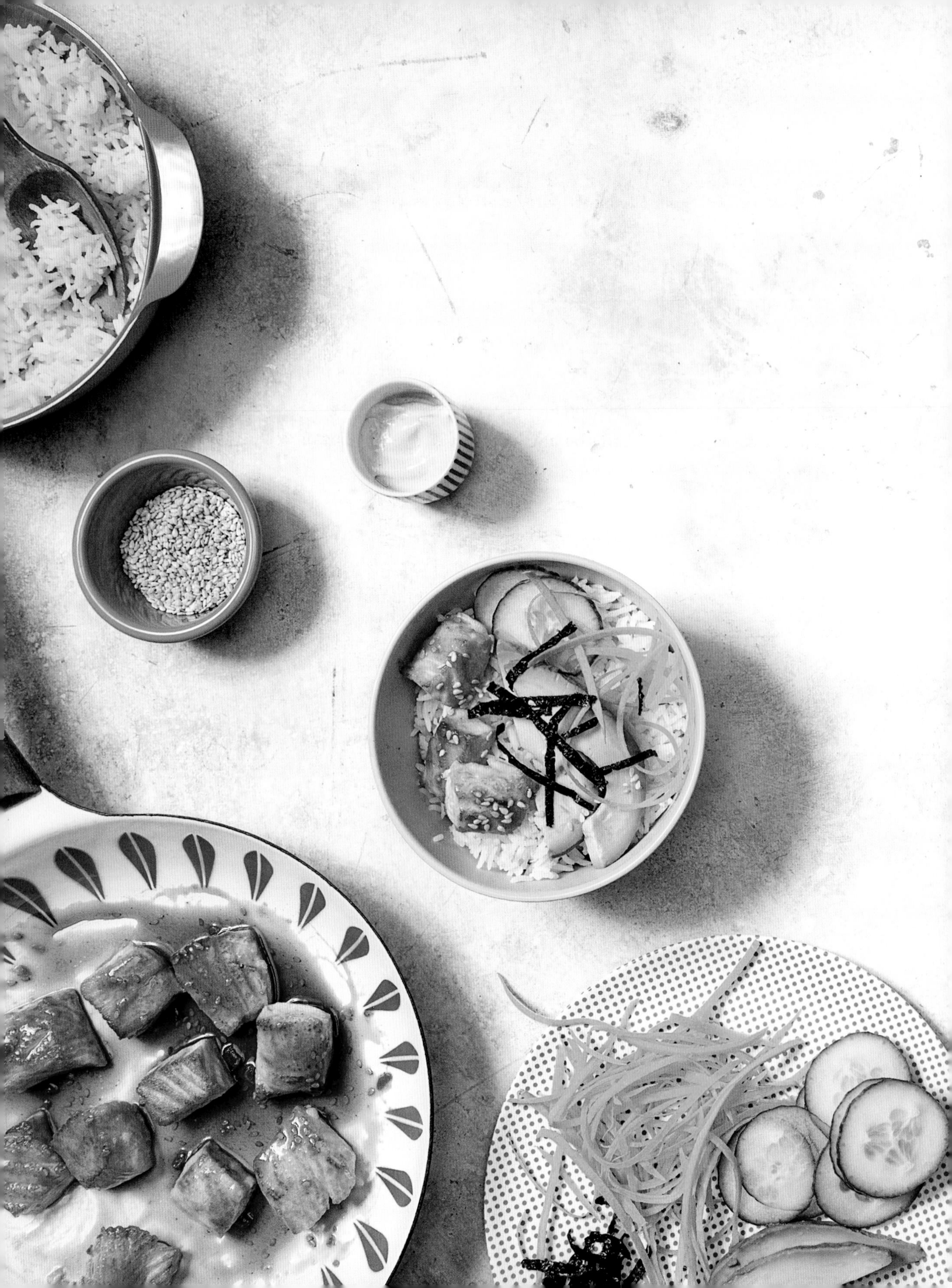

mostly homemade

You probably bought this cookbook for the new and original recipes to feed your whole family. You might have also wanted tips on how to streamline the cooking process, simplify mealtime, and stop feeling like a short-order chef.

Well, let's start with one of our primary tips: use modern conveniences to take shortcuts, without sacrificing on nutrition, flavor, or quality. Premade foods and products quicken the process while adding nutrients and flavor—and time back into your day. It's cooking smarter, not harder.

There are jarred pasta sauces out there that are better than anything I could make at home and they save so much time, it's a no-brainer to pick them up. As much as I'd love to slowly simmer a Sunday sauce, with toddlers running around, that isn't always an option. Sometimes, when I'm making meatballs, I go for *mostly* homemade, like in our Zucchini Lamb Meatballs with Orzo and Feta (page 207), which uses store-bought marinara.

In this chapter, we'll suggest the following premade foods to make life easier and so we can still create delicious, balanced, and inviting meals for our families:

- Jarred pasta sauce
- Flatbreads and frozen pizza crusts
- Canned refried beans
- Oven-ready flaky biscuits
- Seaweed snacks
- Precooked lentils
- Frozen hashed browns
- Salsa
- Baked beans

Mostly homemade is the new homemade—it's time to make life easier for yourself.

freeze-ahead breakfast burritos

time to prep: 20 minutes / time to cook: 10 minutes / makes: 6 burritos

Before you have a baby, people tell you to prep freezer meals. Some expectant parents are all about this, while others can't fathom adding one more thing to their plate, literally. I get it, but hear me out: If you *are* going do it, why not prep some easy breakfast burritos? Yes, casseroles and soups are warming and nutritious, but after I had my first kid, breakfast was the one meal of the day that I looked forward to. I'd wake up foggy after a sleepless night, absolutely ravenous. All I wanted was a big, warm, filling breakfast to satiate my unquenchable postpartum hunger—but the last thing I needed was to cook one. When I was pregnant with my second child, I had learned my lesson. I didn't prep a single meal except a triple batch of freezer breakfast burritos, and let me tell you: game changer. These burritos are filled with hashed browns for extra carb fuel, without the painstaking shredding of potatoes, thanks to bagged frozen seasoned hashed browns. Frankly, I'm still hungry and sleepless from everyday life with kids (will I ever sleep again?!), and these burritos have never let me down.

10 large eggs, beaten

2 tablespoons extra-virgin olive oil

1-pound bag frozen seasoned hashed browns

½ teaspoon chili powder

Cooking spray, for the aluminum foil

6 large burrito-sized wraps/tortillas

2 avocados, peeled, pitted, and mashed (or ¾ cup guacamole)

Heat a large nonstick skillet over medium heat. Once the skillet is hot, add your eggs and scramble. Set aside. Using the same skillet used to cook the eggs, place the olive oil over medium heat. Once the oil is hot, add the hashed browns and season with the chili powder. Cook until crispy, about 7 minutes. Remove from the heat and set aside.

Tear off 6 pieces of aluminum foil large enough to roll up the burrito. Have all your burrito ingredients nearby for easy assembly. Spritz the foil pieces with cooking spray. Place a tortilla on top of a piece of foil. On the end of the tortilla closest to you, spread out some avocado. Top with eggs, then cheese, pico de gallo, and hashed browns.

Roll the burrito tightly by folding the sides over the filling, then rolling tightly from the bottom up. Wrap the burrito tightly in the aluminum foil. Repeat this with the remaining tortillas and filling ingredients.

¾ cup shredded Mexican cheese blend (cheddar is fine, too)

¾ cup pico de gallo

For best results, freeze the burritos in a single layer on a baking sheet. Once frozen, you can transfer to a gallon-sized zip-tight freezer bag.

To reheat, unwrap from the foil, and warm in the oven at 400°F for 15 to 20 minutes, or microwave on high for 1 minute covered with a paper towel, flip, and microwave another 1½ minutes.

INSPIRALIZED TIP

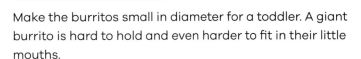

If you are unable to find preseasoned hashed browns, season plain frozen hashed browns with ½ teaspoon of onion powder, 1 teaspoon of garlic powder, and salt and pepper to taste.

FEEDING LITTLES TIP

Make the burritos small in diameter for a toddler. A giant burrito is hard to hold and even harder to fit in their little mouths.

teriyaki salmon bite bowls

time to prep: 30 minutes / time to cook: about 30 minutes / serves: 4

I can't explain the toddler mindset, but for whatever reason, when I make these salmon bites instead of cutting a salmon fillet into pieces, they're better received. It must have something to do with how approachable the pieces look at this mini size. I love them, too, because there is more surface area for the teriyaki sauce to cover and more flavor in every bite. Serve this deconstructed or combined in a bowl.

- **1½ cups dry white rice**
- **1 pound boneless, skinless salmon, cut into 1-inch cubes**
- **½ cup bottled teriyaki sauce (a thick sauce, not a watery marinade)**
- **¼ cup mayonnaise (egg-free works well)**
- **1 tablespoon sriracha**
- **½ tablespoon freshly squeezed lime juice**
- **1 pinch garlic powder**
- **Salt**
- **2 ripe avocados, pitted, peeled, and sliced**
- **½ cup thinly sliced cucumber**
- **1 cup shredded carrots**
- **1 package (0.35 ounces) seaweed snacks, sliced into strips**
- **Sesame seeds, for garnish**

Combine the rice with 3 cups of water in a medium pot and bring to a boil. Reduce the heat to a simmer, cover, and cook for 30 minutes, or until fluffy or according to the package instructions.

While the rice cooks, place the salmon in a bowl and cover with teriyaki sauce. Let it marinate for 20 minutes.

Heat a large skillet over medium heat. Once the pan is hot, add the salmon and cook for 5 minutes per side or until it is opaque on the inside, about 10 minutes.

While the salmon cooks, prepare the sriracha mayo. In a small bowl, whisk together the mayo, sriracha, lime juice, garlic powder, and salt to taste. Set aside.

Once the rice and salmon are done cooking, assemble the bowls. Divide the rice into bowls and top evenly with salmon. Add the avocados, cucumber, carrots, and seaweed. Garnish with sesame seeds and drizzle with the sriracha mayo. Serve.

INSPIRALIZED TIP

Try roasted or dried seaweed for the young eater, and they may surprise you at how much they love this flavor and texture. If your little one likes a certain seaweed snack, use that one in this recipe.

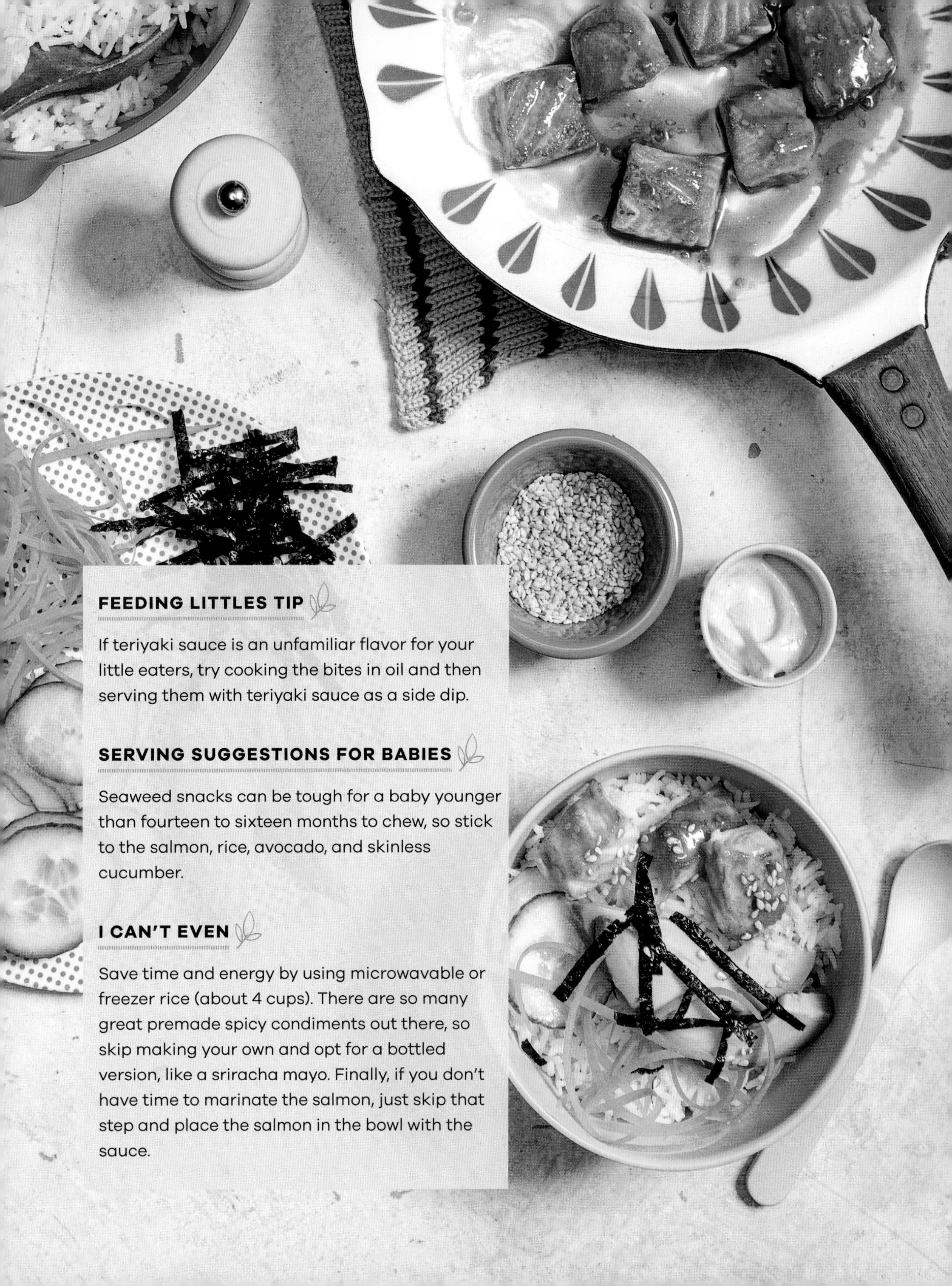

FEEDING LITTLES TIP

If teriyaki sauce is an unfamiliar flavor for your little eaters, try cooking the bites in oil and then serving them with teriyaki sauce as a side dip.

SERVING SUGGESTIONS FOR BABIES

Seaweed snacks can be tough for a baby younger than fourteen to sixteen months to chew, so stick to the salmon, rice, avocado, and skinless cucumber.

I CAN'T EVEN

Save time and energy by using microwavable or freezer rice (about 4 cups). There are so many great premade spicy condiments out there, so skip making your own and opt for a bottled version, like a sriracha mayo. Finally, if you don't have time to marinate the salmon, just skip that step and place the salmon in the bowl with the sauce.

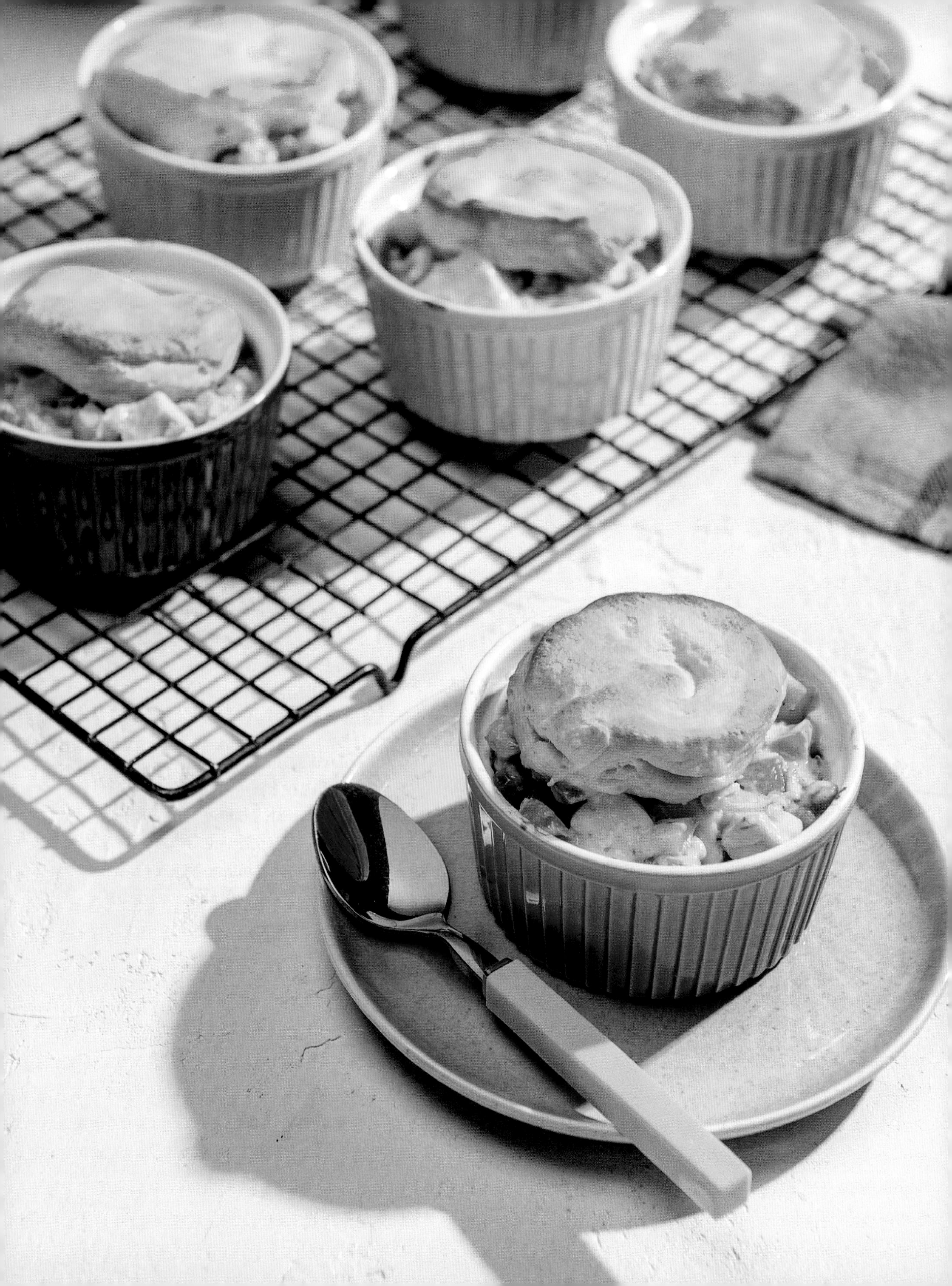

mini biscuit turkey potpies

time to prep: 15 minutes / time to cook: 25 minutes / makes: 6 potpies

Potpies are nostalgic, cozy, and comforting. However, making your own crust or even maneuvering a premade one to cover the fillings can be a Herculean task. The solution? Make mini potpies by spooning the turkey filling into ramekins or a jumbo muffin pan and topping with . . . flaky biscuits! They lend a sweeter flavor and fluffier consistency to the dish, and they're just so easy. They look cute, too.

Cooking spray, for greasing the ramekins

1 container (16 ounces) flaky biscuits

2 tablespoons extra-virgin olive oil

2 garlic cloves, minced

⅓ cup diced yellow onion

½ cup diced celery

½ cup peeled and diced carrot

1 teaspoon dried thyme

1 teaspoon salt, plus more to taste

Pepper

2 tablespoons arrowroot powder (or cornstarch)

1 cup low-sodium chicken broth

½ cup full-fat coconut milk or heavy cream

2 cups diced roasted turkey or rotisserie chicken

½ cup frozen peas

Preheat the oven to 400°F. Place six 6-ounce ramekins on a baking sheet, grease with cooking spray, and set aside. Or you can use a jumbo muffin pan with 6 cavities.

Halve 3 of the biscuits to create 6 biscuits that are thinner. Reserve the rest of the premade biscuits or bake and freeze them for future use.

Heat the oil in a large pot or wide skillet over medium heat. Once the oil is shimmering, add the garlic, onion, celery, carrot, and thyme, and season generously with salt and pepper. Cook, stirring, until the veggies are softened, about 7 minutes.

Sprinkle in the arrowroot powder and stir into the veggies until well combined. While stirring, slowly pour in the broth. While continuing to stir, slowly pour in the coconut milk. Cook, uncovered, and stir frequently, until the contents are thick and creamy, about 5 minutes. Remove from the heat, season with the teaspoon of salt, and stir in the turkey and peas.

Divide the filling evenly among the ramekins or muffin cavities and top each with a biscuit. Transfer to the oven and bake for 10 minutes or until the biscuits are golden on top. If using ramekins, wait 10 minutes before serving, until the ramekins are cooler to the touch. If using a muffin pan, scoop out the biscuit on top, place in a bowl,

(recipe continues)

and scoop out the filling and place into the bowl with the biscuit, repeating for the remaining potpies.

INSPIRALIZED TIP

For a more traditional potpie flavor, replace the oil with a tablespoon of unsalted butter.

FEEDING LITTLES TIP

For the sake of novelty, try serving this in the muffin pan you baked it in (once it has cooled). Remove all but one mini potpie from the muffin pan, let it cool, and offer a side dish in another one of the muffin pan's cavities. Your kid will think it's funny, and you'll have one less plate to clean.

PREP AHEAD

The filling can be prepared ahead and then reheated in a skillet before spooning into ramekins or muffin pans, topping with the biscuits, and baking in the oven.

turkey bolognese with spaghetti squash

time to prep: 15 minutes / time to cook: 60 minutes (halve this time if you cook your spaghetti squash in a pressure cooker) / serves: 4

As an Italian American, I used to cringe when I admitted that I used jarred sauce in my Bolognese. My grandparents made fresh Sunday sauce all the time, why couldn't I? Well, times have changed, and I don't feel any shame about using convenience condiments. Some of them are even better than any I could possibly make at home. I'm always looking to cut corners and save time without sacrificing on flavor, ingredients, or quality, and this recipe is a solid example. Now when I share my recipes that used jarred sauces, I smile confidently with the knowledge that I'm making something nutritious and delicious, while gaining a little extra time to spend on my family—or myself.

1 large spaghetti squash

1 tablespoon extra-virgin olive oil, plus more for the squash

Salt and pepper

½ cup peeled and diced carrot

1 small red onion, diced

⅓ cup diced celery

¼ teaspoon red pepper flakes

2 garlic cloves, minced

1 pound ground turkey

2 teaspoons dried oregano

1 jar (24 ounces) tomato basil sauce

Grated Parmesan cheese, for garnish (optional)

Cook the spaghetti squash. You can do this either in the oven or a pressure cooker for quicker results. First, slice the spaghetti squash in half and then scoop out its seeds. Place the steamer basket in the bottom of the pressure cooker pot and arrange the squash, cut sides down. Cook on High pressure for 7 minutes, and then manually release. Open the cooker and carefully remove the squash and, using forks, shred the insides into spaghetti strands. If baking in the oven, preheat the oven to 400°F and rub the insides of the spaghetti squash with a little bit of olive oil, season with salt and pepper, and place the squash cut sides down on a sheet pan. Bake for 40 to 60 minutes until fork-tender. Use forks to shred the insides into spaghetti strands.

While the spaghetti squash cooks, prepare the Bolognese. Heat the 1 tablespoon of oil in a large skillet over medium-high heat. Once the oil is shimmering, add in the carrot, onion, and celery. Cook until the vegetables soften, about 7 minutes, and then add in the red pepper flakes, half of the garlic, and let cook for 30 seconds or until fragrant.

(recipe continues)

Push the veggies to one side of the skillet and then add in the ground turkey, crumbling with a wooden spoon. Season the meat with the oregano, salt, pepper, and the rest of the garlic. Cook the meat until browned, and then combine the veggies with the meat.

Pour the tomato basil sauce over the meat and veggie mixture and stir until combined. Season again with salt and pepper. Let cook for 5 to 7 minutes to let the veggies and meat soak up the sauce and the flavors to develop.

Divide the cooked spaghetti squash into bowls and top with the Bolognese. Garnish with Parmesan cheese, if using.

INSPIRALIZED TIP

Turn this into a cheesy situation by spreading the spaghetti squash out in a 10-inch skillet, topping with the sauce, and sprinkling with shredded mozzarella cheese. Broil or bake at 425°F until melted.

FEEDING LITTLES TIP

If spaghetti squash is overwhelming to your tot, especially if meat sauce is also new to them, try serving the Bolognese over pasta or with crusty bread. You can always put the spaghetti squash on the side.

I CAN'T EVEN

Save extra time by buying frozen mirepoix (carrots, celery, and onions) and use about 2 cups.

PREP AHEAD

This whole meal can be prepped entirely ahead. Store the Bolognese separately from the spaghetti squash. Use the microwave or the stovetop to separately warm the squash and the sauce, and then combine and top with cheese, if using.

zucchini lamb meatballs with orzo and feta

time to prep: 20 minutes / time to cook: 20 minutes / serves: 4

Meatballs aren't just for serving over pasta. If you've been stuck in a spaghetti and meatball rut, try serving them with orzo instead. OK, fine, orzo *is* a type of pasta, but the texture is more like rice, and the familiar consistency will be easier for young eaters to maneuver with utensils. These meatballs are a departure from the classic Italian version and will expose your family to tasty Moroccan-inspired flavors. With every bite, you'll get a little orzo, a little meatball, and a little feta—what's not to like? Plus, the meatballs are extra moist thanks to shredded zucchini, adding some extra veggies into the meal—which is always a win.

⅓ cup finely grated zucchini

1 pound ground lamb

1 large egg, lightly beaten

3 garlic cloves, minced

2 teaspoons dried parsley

2 teaspoons dried oregano

1 teaspoon ground cumin

¼ teaspoon onion powder

1 teaspoon salt

Pepper, to taste

Cooking spray, for the meatballs

1¼ cups orzo pasta

1 jar (24 ounces) tomato basil sauce

(ingredients continue)

Preheat the oven to 425°F. Line a large baking sheet with parchment paper.

Place the zucchini in a cheesecloth or paper towel and squeeze out any excess moisture. Place it in a large mixing bowl with the lamb, egg, garlic, parsley, oregano, cumin, onion powder, salt, and pepper. Using dampened hands, stir the meatball mixture until combined. Form the mixture into about 16 meatballs and place on the prepared baking sheet. Spritz the meatballs with cooking spray and bake until golden brown, about 15 minutes.

While the meatballs bake, cook the orzo. Combine the orzo and 2½ cups of water in a medium pot and bring to a boil. Once boiling, reduce the heat to a simmer and let cook until all of the liquid is absorbed, about 15 minutes.

Meanwhile, pour the tomato basil sauce into a large, deep skillet and place over a burner. When the meatballs are 5 minutes from being done cooking, raise the heat to medium, and bring the sauce to a simmer. Once the meatballs are done, wipe away any fat buildup, place them in the sauce, and spoon the sauce over the meatballs to cover. Let cook for another 2 to 3 minutes to allow the

(recipe continues)

½ cup crumbled feta cheese

Chopped fresh parsley, for serving

meatballs to absorb some sauce. Remove from the heat and sprinkle with the feta and parsley.

Divide the orzo onto plates and spoon over 4 meatballs per plate.

INSPIRALIZED TIP

Ground turkey works well, too, if you want to change up the protein.

FEEDING LITTLES TIP

Mix the orzo and feta together to give it a little more grip for little hands learning to pick up small pieces.

I CAN'T EVEN

There are some quality frozen meatballs out there. Just sayin'.

PREP AHEAD

Make these meatballs ahead of time and store them in the sauce. When you're ready to eat, heat up the meatballs in sauce in a pot on the stove over medium heat while you cook the orzo. Garnish with the feta and parsley and serve.

mama's trees and sausage pizza

time to prep: 10 minutes / time to cook: about 30 minutes / makes: 2 pizzas, 8 slices each

Let's be real: this is your basic roasted broccoli and sausage pizza. However, with a little rebranding, my pickiest kiddo, Luca, is more likely to eat his greens. As I mentioned in the introduction, in an effort to encourage Luca to eat broccoli, Judy recommended I let him play around with his food and feed his toy dinos some "trees." I haven't stopped calling broccoli "mama's trees" ever since. Now, it doesn't take much to convince anyone to eat pizza, but this is the winning combo in my house, and it comes together quickly, thanks to a premade crust.

5 cups broccoli florets

1 teaspoon extra-virgin olive oil, plus more to drizzle

½ teaspoon garlic powder

Salt and pepper

3 to 4 Italian sausage links

1⅓ cups marinara sauce (or just enough to cover the pizza crusts)

2 frozen (9- to 10-inch) pizza crusts

2 cups shredded mozzarella cheese

Preheat the oven to 400°F, or according to your pizza crust package's instructions.

Place the broccoli on a sheet pan and drizzle generously with olive oil. Toss to coat, and season with the garlic powder and salt and pepper. Bake for 20 minutes or until the broccoli is browned but not burnt. Once cooked, chop the broccoli into small pieces.

Meanwhile, cook the sausage links. First, decase them. Heat the 1 teaspoon of oil in a large skillet over medium heat. Once the oil is shimmering, add the sausage and crumble with a wooden spoon or spatula. Cook until no longer pink, about 7 minutes. Set aside.

Spread the marinara sauce out on the crusts. Sprinkle each pizza with ½ cup mozzarella cheese. Top each pizza equally with broccoli and sausage. Sprinkle the remaining cheese over the pizzas and bake for 10 minutes or until the cheese melts (or according to the package instructions).

Remove from the oven, slice, and serve.

(recipe continues)

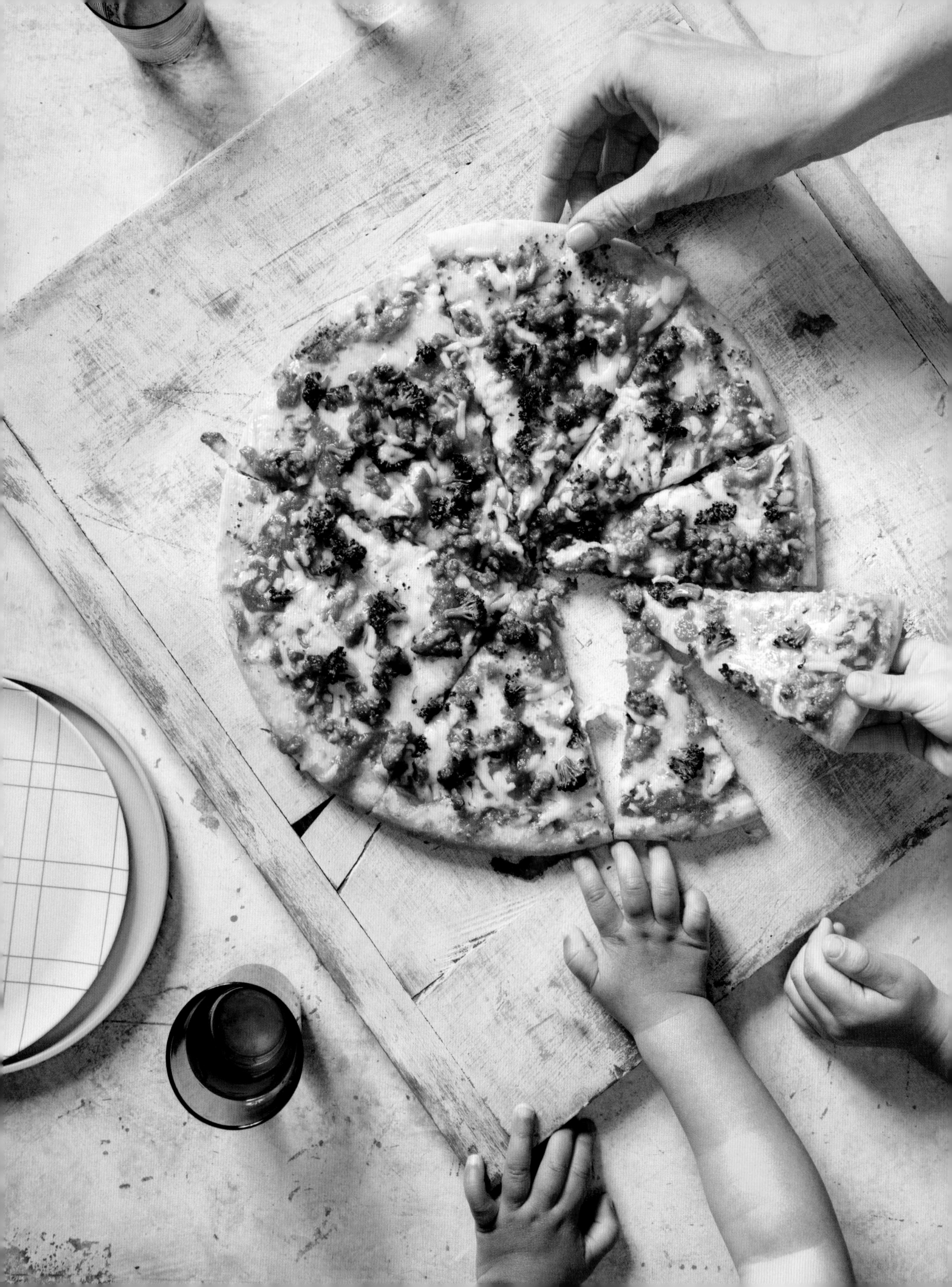

INSPIRALIZED TIP

If your family members are wary of broccoli, make sure you finely dice it after it roasts, so they don't get large chunks in their pizza bites. I first made this pizza with a sprinkling of the chopped broccoli and gradually increased the amount; now, I can pretty much cover it in broccoli, because it has become a familiar food on pizza Fridays. Small exposures like this help reluctant eaters get used to new foods.

FEEDING LITTLES TIP

Let your kid help you slice the pizza with a pizza cutter. They might come up with a more creative shape than you expected, but they're also more likely to eat it if they have interacted with it. Marinara makes for a great dipping sauce here.

I CAN'T EVEN

Skip baking the broccoli and instead boil frozen broccoli in ½ inch of water in a skillet until warmed, about 5 minutes, then season with the garlic powder, salt, and pepper. To save even more time, use precooked sausage links. No need to warm them up; they'll warm as you bake the pizza.

PREP AHEAD

Find some time earlier in the day to cook the sausage and broccoli, so that when it comes to mealtime, all you have to do is build the pizza and bake it.

baked bean rice bowls with barbecue chicken

time to prep: 10 minutes / time to cook: about 40 minutes / serves: 4

This recipe was invented on the fly on a "I don't have anything to make for dinner" kind of night. I opened my pantry, saw a can of baked beans in the way back, and remembered that I had some chicken thighs in the freezer. Since I always have rice on hand, I decided to make a barbecue chicken rice bowl with avocado, because I had a lonely, browning avocado on the countertop that needed to be used up. Well, it turned into one of my family's favorite meals and is now my secret weapon when I need something fast and crowd pleasing. Our recipe testers agreed—this was unexpectedly one of their top-rated (unexpectedly easy) combos. We hope you love it, too.

2 pounds boneless, skinless chicken thighs

1 cup barbecue sauce

Salt and pepper

1 cup dry brown short-grain rice

2 cans (16 ounces each) vegetarian baked beans

2 avocados, peeled, pitted, and sliced, for serving

Preheat the oven to 425°F.

Place the chicken thighs in a large bowl with the barbecue sauce and toss to coat. Let them marinate in the sauce while the oven preheats. Once the oven is preheated, transfer the chicken thighs, using tongs, to a baking sheet and season with salt and pepper. Bake for 35 minutes or until they are no longer pink on the inside. Turn the oven to broil and let the chicken broil for 3 to 5 minutes, to slightly brown the tops and edges of the chicken.

While the chicken bakes, place 2¼ cups of water and the rice in a medium pot over high heat and bring to a boil. Reduce the heat to a simmer, cover, and simmer for 30 minutes or until the rice is fluffy, adding water as needed.

While the chicken and rice cook, pour the beans in a medium pot, set over medium-high heat, and bring to a slight boil. Once boiling, reduce the heat to medium-low, cover, and let simmer for 10 minutes. Turn off the heat and keep warm.

Divide the cooked rice into bowls and top evenly with the chicken, baked beans, and avocados. Serve.

INSPIRALIZED TIP

If you want to add a vegetable to this meal, sautéed spinach, steamed broccoli, or sautéed string beans would work nicely.

FEEDING LITTLES TIP

Canned beans are an inexpensive nutritional powerhouse that offer protein, folate, and fiber. They also are good practice for babies working on their pincer grasp or toddlers trying to master utensils.

I CAN'T EVEN

Save time with microwavable rice.

PREP AHEAD

The rice and chicken can be made ahead of time, so that all you have to do is heat everything up along with the beans and then top with the avocados. If you do this, you may want to heat up the chicken with a little more barbecue sauce, for extra flavor.

refried bean flatbreads

time to prep: 10 minutes / time to cook: about 15 minutes / makes: 3 flatbreads

When you want a pizza but even defrosting a premade crust sounds like too much work, make a flatbread instead. I prefer to use naan because it's a little fluffy, so it gives this a fresh-out-of-the-oven consistency. It's also less doughy and lighter than a traditional crust, but it gets the job done as a vessel for your desired toppings. And don't forget the refried beans, which are perfectly spreadable as a base, and the canned variety usually comes well-seasoned for plenty of flavor.

3 whole wheat naan

1 can (16 ounces) refried black beans, low-sodium

1 cup shredded Mexican cheese blend

6 tablespoons frozen corn

1 small Roma tomato, diced

¾ cup sliced black olives

Chopped cilantro, for garnish

Preheat the oven to 425°F. Place the naan directly on the oven rack and let it toast for 5 minutes until slightly crispy.

Place the toasted naan on a baking sheet and spread each evenly with about ½ cup of the refried beans. Then top each evenly with a third of the cheese, 2 tablespoons of the corn, a third of the tomato, and ¼ cup olives.

Bake for 5 to 10 minutes or until the cheese melts. Garnish with cilantro, slice into 4 pieces each, and serve.

INSPIRALIZED TIP

Make this dairy-free by omitting the cheese and letting the refried beans do all the talking.

FEEDING LITTLES TIP

Don't panic if your kids don't like cilantro: a good portion of the population has a gene receptor that makes the herb taste soapy. No amount of nudging or gradual exposures will convince them otherwise—that's OK.

lentil gyro wraps with tzatziki and avocado

time to prep: 15 minutes / time to cook: 30 minutes / makes: 4 wraps

This vegetarian gyro uses lentils in a patty form in place of the more traditional meat filling. Lentil cakes are dense, hearty, and protein packed, so they easily satisfy and fill you up. The cumin, thyme, and rosemary will give you a Greek-inspired flavor in every bite.

1 cup dry brown lentils

1 bay leaf

2 ripe avocados

1 beefsteak tomato

8 pieces romaine lettuce

1 tablespoon extra-virgin olive oil

½ cup chopped red onion

2 garlic cloves, minced

¾ cup rolled oats

2 large eggs

1 teaspoon dried oregano

½ teaspoon ground cumin

¼ teaspoon dried thyme

¼ teaspoon dried rosemary

Salt and pepper

Grapeseed oil, for frying

4 large whole wheat wraps (burrito size)

1 cup tzatziki sauce

Place the lentils, 3 cups of water, and the bay leaf in a medium pot and bring to a boil. Once boiling, reduce the heat to medium-low and let cook until no water remains and the lentils are tender, 15 to 20 minutes. Discard the bay leaf.

While the lentils cook, prep the avocados, tomato, and lettuce. Peel, pit, and slice the avocados. Slice the tomato into ¼-inch-thick rounds. Trim and chop the romaine into 2-inch pieces. Set all the prepped ingredients aside.

Heat the olive oil in a medium skillet over medium heat. Once the oil is shimmering, add the onion and garlic and cook until softened, about 5 minutes.

Once the lentils, onion, and garlic are all cooked, transfer to a food processor along with the rolled oats, eggs, oregano, cumin, thyme, and rosemary, and season with salt and pepper. Pulse until the mixture can be easily molded into patties, stopping to scrape down the sides. With damp hands, shape the mixture into 12 small 2½-inch patties.

Heat about a tablespoon of the grapeseed oil in a large skillet over medium-high heat. Once the oil is shimmering, add the lentil cakes and fit as many as you can in the pan without them touching. Cook for 3 to 5 minutes, flip, and cook for another 3 to 5 minutes or until they are firm and browned. Repeat with more oil and lentil mixture until all of the cakes are cooked.

(recipe continues)

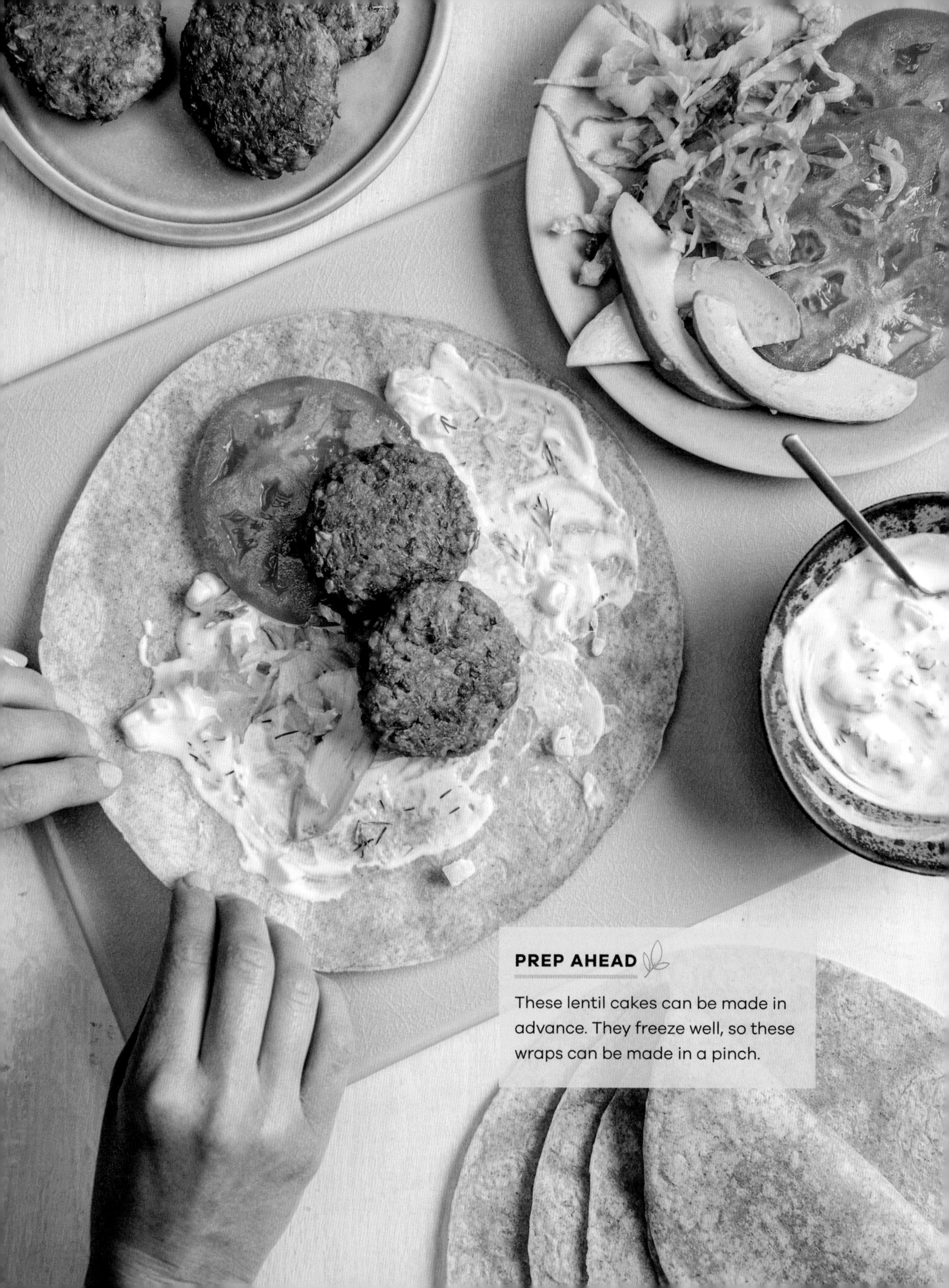

PREP AHEAD

These lentil cakes can be made in advance. They freeze well, so these wraps can be made in a pinch.

Build your gyros. Place down a wrap. Spread with some tzatziki, if you wish, or save it for drizzling. About 2 inches from the edge of the wrap (closest to your body), place avocado slices and top with 3 lentil patties, tomato, and lettuce, and then drizzle with tzatziki sauce. Fold the sides of the wrap in and roll tightly like a burrito. Slice and secure with toothpicks or simply place seam side down to keep closed. Repeat with the remaining wraps and fillings. Serve.

INSPIRALIZED TIP

The star of this recipe is the lentil cake. Our family loves lentil cakes and uses them in many different ways. For a milder taste, just use oregano and omit the other spices.

FEEDING LITTLES TIP

Plain lentils are small and hard to pick up, but lentil cakes solve that problem, and this recipe will help your baby learn to love the flavor of lentils without the frustration. If there are scattered lentils, just roll them into a small ball or other shape and offer those to small hands.

I CAN'T EVEN

Precooked packaged or canned lentils are your friend—use them! Substitute 18 ounces of steamed brown lentils instead of cooking them yourself.

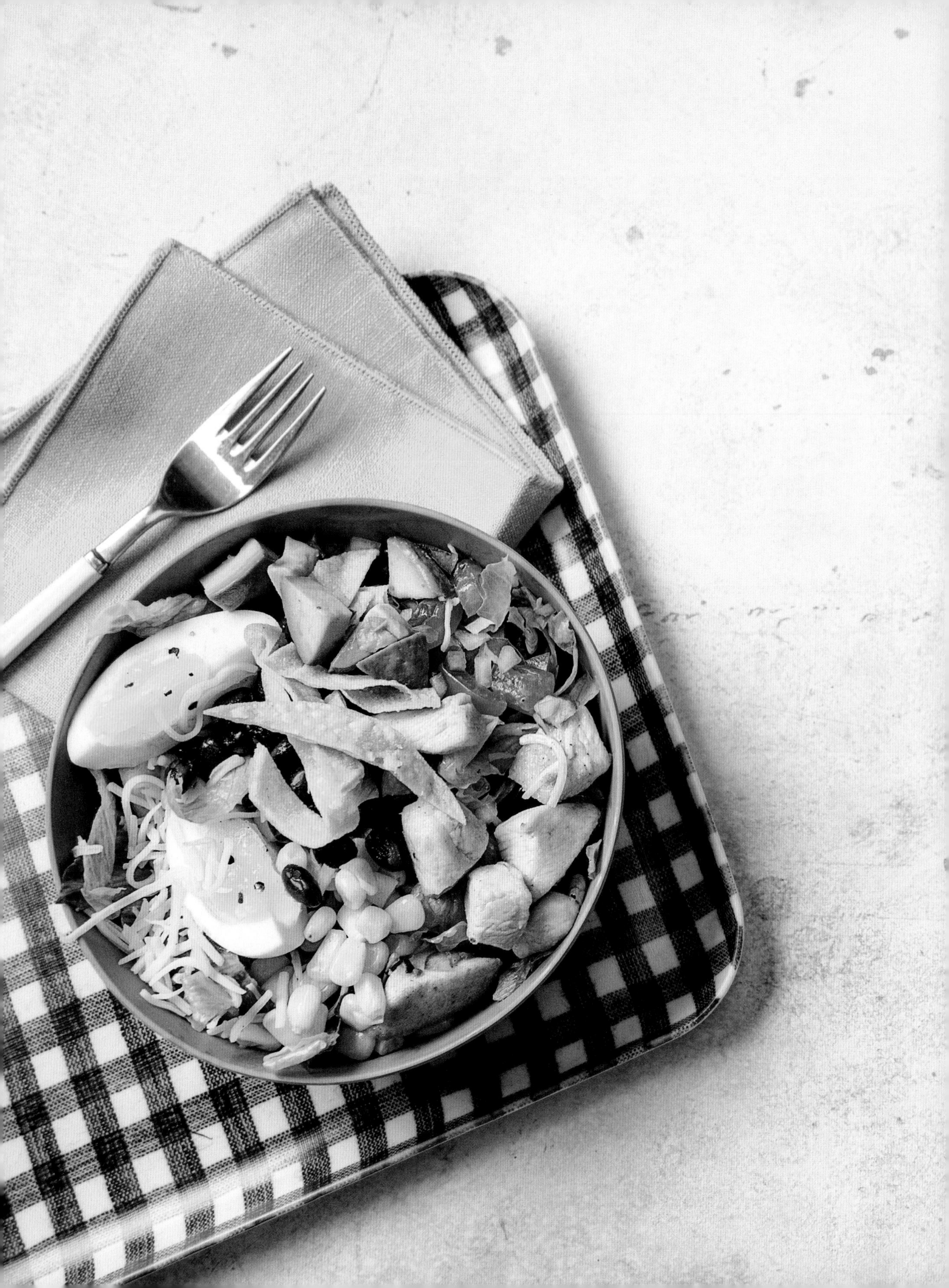

serious green salads

You know when you're in the mood for a refreshing pile o' greens, but making a salad for yourself means making a separate meal for your kids? Well, what if you could make a salad that had enough hearty toppings that your child would dive right in? Many kids love salads *now*, but it may have taken time to get there. Have your cake—err, salad—and eat it, too, with these fun, filling dishes.

The recipes here not only will satiate a hungry adult but also are built with a kid's palate in mind. When children start eating solids at around six months, they can start with the toppings (appropriately served). As they progress to around fourteen to sixteen months and beyond, you can also offer crunchy raw lettuce, which is easier for them to feel in their mouths than softer raw greens. If your child is doing well with the lettuce, try other types of leafy greens. Serve dressing as a dip or drizzled on top. Pretty soon, your kiddo might be eating full-blown salads with you. Just remember that this is a process that looks different in every family, and if they're not into salads now, it doesn't mean they won't be eventually.

Here are some tips for building a hearty salad that can be served as a stand-alone meal or on a kid's plate:

- Try a creamy dressing served as a dip (like with the Summer Steak and Peach Salad with Greek Yogurt Balsamic, page 236).
- Include a protein—salmon, steak, chicken, beans, eggs, tofu, and other hearty proteins are easy to serve (try the Grilled Salmon Niçoise Salad with Fingerlings, page 224).

- If your child is fourteen months or older, romaine works great as a starter lettuce (like a Caesar or Cobb salad; see page 221).
- Top with both raw and cooked vegetables, depending on the child's age. In infancy, any hard veggie should be cooked. Once your child is fourteen to sixteen months old, try thinly sliced raw veggies like shaved carrot or chopped raw broccoli.
- Add some pasta to your salad. It's a filling way to make a salad kid-approved (try our Tuna, Broccoli, and Kale Caesar Pasta Salad, page 230).
- Beans and other legumes are a quick and easy way to add variety on a kid's plate (try the Greek-ish Salad with Lemony Shrimp and Pita, page 227).

These are just a few pointers to get you started, but you get the idea: all types of foods and meals are appropriate for kids, not just the obvious classics like casseroles and burgers. You'll be happy to bring salads back into the rotation if you had given up on them or reserved them for adult-time only.

chicken cobb salad with cilantro-lime dressing

time to prep: 10 minutes / time to cook: 15 minutes / serves: 4 adults (2 adults and 2 to 4 children)

If a burrito bowl and a Cobb salad met at a bar, this would be the meal they'd make together. Place a sticky note right over the cilantro-lime dressing, because it will become your go-to dressing for Mexican-inspired meals. It's delicious over rice and salads, and as a marinade for meat or tofu. Above all else, it's the best dressing for this salad, tossed with crunchy romaine and topped with approachable ingredients for a baby or toddler's plate: hard-boiled eggs, chicken, avocados, cheese, black beans, and corn. Even if they haven't seemed interested in salad yet, keep serving it to them in small amounts. They have to see it again and again to try it. I love a packed salad bowl that I can eat alongside my little ones.

¼ cup plus 1 tablespoon extra-virgin olive oil

2 boneless, skinless chicken breasts, chopped into ½-inch cubes

1 teaspoon taco seasoning

Salt and pepper

2 tablespoons freshly squeezed lime juice

¼ cup cilantro leaves, roughly chopped

8 cups chopped romaine lettuce

4 hard-boiled eggs, sliced

½ cup pico de gallo, or mild salsa

(ingredients continue)

In a medium bowl, place 1 tablespoon of the olive oil, the chicken, and the taco seasoning, and season with salt and pepper. Toss to thoroughly coat the chicken.

Heat a large skillet over medium-high heat. Once heated, add the seasoned chicken along with any juices and cook for 10 minutes or until the chicken is no longer pink on the inside.

While the chicken cooks, whisk together in a large mixing bowl the remaining ¼ cup of olive oil, the lime juice, and cilantro, and season with salt and pepper. Add the romaine lettuce and toss well to combine. Divide the lettuce onto plates. Top each plate evenly with the chicken, eggs, pico de gallo, avocados, cheese, black beans, and corn. Top with tortilla strips. Serve.

INSPIRALIZED TIP

Switch up the protein by using shrimp, or omit the animal protein completely and serve it vegetarian.

(recipe continues)

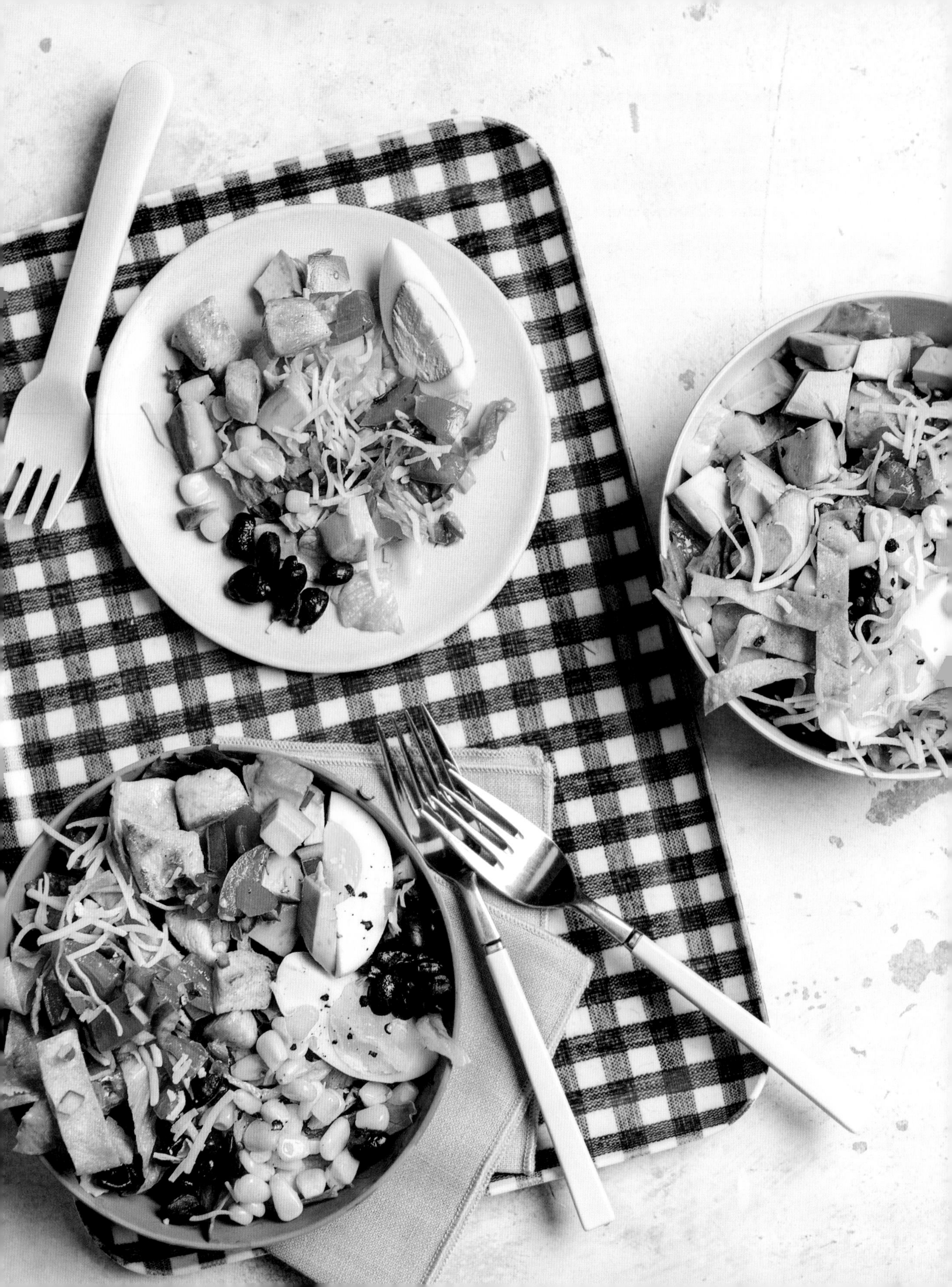

2 ripe avocados, peeled, pitted, and cubed

½ cup shredded Monterey Jack cheese (any Mexican cheese blend works)

1 cup canned black beans, drained and rinsed

1 cup corn (frozen works, but make sure it's fully defrosted before using)

Crunchy tortilla strips, for serving (crushed for kids under 4)

FEEDING LITTLES TIP

To add to the fun, serve each topping in a muffin pan or ice cube tray compartment and allow your kid to pick and choose. If using corn on the cob, you can serve the entire cob to your baby or toddler.

I CAN'T EVEN

Buy premade hard-boiled eggs to save time on the boiling. Use precooked chicken or chop up a rotisserie chicken and heat it in a skillet with the taco seasoning and some oil.

PREP AHEAD

The chicken and dressing can be prepared ahead of time so this salad can be more quickly assembled.

grilled salmon niçoise salad with fingerlings

time to prep: 10 minutes / time to cook: 20 to 30 minutes / serves: 4

The ultimate fancy salad: the niçoise. It originated in the city of Nice and is traditionally made with tomatoes, hard-boiled eggs, Niçoise olives, and tuna, simply dressed with olive oil. Somewhere along the line, someone got ahold of the recipe, and now it might as well be a full plated entrée. It's the salad you make when you want a bright, satisfying salad. And it includes so many familiar foods that it has worked wonders for my kids, who have always been shy about eating lettuce. When I first made this recipe, my littlest was seven months old and didn't have a pincer grasp, and so I found fingerling potatoes at the farmers market and never looked back. Now it's fingerlings or bust.

1 pound fingerling potatoes, halved

Olive oil, to drizzle

¼ teaspoon garlic powder

Salt and pepper, to taste

8 ounces green beans

4 (3-ounce) boneless, skinless salmon fillets

1 pound bibb lettuce

4 hard-boiled eggs, sliced into thin rounds

⅔ cup halved cherry tomatoes

½ cup pitted Kalamata olives

(ingredients continue)

Preheat the grill to about 450°F.

Place the fingerling potatoes in a large bowl. Toss the potatoes with olive oil, the garlic powder, salt, and pepper. Place in a grill basket. Set aside. In the same large bowl, toss the green beans with more olive oil, salt, and pepper. Place in another grill basket. Note: if you don't have enough grill baskets, you can always make foil pouches to hold the vegetables.

Place the vegetables on the grill, leaving room for the salmon. Let the vegetables cook for 20 minutes, uncovering the grill every 5 minutes to toss, until the vegetables are fork-tender, removing them as they're ready.

Rub the salmon with olive oil and season with salt and pepper. If you have a fish grill basket or something similar, place the salmon on the basket. If not, place the salmon directly on the grill racks, but first make sure they are clean and oiled to ensure the salmon doesn't stick. Cook the salmon for 6 to 8 minutes, flip, and cook for another

(recipe continues)

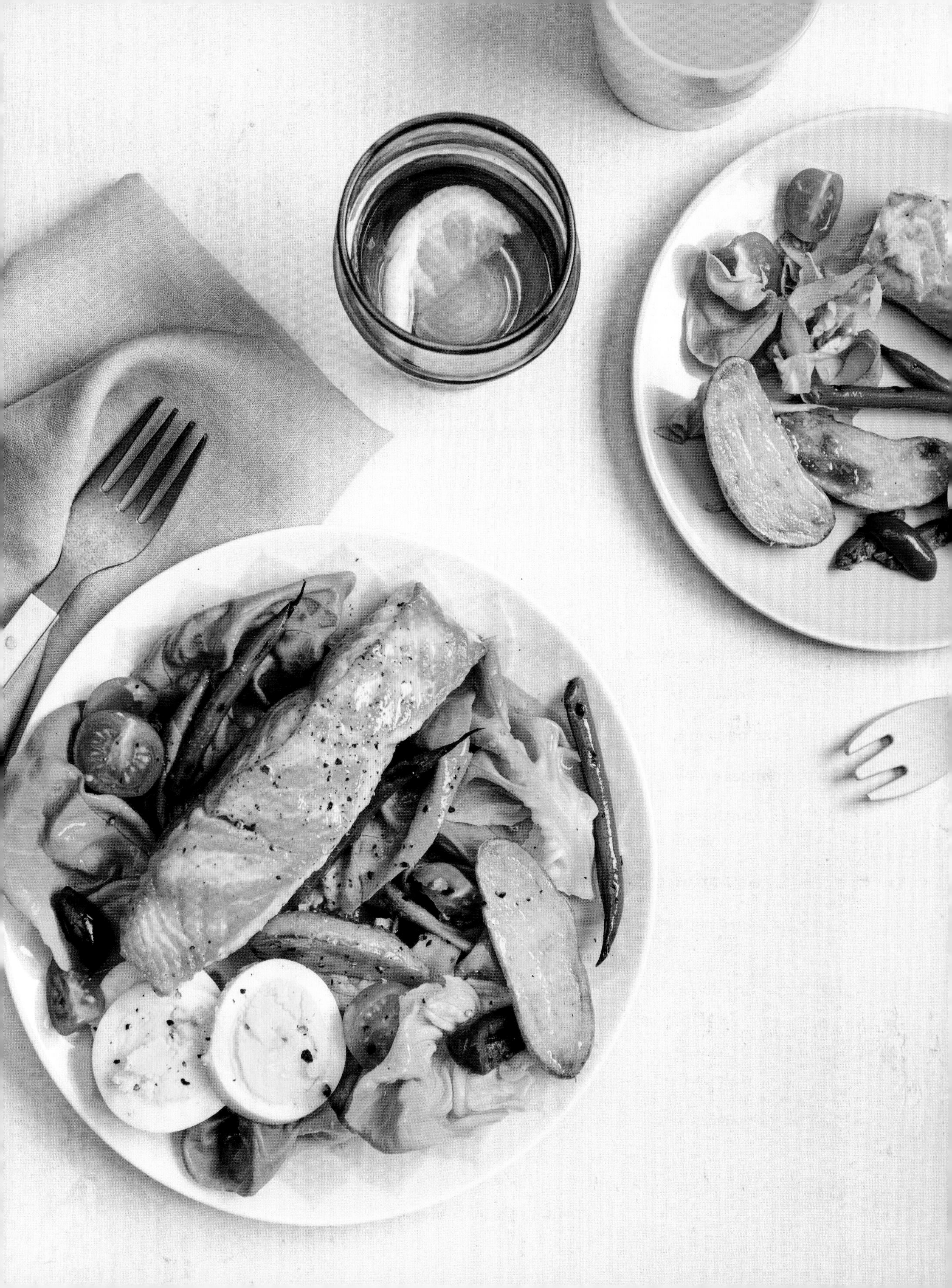

For the vinaigrette

¼ cup extra-virgin olive oil

2 tablespoons white wine vinegar (or red wine vinegar)

2 teaspoons freshly squeezed lemon juice

2 teaspoons coarse ground mustard

2 teaspoons fresh thyme leaves

1 tablespoon minced shallot

Salt and pepper, to taste

4 minutes, or until the fish registers 130°F or is no longer raw on the inside.

While the vegetables and salmon cook, whisk all the ingredients for the vinaigrette together and set aside.

Assemble your salads: set down four plates or bowls. Divide the lettuce between the plates. Then, top each plate with the potatoes, green beans, salmon, eggs, cherry tomatoes, and olives. Drizzle each plate with the vinaigrette and serve.

INSPIRALIZED TIP

If you don't have access to a grill, cook the vegetables and salmon on two separate sheet pans at 425°F. For the salmon, cook for 10 to 15 minutes or until done to your preference. For the vegetables, spritz with cooking spray and cook for about 30 minutes or until fork-tender.

FEEDING LITTLES TIP

Interestingly, Judy uses tangy vinaigrettes like the one in this recipe to help "wake up" her clients' mouths when they're struggling to feel food in their mouths appropriately. If your child doesn't chew food well or pockets food, try using this dressing as a dip for the other ingredients. It might help your child chew a little more skillfully.

I CAN'T EVEN

Buy premade hard-boiled eggs and use canned tuna or canned salmon instead of fresh fish. To skip the vinaigrette, substitute a bottled red wine vinaigrette.

PREP AHEAD

You can cook the green beans and potatoes and hard-boil the eggs ahead of time.

greek-ish salad with lemony shrimp and pita

time to prep: 15 minutes / time to cook: 5 to 7 minutes / serves: 4

I'd say this is a "Greek-ish" salad, because as anyone who has visited the Santorini coast knows . . . this isn't an authentic Greek salad. However, it's definitely Greek-like, made with Kalamata olives, cucumber, bell pepper, tomatoes, onion, and feta, then bulked up with romaine lettuce, chickpeas, shrimp, and pita bread. The dippable dressing and seasonings bring all the flavors together, and it's foolproof to plate for a baby or toddler, as there are many components to work with. If you're making this in the summertime, grill the pita and shrimp—trust me.

For the vinaigrette

¼ cup extra-virgin olive oil

3 tablespoons red wine vinegar

1 tablespoon freshly squeezed lemon juice

1 garlic clove, minced

1 teaspoon Dijon mustard

½ teaspoon dried oregano

Salt and pepper

For the salad

2 pieces pita bread

8 cups chopped romaine lettuce

½ cup pitted and quartered Kalamata olives

(ingredients continue)

In a small bowl, whisk together the olive oil, vinegar, lemon juice, garlic, Dijon mustard, and oregano, and season with salt and pepper. Set aside.

Place the pita bread in the oven or toaster, just until warmed through and slightly toasted. Cut into 8 triangular pieces.

Divide the lettuce onto 4 plates. Top with 4 pita triangles per salad. Top with the olives, cucumber, bell pepper, onion, chickpeas, and tomatoes, and set aside.

Place the shrimp in a bowl, drizzle with olive oil, and season with the garlic powder and salt and pepper. Set aside.

Heat a grill pan or skillet over medium heat. Once the pan is hot, add the shrimp and cook for 2 minutes, flip, pour the lemon juice on top, and cook for another 2 to 3 minutes or until the shrimp are opaque.

Pour the prepared dressing evenly over the salads and top evenly with shrimp. Sprinkle the feta over all. Serve.

(recipe continues)

INSPIRALIZED TIP

This salad is filling enough without the shrimp, so keep that in mind if you don't have any on hand—no biggie.

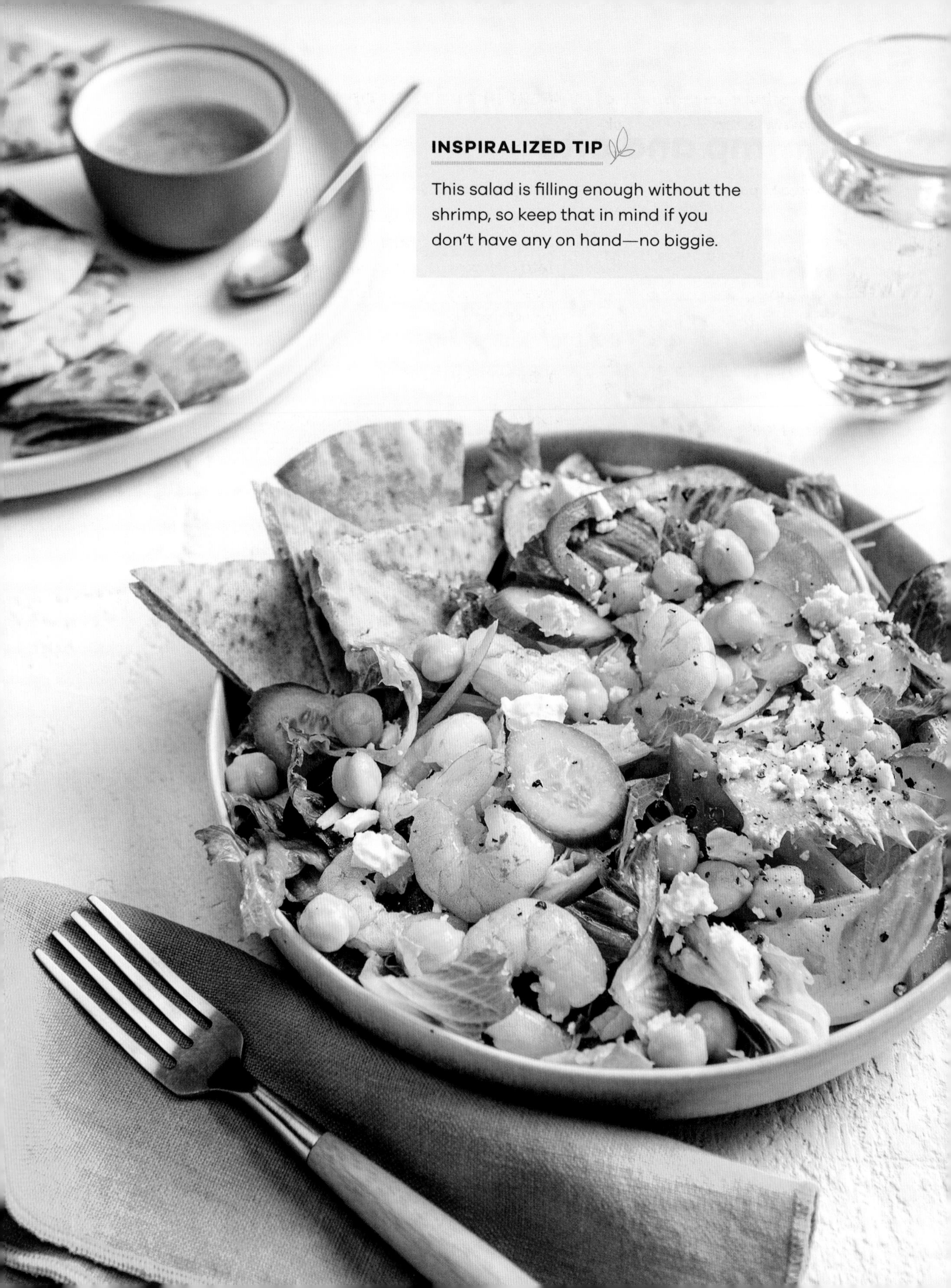

½ seedless cucumber, sliced crosswise into ⅛-inch-thick rounds

1 red bell pepper, seeded and thinly sliced

½ small red onion, sliced

1 can (15½ ounces) chickpeas, drained and rinsed

2 Roma tomatoes, cut into wedges

1 pound medium shrimp, shelled and deveined

Extra-virgin olive oil, to drizzle

½ teaspoon garlic powder

Salt and pepper

½ lemon, juiced

½ cup crumbled feta

FEEDING LITTLES TIP

To serve this to a baby, cut the cucumber into strips (remove the skin and seeds) and cut the tomato into wedges. Serve with a strip of toasted pita bread and some cooked shrimp. To help babies pick up chickpeas and quartered olives, serve them on a loaded fork. Serve feta as strips. Drizzle olive oil or the prepared dressing over each component for some extra flavor and brain-boosting fat.

I CAN'T EVEN

Defrost precooked frozen shrimp and use that instead. There are plenty of delicious bottled Greek dressings, so check those out if you're in a pinch.

PREP AHEAD

Prep the dressing and raw veggies and put them in a zip-tight bag so when you're ready to throw everything together, all you need to do is cook the shrimp and assemble.

tuna, broccoli, and kale caesar pasta salad

time to prep: 15 minutes / time to cook: 20 minutes / serves: 4

I know what you're thinking: so is this a pasta, salad, or pasta salad? It's kind of all three. It's creamy and there's that rotini, so it's a pasta salad, but it's definitely a *salad* salad, because, well, kale. However you want to classify it, this dish is brimming with flavor and nutrients, with plenty of consistencies and ingredients to pull out for a baby or toddler. It's also the kind of salad you might make when it's cold outside or you just want something heartier. All of the parts work in delightful harmony but can be easily deconstructed, too, making it an ideal meal for you and your little ones.

1 box (8 ounces) rotini pasta

1 tablespoon extra-virgin olive oil

3 cups broccoli florets

Salt and pepper

1 bunch lacinato kale, finely sliced

3 cans (5 ounces each) wild albacore tuna in water, drained and broken up

¼ cup Caesar dressing

½ cup sliced Parmesan cheese, for serving

Fill a large pot halfway with water and bring to a boil. Once boiling, add the pasta and cook until al dente, according to the package instructions. Drain the pasta into a colander.

While the pasta cooks, cook the broccoli. Heat the oil in a large skillet over medium-high heat. Once the oil is shimmering, add the broccoli and season with salt and pepper. Cook for 10 minutes or until the broccoli is tender and browned. Set aside.

Toss together the kale, tuna, cooked pasta, and Caesar dressing in a large mixing bowl. Divide the mixture onto four plates and top with the broccoli and sliced Parmesan.

INSPIRALIZED TIP

Try chicken or chickpeas as a substitute for the canned tuna.

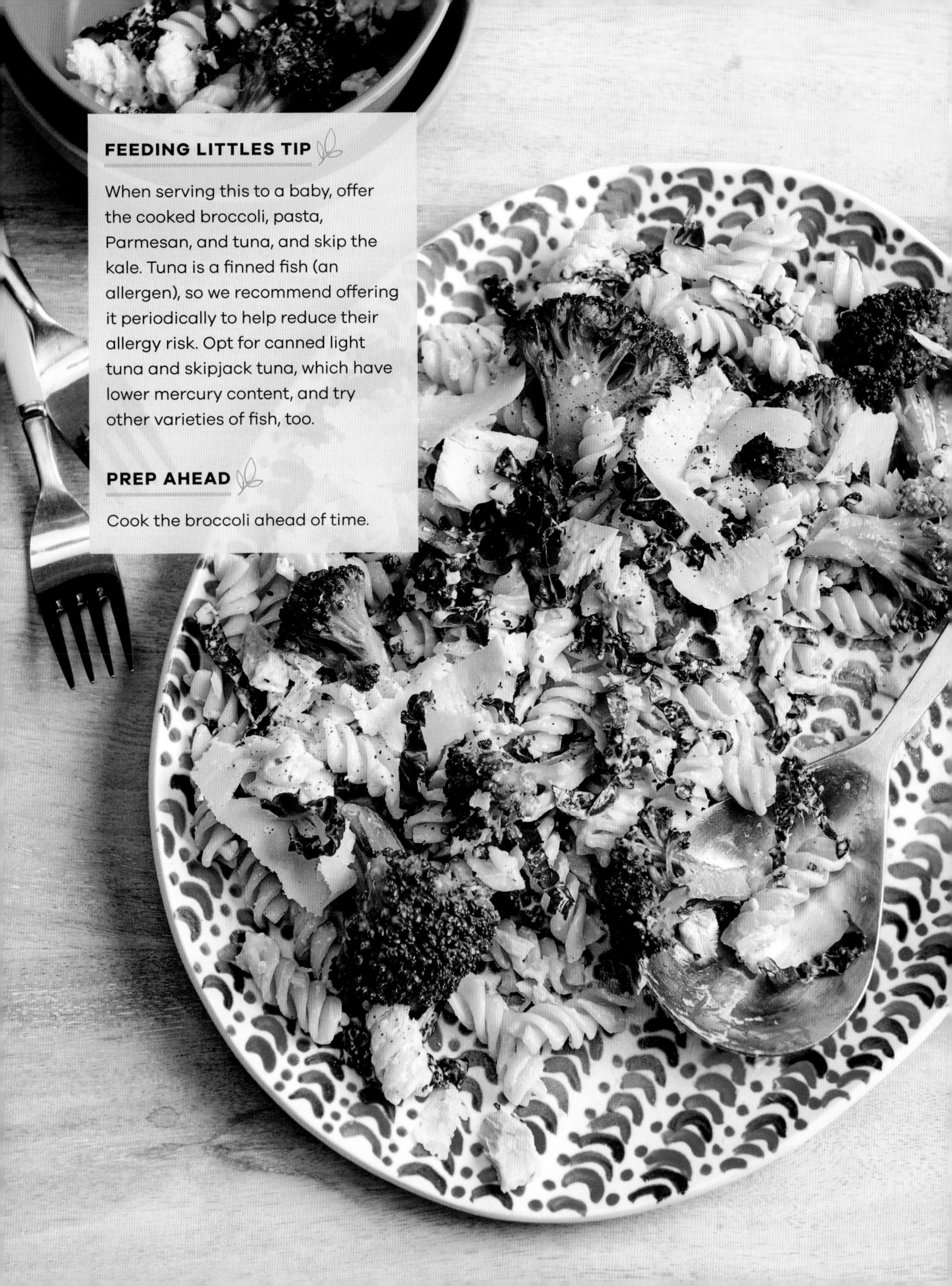

FEEDING LITTLES TIP

When serving this to a baby, offer the cooked broccoli, pasta, Parmesan, and tuna, and skip the kale. Tuna is a finned fish (an allergen), so we recommend offering it periodically to help reduce their allergy risk. Opt for canned light tuna and skipjack tuna, which have lower mercury content, and try other varieties of fish, too.

PREP AHEAD

Cook the broccoli ahead of time.

sweet potato, quinoa, and lentil arugula salad

time to prep: 20 minutes / time to cook: 30 minutes / serves: 4

At first glance, you may be wondering, "How will my child ever eat something like this?" Well, don't turn the page just yet—let me explain. What I love most about this salad is that it's chunky and creamy, consistencies that babies and toddlers tend to love. You can serve the sweet potatoes, quinoa, lentils, and avocados mixed together with the tahini dressing as a bowl meal or completely deconstructed, with the tahini dressing as a dip. There are many ways this salad can be assembled for your little ones, and I know that you will crave it, too, especially the way the herbed tahini and almond crunch come together in every hearty bite.

3 cups cubed sweet potatoes

Cooking spray, for the sweet potatoes

Salt and pepper

¼ cup dry quinoa (or 1 cup cooked)

½ cup dry black lentils (or 1¼ cups cooked)

2 avocados

1 box (5 ounces) baby arugula

¼ cup blanched and slivered almonds

For the tahini dressing

½ cup tahini

¼ cup cilantro

¼ cup fresh parsley

Preheat the oven to 425°F. Line a baking sheet with parchment paper and lay out the sweet potatoes. Spray the sweet potatoes with cooking spray to coat, and season with salt and pepper. Bake the sweet potatoes for 25 minutes or until fork-tender.

Meanwhile, cook the quinoa (if using dry). Place the quinoa and ½ cup of water in a medium pot and bring to a boil. Reduce the heat to low and let simmer for 15 to 20 minutes or until the quinoa is fluffy.

At the same time, cook the lentils (if using dry). Place the lentils and 2 cups of water in a medium pot and bring to a boil. Once boiling, reduce the heat to low and let simmer for 15 to 20 minutes or until the lentils are soft.

While the quinoa and lentils cook, peel, pit, and cube the avocados. Set aside. Also, prepare the dressing. In a food processor, combine the tahini, cilantro, parsley, garlic powder, lemon juice, honey, ¼ cup of water, and salt and pepper. Pulse until the dressing is green with only small flecks of the green herbs.

⅛ teaspoon garlic powder

3 tablespoons freshly squeezed lemon juice

1 teaspoon honey (remove if serving to babies under 1 year)

Salt and pepper, to taste

Transfer the cooked quinoa and lentils to a large mixing bowl along with the cooked sweet potatoes and avocados. Stir to combine, fold in the arugula and ⅓ cup of the dressing, and toss well to combine. If you'd like more dressing, add more. Reserve leftover dressing for future meals.

Divide the salad onto plates and top with the almonds. Serve.

INSPIRALIZED TIP

If you want to switch it up, cubed butternut squash is a good substitute for the sweet potatoes..

FEEDING LITTLES TIP

To serve this to a baby, mix the sweet potatoes, quinoa, lentils, and avocados with the dressing so it's easier to grip. Serve it on a loaded spoon or fork, or see if your baby can pick it up—or roll it into a shape and hand to your baby.

I CAN'T EVEN

Use frozen sweet potatoes and steam them instead of roasting. Use microwavable quinoa and precooked lentils in a package or can. To simplify the dressing, use dried herbs instead of fresh; a good rule of thumb is 1 tablespoon of fresh herbs to 1 teaspoon of dried herbs.

PREP AHEAD

Prep the sweet potatoes, quinoa, lentils, and dressing ahead of time so that all you need to do is assemble them when it's time to eat. If you're refrigerating the dressing, add another tablespoon or so of water to thin it out, as it thickens after storing.

brussels sprouts and bacon harvest kale salad

time to prep: 20 minutes / time to cook: about 30 minutes / serves: 4

The secret to making this salad stand out is to let the Brussels sprouts roast until crispy, so there's a bit of smoky crunch to complement the bacon. Even if yours don't crisp up, this salad is still a must-make during the fall and winter months, when you want a warm, comforting, and nourishing bowl of food that's still light. I use this apple cider vinegar dressing over and over during the colder months of the year, because it's like a sweet little hug. Combined with salty bacon, pecans, cranberries, goat cheese, and those savory, tender Brussels sprouts, this salad feels like a special meal. If your little ones don't love Brussels sprouts just yet, this may be the meal that convinces them.

1 pound Brussels sprouts, trimmed and sliced into ¼-inch pieces

2 tablespoons extra-virgin olive oil, plus more to drizzle

Salt and pepper

2 tablespoons apple cider vinegar

1 teaspoon honey (remove if serving to babies under 1 year)

8 cups finely shredded Siberian or lacinato kale (stems removed first)

6 strips bacon

½ cup chopped pecans

⅓ cup dried cranberries

⅓ cup crumbled goat cheese

Preheat the oven to 425°F. Line a baking sheet with parchment paper. Spread out the Brussels sprouts on the baking sheet, drizzle with olive oil, toss to coat, and then season with salt and pepper. Roast for 25 minutes, shaking the pan halfway through, until fork-tender and some leaves are crispy.

Meanwhile, prepare the dressing and kale. In a large mixing bowl, whisk together the 2 tablespoons of oil, the vinegar, and the honey, and season with salt and pepper. Add the kale and toss well, massaging with your fingers for 1 to 2 minutes, which softens it to make it more palatable for all eaters. Once the kale is coated with the dressing, set aside.

Cook the bacon. Place the bacon in a large skillet and heat to medium. Cook the bacon until crispy, flipping the strips as the bacon curls. Transfer to a paper towel–lined plate and break the cooked bacon into pieces.

Once the Brussels sprouts are done roasting, add them to the bowl with the kale, along with the bacon, pecans, cranberries, and goat cheese. Toss well to combine. Divide the salad into bowls and sprinkle with any remaining fixings in the mixing bowl. Serve.

INSPIRALIZED TIP

Serve this salad with buttered crusty bread, especially if there are too many unfamiliar foods in the dish for your little one.

FEEDING LITTLES TIP

This recipe contains a lot of sophisticated ingredients and flavors. Remember, sometimes it's all about exposure. This salad can be a satisfying meal for adults, but if you're serving it to kids you might want to offer it on the side of a preferred main dish. Don't get discouraged—this takes time. Note: this might not be a great recipe for babies just yet—you can offer the Brussels sprouts and finely chopped bacon mixed with goat cheese from the salad alongside leftovers or another component of your meal.

I CAN'T EVEN

Buy pre-shredded Brussels sprouts instead of slicing them yourself—they'll cook more quickly, because they're shredded instead of sliced, but the flavor will still be right.

PREP AHEAD

Cook the Brussels sprouts and prepare the dressing ahead of time.

summer steak and peach salad with greek yogurt balsamic

time to prep: 15 minutes / time to cook: about 10 minutes / serves: 4

Does anything scream summer more than peaches and corn? Next time you drive past a farmstand (or hit the grocery store), grab yourself salad greens, corn, and peaches, and swing by the butcher for steak—you'll feel like you're winning an episode of *Chopped*. The star here is the Greek yogurt balsamic, which has just enough tang and sweetness to complement the steak. I joke that my children are fruitarians because whenever a meal includes fruit, I know they'll be more adventurous with the other ingredients. As Judy and Megan have taught me, eating begets eating.

1 pound New York strip steak

Salt and pepper

Avocado oil, to drizzle

2 cups sliced ripe peaches (can use frozen if you're making this out of season)

2 cups fresh corn kernels (can use frozen if you're making this out of season)

½ cup plain Greek yogurt

¼ cup balsamic vinegar

4 teaspoons Dijon mustard

4 teaspoons honey

10 ounces mixed greens

Season the steak generously with salt and pepper on both sides. Drizzle both sides of the steak with avocado oil.

Heat a cast-iron pan over high heat. Once the pan is hot, add the steak and sear for 3 minutes, flip, and sear for another 2 to 3 minutes more. Transfer the steak to a cutting board and let it rest.

While the steak rests, add the peaches and corn to the skillet over medium heat and let them cook for 5 minutes, stirring to cook evenly. Turn off the heat.

Prepare the dressing. In a medium bowl, whisk together the Greek yogurt, balsamic vinegar, Dijon mustard, and honey, and season with salt and pepper. Set aside.

Slice the steak against the grain crosswise into ¼-inch-thick pieces.

Divide the mixed greens into bowls or onto plates. Top evenly with the steak, peaches, and corn, and drizzle with the dressing.

INSPIRALIZED TIP

If you're in the midst of summer or have access to fresh corn, grill or boil ears of corn and shave the cooked kernels over the salad.

FEEDING LITTLES TIP

We recommend serving steaks cooked to 145°F for young children. If you like your steak a little less done, cut off slices and microwave them for 10 seconds at a time until desired doneness. If the steak is too tough to pass the "squish test," it's not safe for your baby or young toddler. Note: since the dressing contains honey, omit for babies.

I CAN'T EVEN

Use a bottled creamy balsamic dressing instead of making your own.

PREP AHEAD

Cook the steak, peaches, corn, and make the dressing all ahead of time. Then, assemble—it'll be a colder salad, but just as tasty.

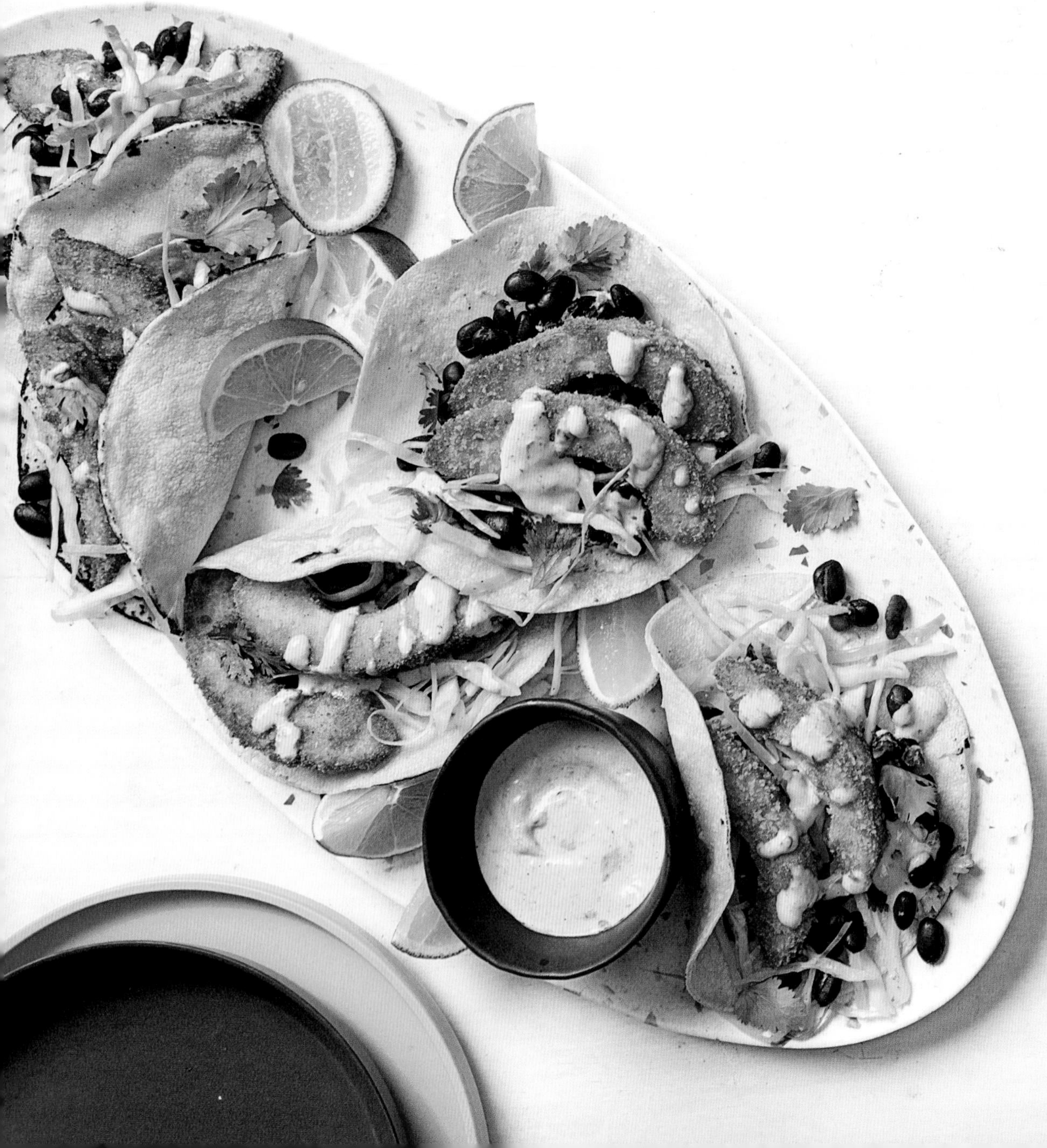

set it and forget it

Whether you have children at home or not, the following devices are lifesavers: the air fryer, slow cooker, and pressure cooker. As the chapter title suggests, you'll find recipes here that you can "set" (in a device) and "forget" (until it's ready to be served). We love these meals because all the work happens *in the machine*. You can still feel like a champ when dinner's on the table with the secret knowledge that all you had to do was put the ingredients in the pot.

If you don't know these robot friends, here are the basics:

The air fryer: this device fries food without the messy stovetop. You won't believe the crunch on our Crispiest Chicken Nuggets (page 274) or Salmon Fish Sticks with Mustard Sauce (page 266). The air fryer also cooks vegetables—you'll never eat Brussels sprouts any other way—and saves time doing it. If a vegetable typically takes 25 to 30 minutes, the air fryer will get it done in 7 to 15 minutes, depending on what you're cooking.

The slow cooker: this popular device enables you to time your meals so that when you're ready to eat, the food is ready. The slow cooker works wonders for meats, as its low and consistent temperatures retain moisture—ideal for young eaters. Check out the tender and robust flavor of the Tuscan-Style Short Ribs (page 272) for proof.

The pressure cooker: another busy weeknight must-have, the pressure cooker prepares your meats, soups, grains, and vegetables in one pot, in a matter of minutes. It's kind of like a slow cooker, just... faster. Note that because it cooks by building up pressure first, it can sometimes take longer than expected, so keep that in mind when you're timing your meals. Try our Curried Lentils and Carrots with Rice (page 256) for a tasty (and easy) way to introduce lentils and curry flavors to your family.

All that said, fancy gadgets aren't necessary to cook nourishing meals for your family—any recipes you see in this chapter can be cooked in the oven or on the stovetop—but they can save time and reduce mess.

pressure cooker aloo gobi with chickpeas

time to prep: 20 minutes / time to cook: 20 minutes / serves: 4

Aloo gobi is one of the first Indian dishes I remember eating, and it was the gateway meal to my love affair with Indian spices. A hearty vegetarian dish with bold seasonings, this flavorful meal is welcoming to young tastebuds. It isn't traditionally made with chickpeas, but I love the burst of protein that makes the dish a bit heartier. We eat this with toasted naan or white basmati rice (or both), which soaks up the aloo gobi's ingredients in each sumptuous, aromatic bite.

- **½ tablespoon extra-virgin olive oil**
- **1 small onion, finely chopped**
- **1 garlic clove, minced**
- **1 tablespoon peeled and minced ginger**
- **1 can (14 ounces) diced tomatoes**
- **½ teaspoon chili powder**
- **¼ teaspoon turmeric powder**
- **½ teaspoon garam masala**
- **¼ teaspoon ground coriander**
- **½ teaspoon ground cumin**
- **1 bay leaf**
- **1 can (14 ounces) lite coconut milk (or ½ can full-fat coconut milk + half can water)**

Heat the olive oil in a pressure cooker set to the Sauté function. Once the oil is shimmering, add the onion, garlic, and ginger, and cook until the onion is translucent, 3 to 5 minutes. Add the tomatoes, chili powder, turmeric powder, garam masala, coriander, and cumin. Stir well to combine and coat the tomatoes in the spices. Add the bay leaf, coconut milk, and vegetable broth. Stir well. Add in the potatoes and cauliflower, season with salt and pepper, stir, and place the top on the pressure cooker. Cook on High pressure for 10 minutes. Release the pressure manually, remove the bay leaf, and stir in the chickpeas.

Divide the mixture into bowls and garnish with the cilantro. Serve with rice or naan.

3 cups low-sodium vegetable broth

3 medium red potatoes, cubed

1 large cauliflower head, chopped into florets (about 5 cups florets)

Salt and pepper

1 can (15½ ounces) chickpeas, drained and rinsed

2 tablespoons chopped cilantro, for garnish

Cooked rice or naan, for serving

INSPIRALIZED TIP

For extra veggies, stir in some chopped spinach for 1 minute or until wilted at the end of cooking.

FEEDING LITTLES TIP

Herbs and spices are full of nutrition and disease-fighting compounds. Yes, babies can have spices and even spicy foods (you just want to go easy on the salt). Some babies and toddlers love spicy foods while others cannot handle them, so start slowly and build up as your child tolerates it.

I CAN'T EVEN

Buy cauliflower florets in a bag instead of having to chop them up.

PREP AHEAD

This entire dish can be prepared ahead of time.

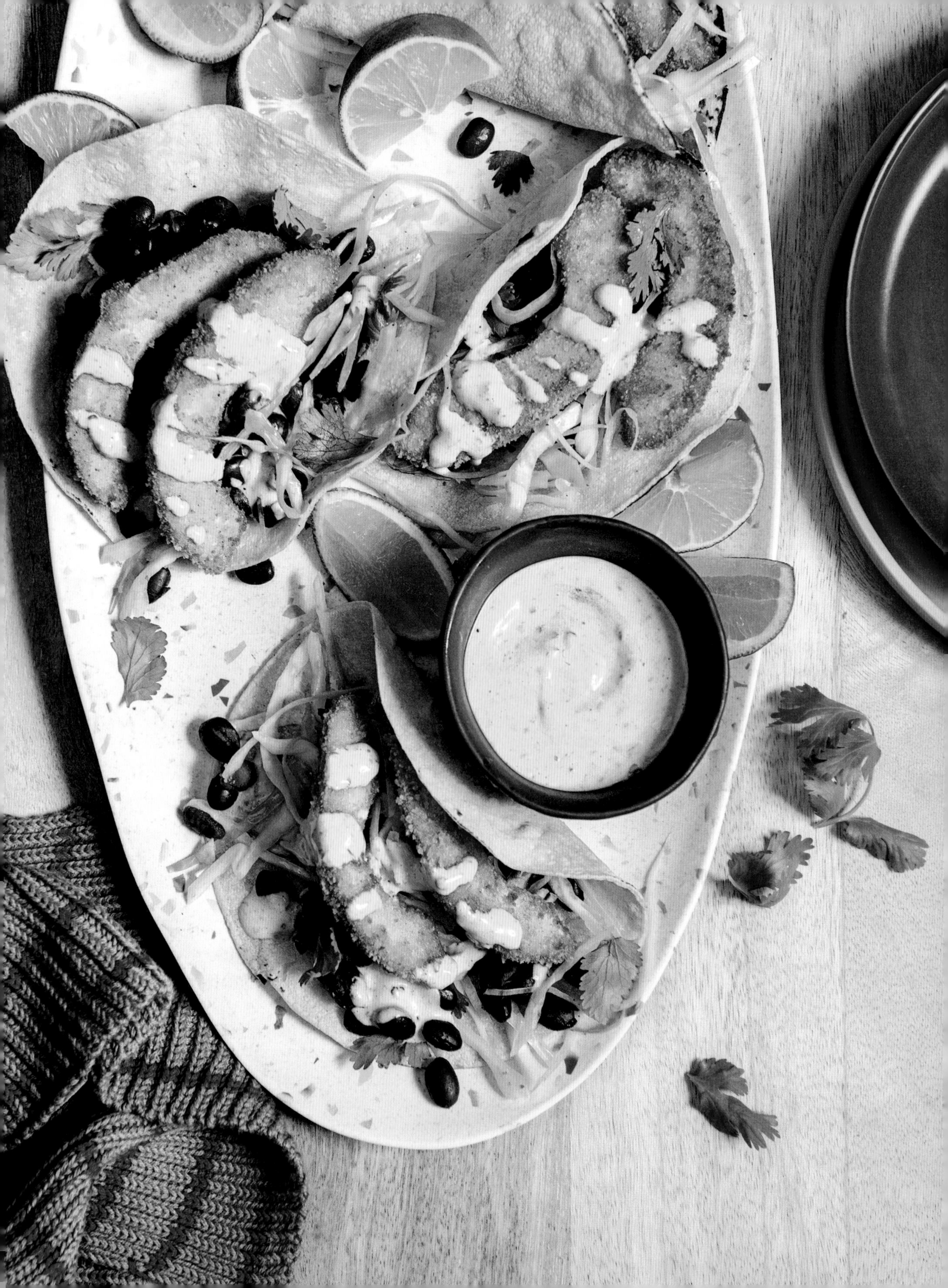

crispy avocado and black bean tacos with chipotle crema

time to prep: 25 minutes / time to cook: 15 to 30 minutes / serves: 3 (2 tacos per serving)

Vegetarian tacos are often underwhelming—I'm talking just slaw and veggies, maybe a dab of hot sauce or some cheese. I've rarely been pleasantly surprised, so as someone who eats primarily plant-based, it's my mission to make the dreamiest vegetarian taco out there. I don't want to get ahead of myself, but let's just say: mission accomplished. In a twist, the avocado is lightly breaded and toasted in the air fryer, which gives the taco the substantial consistency needed to make a filling entrée (and let's not forget the black beans, crunchy slaw, and chipotle crema!). Every bite will turn you into a believer, too.

For the chipotle crema

½ cup mayonnaise

1 chipotle pepper in adobo sauce, plus 1 teaspoon sauce from can

½ teaspoon minced garlic

1 tablespoon freshly squeezed lime juice

Salt and pepper, to taste

For the tacos

1 large egg

⅓ cup whole wheat breadcrumbs

1 teaspoon taco seasoning

2 medium avocados

(ingredients continue)

Preheat an air fryer to 400°F. Prepare the chipotle crema. Combine the mayonnaise, chipotle pepper and sauce, garlic, lime juice, and salt in a food processor and process until smooth. Set aside.

Once the air fryer is preheated, line a plate with parchment paper and set aside. Whisk the egg in one small shallow bowl or plate. Add the breadcrumbs to another similar bowl or plate and sprinkle with the taco seasoning and mix to combine. Peel and pit the avocados and slice lengthwise into ½-inch-thick strips, yielding about 6 slices per avocado. Dip one avocado in the egg and then roll in the breadcrumbs and transfer to the parchment paper. Continue until all the avocados are coated.

Place the avocados in the air fryer, spritz with cooking spray, and cook them for 15 minutes or until browned and crispy, cooking in batches if necessary.

In a medium bowl, place the coleslaw, cilantro, oil, lime juice, and salt and pepper, and toss to coat. Set aside.

(recipe continues)

Cooking spray, for the air fryer

2 cups coleslaw or shredded cabbage

¼ cup packed cilantro leaves

1 tablespoon extra-virgin olive oil

1 ripe lime, juiced

Pepper, to taste

6 tortillas

1 can (15 ounces) black beans, drained and rinsed

While the avocados cook, place a large skillet over medium-high heat. Once the pan is hot, warm the tortillas, adding each into the skillet and warming for about 30 seconds per side. Divide the warmed tortillas onto plates. Immediately add the beans to the same skillet. Stir for 2 to 3 minutes or until warmed through.

Build your tacos. Divide the black beans among the warmed tortillas, mashing some on the tortillas with the back of a fork. Top each tortilla with 2 avocado slices, the coleslaw mixture, and drizzle with the chipotle crema. Serve.

INSPIRALIZED TIP

When I introduced these tacos to my kids, I made a cheese quesadilla with the tortilla and served it alongside the black beans and avocados. Slowly but surely they tried the other components of the meal independently.

FEEDING LITTLES TIP

Get creative with your tortillas—there are so many on the market. Corn, whole wheat, even cassava flour all lend different nutrients, flavors, and textures. Check out the options the next time you're at the store.

I CAN'T EVEN

Buy a premade chipotle mayo. If you're really in a pinch, skip breading the avocados and just serve them sliced.

pressure cooker chicken teriyaki and rice bowls with broccoli

time to prep: 15 minutes / time to cook: 30 minutes / serves: 4

When I was in high school and a bit into college, I worked on Friday and Saturday nights at a Japanese restaurant in my hometown. Working nights meant that I would eat at the restaurant on a quick break, and for whatever reason, all I ever wanted was white rice smothered in teriyaki sauce. This pressure cooker chicken teriyaki with rice is my adult version, made complete with a protein and veggie. The sweet smells of teriyaki steaming in the pressure cooker will call your whole family into the kitchen for dinner.

1¼ cups dry white rice

1 tablespoon sesame oil

5 cups broccoli florets

Pepper

½ cup low-sodium soy sauce

2 garlic cloves, minced

1-inch knob ginger, peeled and minced

2 tablespoons honey

Pinch red pepper flakes

2 teaspoons white sesame seeds, plus more for garnish

2 tablespoons arrowroot powder (or cornstarch)

1½ pounds boneless, skinless chicken thighs

Cook the rice according to the package directions. When cooked, cover to keep the rice warm.

Set a pressure cooker to the Sauté function and add the oil. Once the oil is shimmering, add the broccoli, season with pepper, and cook, tossing frequently, until the broccoli is browned on the edges, about 5 minutes. Add ¼ cup of water and let the broccoli cook until fork-tender. Using tongs, transfer the broccoli to a bowl and cover to keep warm.

To the pressure cooker pot, immediately add in the soy sauce, garlic, ginger, honey, red pepper flakes, sesame seeds, and 1½ cups of water, and bring to a simmer. Meanwhile, in a small bowl, whisk together the arrowroot powder and 2 tablespoons of water. Once the soy sauce mixture is simmering slightly, add the arrowroot slurry to the pressure cooker pot and stir constantly until combined and the sauce is thickened. Add in the chicken. Cover and set the pressure cooker to High pressure for 12 minutes. Once done, manually release the pressure, uncover, and use a fork and knife to shred the chicken.

Divide the rice into bowls, top evenly with the shredded chicken and broccoli, and drizzle with the remaining teriyaki sauce from the pressure cooker pot. Garnish with sesame seeds and serve.

(recipe continues)

INSPIRALIZED TIP

If you want to make this meal gluten- and soy-free, substitute coconut aminos for the soy sauce.

FEEDING LITTLES TIP

This is a great dish to let your child plate themselves. If your toddler isn't great at scooping, use a hand-over-hand technique to gently guide them. Put sesame seeds into a shaker bottle and ask your kiddo if they want to sprinkle some on. Note: Omit the sauce for babies under twelve months since it contains honey.

I CAN'T EVEN

Use a bottled teriyaki sauce instead of making this one from scratch.

PREP AHEAD

This entire dish can be made and prepped ahead of time.

steak bites and sweet potatoes with chimichurri

time to prep: 15 minutes / time to cook: about 25 minutes / serves: 4

The chimichurri sauce doesn't get as much love as its green cousin, pesto. Chimichurri has a few more ingredients and fresh herbs, but the extra flavor is worth the effort. Here, it's drizzled over steak and sweet potatoes. The potatoes are cooked until they're almost mashed in consistency, with the meat juice flavoring each tasty bite. Perhaps this recipe will make you a chimichurri crusader, too.

2 tablespoons extra-virgin olive oil

2 pounds sirloin steak, cut into 2-inch pieces

Salt and pepper

1½ pounds sweet potatoes, peeled and chopped into 1-inch cubes

4 large garlic cloves, minced

⅔ cup low-sodium beef broth

For the chimichurri

1 cup fresh flat-leaf parsley

1 teaspoon dried oregano

1 cup cilantro

3 garlic cloves

1 serrano chile or jalapeño, seeded and chopped (can use less or more)

(Ingredients continue)

Set a pressure cooker to the Sauté function and add the oil. Season the steak bites with salt and pepper. Once the oil is shimmering, add the steak in a single layer, and cook for 1 to 2 minutes per side, until browned, working in batches if needed. Add all of the steak, sweet potatoes, garlic, and beef broth, and season generously with more salt and pepper. Cook for 10 minutes on High pressure. Manually release the pressure and transfer to a serving dish, using a slotted spoon.

Meanwhile, prepare the chimichurri. Place the parsley, oregano, cilantro, garlic, chile, onion, if using, vinegar, and oil in a food processor, season with salt and pepper, and process until smooth and creamy (not chunky), about 1 minute. Set aside.

Serve the steak and sweet potatoes with the chimichurri.

(recipe continues)

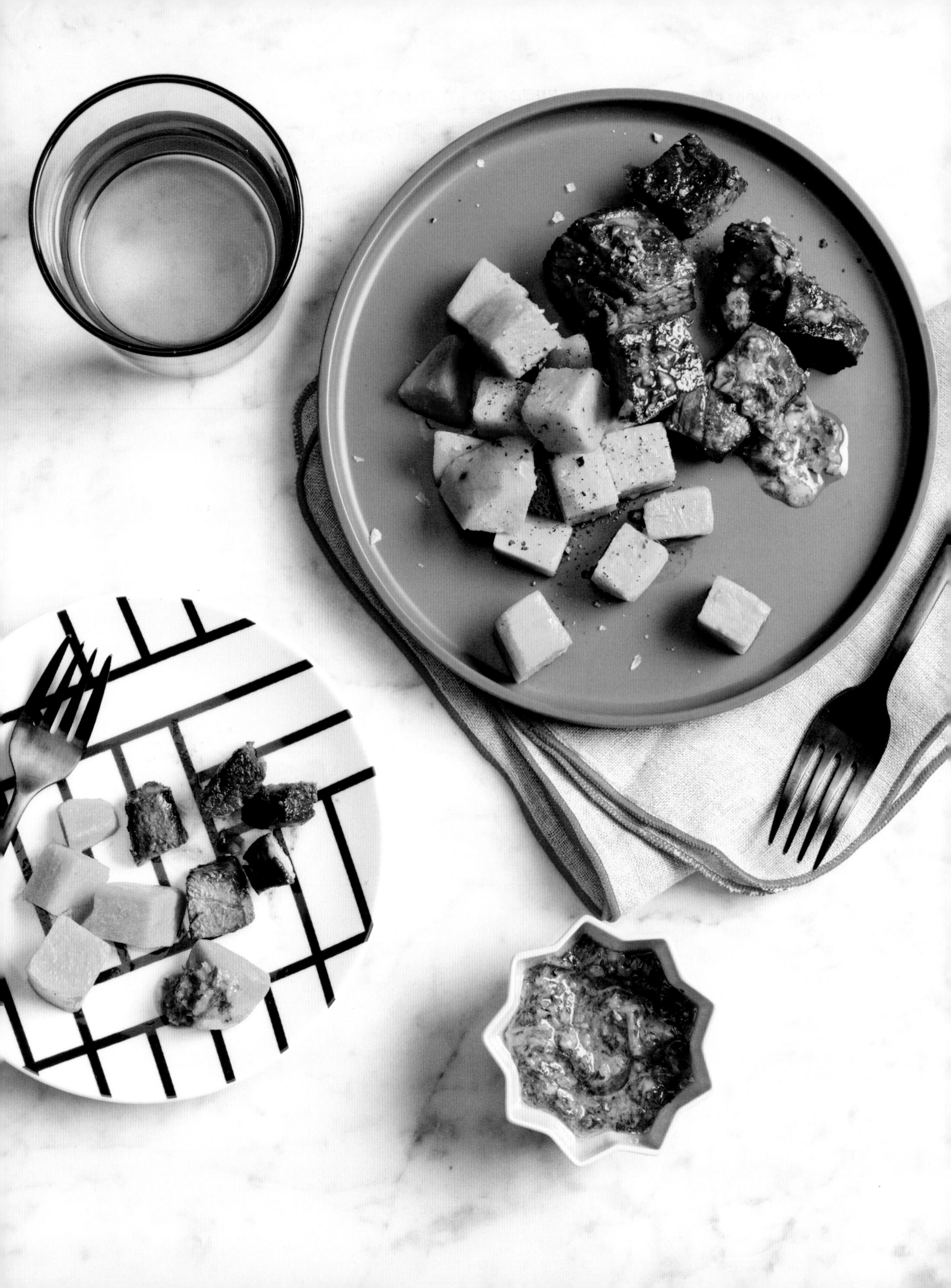

2 tablespoons chopped white onion (can be omitted)

3 tablespoons red wine vinegar

¼ cup olive oil

Salt and pepper

FEEDING LITTLES TIP

If you're serving this dish to a reluctant eater for the first time, make sure to pair it with one or two familiar sides like fruit salad and a whole-grain roll. Encourage your child to dip the roll into the chimichurri as a first step in learning about that flavor.

I CAN'T EVEN

Buy premade chimichurri.

PREP AHEAD

Prep the chimichurri ahead of time.

thai peanut chicken quinoa bowls

time to prep: 15 minutes / time to cook: 20 minutes / serves: 4

These chicken bowls are particularly enticing for early eaters, because they're a tasty way to introduce the nut allergen, and the sauce gives the quinoa something to stick to, so it can be preloaded onto utensils if needed. You can also serve the sauce over rice and noodles, but I especially love it with fluffy, light quinoa.

Take note that, as a general rule, quinoa may test your patience more than most foods. It gets everywhere—you will likely find it in unexpected places for a while—but on the plus side, it's a wonderful sensory experience, a complete protein, and it's easy to prepare and can be built into many different types of meals. Pro tip: serve this one before bathtime.

2 tablespoons sesame oil

1½ pounds boneless, skinless chicken breasts, cut into 1-inch cubes

2 garlic cloves, minced

1 tablespoon peeled and freshly grated ginger

⅔ cup creamy peanut butter

½ cup low-sodium soy sauce (or coconut aminos)

1 tablespoon chili paste (or sriracha)

2 tablespoons freshly squeezed lime juice

2 teaspoons honey (omit for babies younger than 1 or use granulated sugar)

1 cup canned unsweetened full-fat coconut milk

(ingredients continue)

Set a pressure cooker to the Sauté function and add 1 tablespoon of the oil. Once the oil is shimmering, add the chicken, cook for 2 minutes, flip, and cook for another minute just to brown and sear the cubes. Press Cancel.

Add into the pressure cooker (with the chicken) the remaining 1 tablespoon oil, the garlic, ginger, peanut butter, soy sauce, chili paste, lime juice, honey, and coconut milk. Cook on High pressure for 8 minutes. Manually release the pressure, uncover, and let stand for 5 minutes to thicken.

While the chicken cooks, cook the quinoa. Place the quinoa and 2 cups of water in a medium pot and bring to a boil. Once boiling, reduce the heat to low to simmer, cover, and cook for 15 minutes or until fluffy.

Place the edamame in a small pot and cover with water. Bring to a boil and boil until the edamame is cooked and warmed through, about 5 minutes. Drain, place in a food processor with the peanuts, and pulse until chopped. Set aside.

(recipe continues)

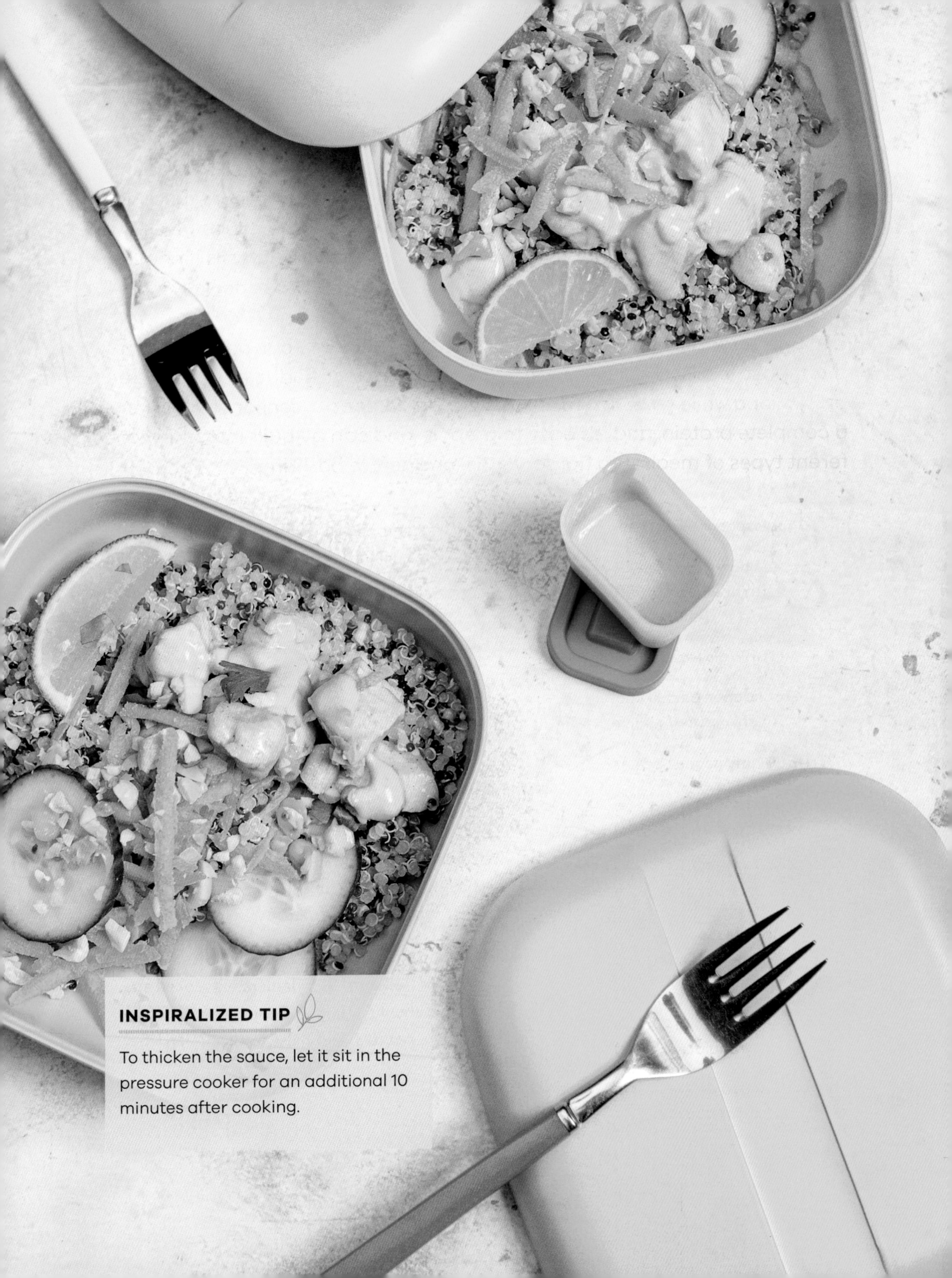

INSPIRALIZED TIP

To thicken the sauce, let it sit in the pressure cooker for an additional 10 minutes after cooking.

1¼ cups dry quinoa

1 cup frozen shelled edamame

¼ cup peanuts

½ seedless English cucumber

2 carrots, peeled

Cilantro leaves, for garnish

Lime wedges, for serving

Thinly slice the cucumber crosswise to make thin rounds. Cut the cucumber in half again for babies and young toddlers. Shred the carrots. Set everything aside.

Once the quinoa and chicken are done cooking, build your bowls. Divide the quinoa into bowls and top with the chicken, cucumber, and carrots. Garnish with the peanut and edamame mixture and cilantro. Serve with lime wedges.

FEEDING LITTLES TIP

Since this is a bit of a complicated dish that can overwhelm new eaters, try deconstructing it. Sometimes a familiar component on the plate—like edamame or chicken—can make the whole meal more approachable.

I CAN'T EVEN

Use microwavable quinoa and a premade bottled peanut sauce.

PREP AHEAD

This meal can be prepped in advance, but separate the quinoa and the peanut chicken for best consistency when serving.

air fryer sweet potato and black bean taquitos

time to prep: 15 minutes / time to cook: 30 minutes / serves: 4 (2 taquitos per person)

Do you love Taco Tuesdays? What about Taquito Tuesdays? I find that taquitos are a kid-friendlier taco, because everything stays together while eating. I've made every kind of taquito under the sun, and I'm here to say that this sweet potato and black bean version is the winner. Sweet potatoes are a familiar food for a lot of kids, and here they add a bit of sweetness. Don't skip the avocado crema, which pulls the meal together and can either be drizzled on top or served alongside the taquitos as a dip. So—are you embracing Taquito Tuesdays, too?

1 medium sweet potato, peeled and cubed

1 tablespoon extra-virgin olive oil

3 garlic cloves, minced

½ cup diced onion

1 can (15 ounces) black beans, drained and rinsed

1 tablespoon taco seasoning

Salt and pepper

2 tablespoons minced cilantro

8 (8-inch) tortillas

Cooking spray, for the air fryer

2 ripe limes

1 large ripe avocado, peeled, pitted, and cubed

½ cup cilantro leaves, plus more for garnish

Pico de gallo, for garnish

Place the sweet potato and ¼ cup of water in a large skillet and bring to a boil. Once boiling, reduce the heat to a medium simmer, cover the pan, and cook the sweet potato until it is fork-tender, about 10 minutes.

Set the sweet potato aside on a plate and immediately add the oil, a third of the garlic, and the onion to the skillet and set heat to medium-high. Cook the vegetables for 5 minutes or until softened. Add the black beans, taco seasoning, and cooked sweet potato, and season with salt and pepper. Stir to combine, and let the mixture cook for 2 minutes to warm up the beans. Lightly mash the sweet potato with the back of a fork and stir so that the sweet potato and black beans are evenly combined, crushing the black beans slightly as well. You still want some sweet potato chunks left, so don't over smash. Remove from the heat and stir in the minced cilantro.

Preheat an air fryer to 400°F.

Lay a tortilla down on a flat, clean surface and place about ¼ cup of the sweet potato mixture down on one side of the tortilla and roll into a tube. Set aside, seam side down to keep it closed. Continue with the remaining filling and

(recipe continues)

tortillas until all are used. Place the tortillas, seam side down, into the tray of the air fryer and spritz with cooking spray. Cook for 15 minutes or until crispy. You may have to do this in batches depending on the size of your air fryer.

While the taquitos air-fry, prepare the crema. Juice the limes into a food processor and then add the remaining garlic, the avocado, the ½ cup of cilantro, and ½ cup of water, and season with salt and pepper. Process until creamy, adding more water by the tablespoon if needed, and set aside.

Place the taquitos on a serving tray, drizzle with crema, and garnish with pico de gallo and cilantro. Serve.

INSPIRALIZED TIP

For added cheesy deliciousness, sprinkle a tablespoon of a shredded Mexican cheese blend into each taquito before rolling up.

FEEDING LITTLES TIP

Since these can get crunchy on the outside like a chip, we recommend cutting off the crunchy ends if you're feeding them to a young toddler. For babies, serve the scooped-out filling.

I CAN'T EVEN

Skip cooking the beans; just mash half of them in a bowl along with the taco seasoning and then add the boiled sweet potatoes, mashing with the back of a fork, and stir well. Use that as your filling.

PREP AHEAD

Prepare the filling ahead of time, so that all you need to do is stuff, roll, and air-fry.

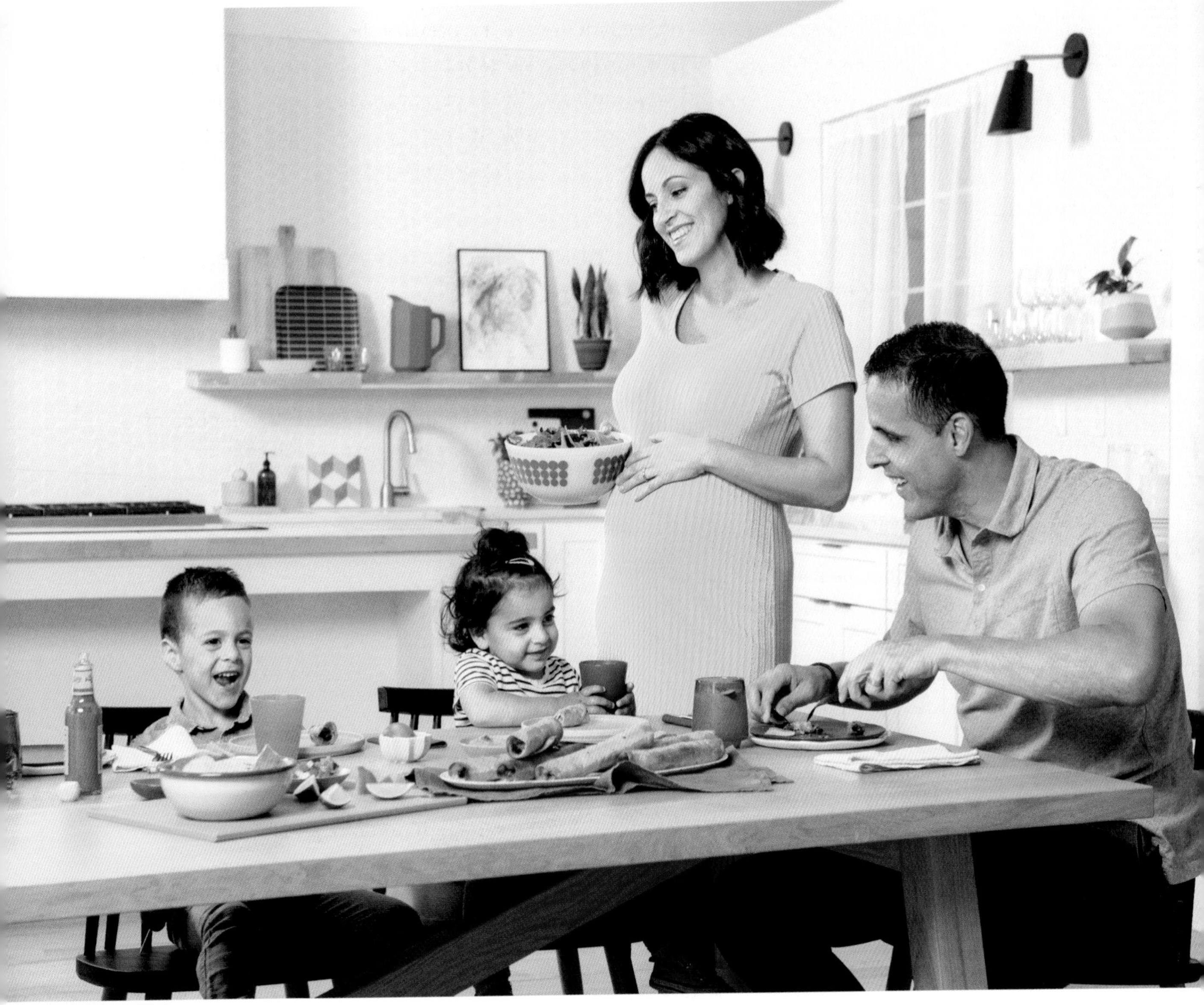

curried lentils and carrots with rice

time to prep: 15 minutes / time to cook: 35 minutes / serves: 5 to 6

This is a carrot-packed version of masoor dal, a popular Indian dish meaning "spiced red lentils." If you're feeding this to your baby as a first food, two things: 1) it's a fantastic introduction to these spices, and 2) buckle up for the cleanup. You may want to make this and document it as part of Megan and Judy's "Messy Mondays," when they encourage parents to embrace the mess in the name of sensory experience. If you're mess-averse, don't let that turn you off this recipe—it's nutritious, filling, and flavorful. The rice soaks it all up and serves as a vessel to preload the lentils onto a utensil.

1½ cups dry jasmine rice

1 tablespoon extra-virgin olive oil

1 medium yellow onion, diced

1-inch knob ginger, peeled and minced

2 garlic cloves, minced

2 medium carrots, peeled and sliced into ¼-inch-thick rounds (if using larger carrots, halve the rounds as well)

1 can (28 ounces) diced tomatoes

2 tablespoons curry powder

½ teaspoon ground turmeric

2 teaspoons ground cumin

½ teaspoon ground coriander

Combine the rice and 3½ cups of water in a medium pot, cover, and bring to a boil. Reduce the heat to a simmer and let cook, covered, until the rice is cooked through and fluffy, about 30 minutes.

While the rice cooks, set a pressure cooker to the Sauté function and add the oil. Once the oil is shimmering, add the onion, ginger, and garlic, and cook for 3 minutes or until the vegetables begin to sweat. Add the carrots, tomatoes, curry powder, turmeric, cumin, coriander, chili powder, salt, and pepper. Stir together well to combine and let cook for 1 minute. Add the lentils, coconut milk, and vegetable broth, and stir well to combine. Press Cancel. Set the pressure cooker to High pressure and cook for 15 minutes. Let the pressure release naturally for 10 minutes, and then manually release any remaining pressure, open, and stir in the lemon juice.

Serve the curry over the rice, garnished with cilantro.

2 teaspoons chili powder (see Note in Inspiralized Tip)

1 teaspoon salt

Pepper, to taste

1½ cups dry red lentils

1 can (14 ounces) lite coconut milk (or ½ can full-fat coconut milk + ½ can water)

1 cup low-sodium vegetable broth

1 tablespoon freshly squeezed lemon juice

Chopped cilantro, for garnish

INSPIRALIZED TIP

Be careful with the spice level. If you're serving this to a very new eater or a toddler who doesn't love spicy foods, reduce the chili powder to ½ teaspoon or 1 teaspoon.

FEEDING LITTLES TIP

If you have young kids at home, remind yourself that one day they won't make a mess while they eat. This is a temporary period of time. The more skilled they become at using utensils and their hands, the more food will actually end up in their mouths. Try to stay patient.

I CAN'T EVEN

Use microwavable rice.

PREP AHEAD

This entire dish can be fully prepped ahead.

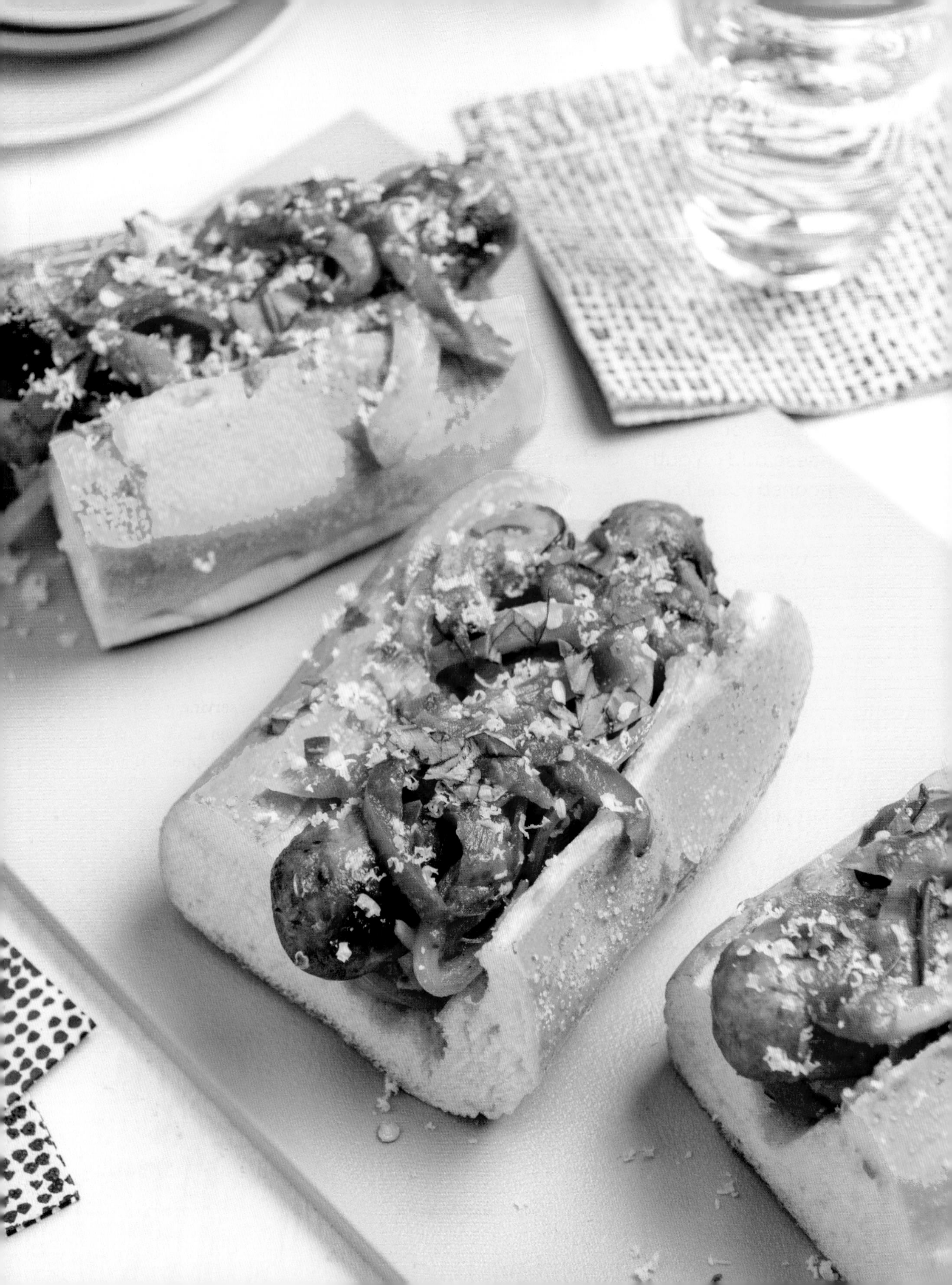

slow cooker sausage and pepper hoagies

time to prep: 15 minutes / time to cook: 6 hours / serves: 6

Growing up with Italian American grandparents, our family either ate freshly made sauce with meatballs or sausage and peppers on Sunday nights. I can practically smell the sausage and peppers as I type, and I wanted to bring this classic back in a more manageable way for anyone with little ones running (or crawling) around. This slow cooker version doesn't exactly replicate that seared flavor, but it gets nourishing, savory sausage and peppers on your family's plates, and the fresh basil and grated Parmesan cheese add an authentic finish. Adults can enjoy it as a hoagie and serve it deconstructed for kiddos.

1 can (28 ounces) crushed tomatoes (no salt added)

3 garlic cloves, minced

1 tablespoon Italian seasoning

¼ teaspoon red pepper flakes, plus more for garnish (optional)

2 tablespoons extra-virgin olive oil

6 Italian sausage links

3 bell peppers, seeded and thinly sliced

1 large onion, sliced

Salt and pepper

2 tablespoons thinly sliced fresh basil

(ingredients continue)

Combine the tomatoes, garlic, Italian seasoning, red pepper flakes, if using, and oil in a slow cooker. Stir in the sausages, peppers, and onion, and season with salt and pepper. Cover and cook on low for 6 hours. Then, press Cancel and stir in the basil.

Cut the sausages into small pieces before serving to kids. Before plating, warm up the rolls in the oven at 400°F for 5 to 7 minutes and serve with the sausages, peppers, onion, and Parmesan.

For the adults or kids who can handle spice, garnish with red pepper flakes.

INSPIRALIZED TIP

If you can't find hoagies, hot dog buns will do the trick. To add a little more flavor and color to the sausages, first sauté them in a skillet over medium heat until browned on all sides, and then start the recipe from the beginning.

(recipe continues)

6 hoagie rolls, for serving

Grated Parmesan cheese, for serving

FEEDING LITTLES TIP

Whole sausages can be a choking hazard for kids younger than four. To make these safer, cut lengthwise into strips and then slice into small pieces. Let your older toddler or big kid add the sausage and pepper filling to their own hoagie or bun using mini tongs. If the whole hoagie is too big for them to hold or bite, cut it into smaller sections to make mini sandwiches.

I CAN'T EVEN

Use a 24-ounce jar of tomato basil sauce as a substitute for the tomatoes, garlic, Italian seasoning, and red pepper flakes. This will save time and offer a similar flavor without all the prep.

PREP AHEAD

This entire dish can be prepped ahead and keeps well in the refrigerator for 3 to 5 days.

pressure cooker chicken salsa kinda-chiladas

time to prep: 30 minutes / time to cook: about 20 minutes / serves: 4 to 6

OK, calling these "enchiladas" is a stretch because enchiladas are made with enchilada sauce . . . and there's no enchilada sauce here. Instead, the chicken, peppers, and onion are pressure-cooked with a jar of salsa (talk about easy), creating a delicious sauce. But they're enchilada *adjacent* in terms of preparation: the tortillas are stuffed with the chicken and veggies and rolled, placed in a baking dish, topped with cheese and extra sauce, and baked until melted and dreamy. Little eaters can eat them deconstructed with sliced avocado and still relish the same flavors. Next time you buy a jar of salsa for your chips, pick up an extra and make these (kinda) enchiladas for dinner.

2 pounds boneless, skinless chicken thighs

2 bell peppers, seeded and sliced thinly

1 small red onion, sliced thinly

1 jar (15 to 16 ounces) salsa

8 tortillas

1½ cups shredded Mexican cheese blend

Chopped cilantro and sliced or diced avocado, for serving

Place the chicken thighs in the bottom of a pressure cooker and top with the peppers and onion. Pour in the salsa and toss lightly until the vegetables and chicken are coated, keeping the chicken on the bottom of the pot. Cook in the pressure cooker for 8 minutes on High pressure. Manually release the pressure. Press Cancel.

Meanwhile, warm your tortillas. Heat the tortillas in a skillet or in the oven until warmed through and pliable. Set aside. Take out a large baking dish.

Once the chicken and veggies are done cooking, preheat the oven to 400°F. Remove the chicken thighs from the pressure cooker pot and place in a bowl. Using two forks, shred the chicken.

Prepare your enchiladas. In the baking dish, pour in enough of the juices from the pressure cooker to cover the bottom (it's OK if you spoon in some peppers and onion). Using tongs, transfer some of the chicken and some of the pepper mixture onto one end of a tortilla. Sprinkle with

(recipe continues)

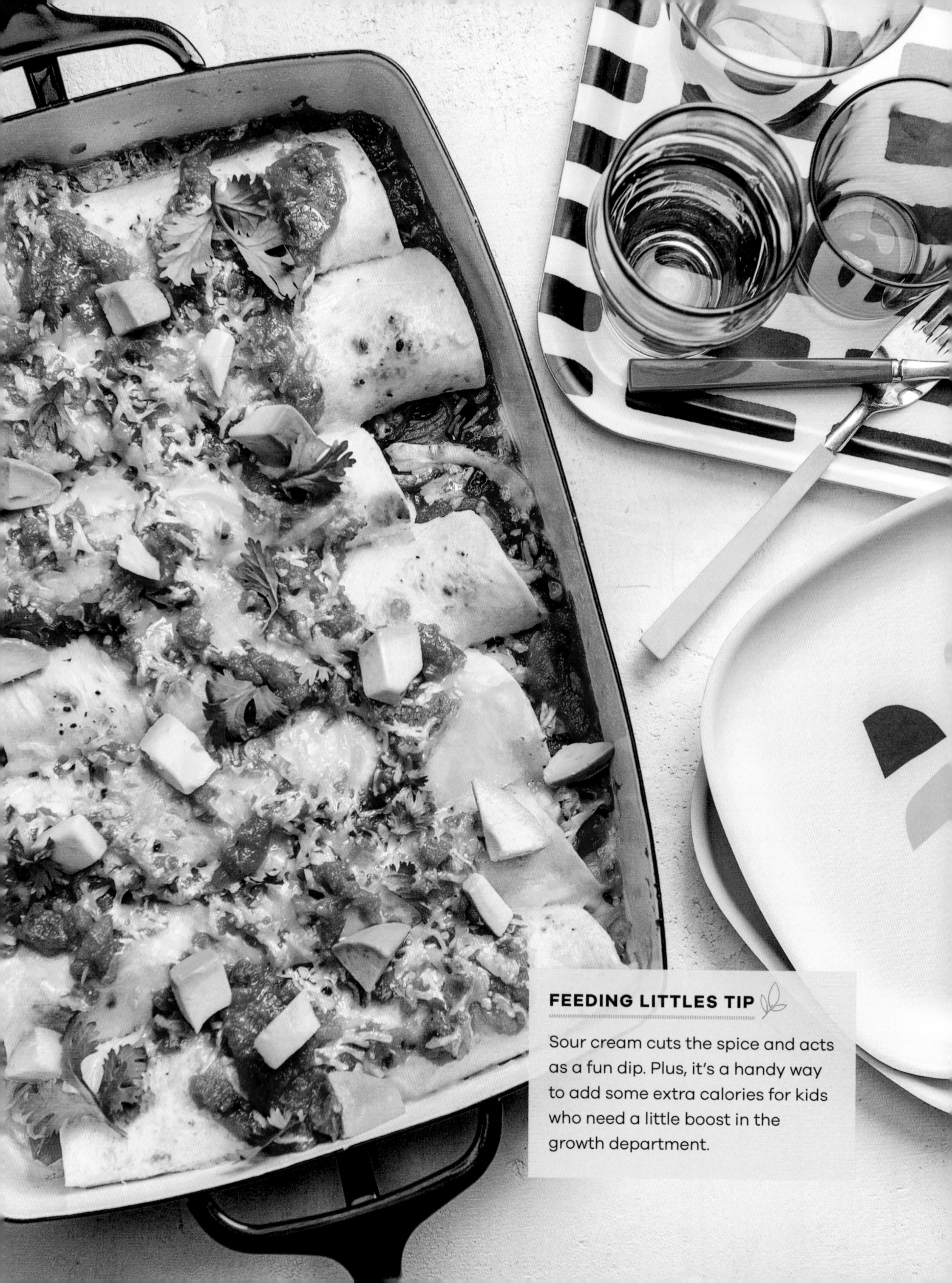

FEEDING LITTLES TIP

Sour cream cuts the spice and acts as a fun dip. Plus, it's a handy way to add some extra calories for kids who need a little boost in the growth department.

2 tablespoons of cheese, roll tightly, and place in the baking dish, seam side down. Repeat with the remaining tortillas, chicken, and pepper mixture.

Pour over some of the remaining juices from the pressure cooker pot to coat the enchiladas and sprinkle with the remaining ½ cup of cheese. Bake for 10 minutes or until the cheese is melted and bubbling. Garnish with cilantro and avocado. Serve.

INSPIRALIZED TIP

For a distinct flavor each time, switch up the type of salsa you use: think salsa verde. Just be careful of the heat levels when serving to little ones.

I CAN'T EVEN

Skip baking and serve fajita-style (deconstructed or separated out) with tortillas, cheese, and avocado.

PREP AHEAD

These can be prepared fully ahead of time, or prepare the chicken and pepper mixture and assemble the enchiladas when ready to eat.

slow cooker turkey and butternut squash enchilada chili

time to prep: 15 minutes / **time to cook: 15 minutes + 4 hours or more in the slow cooker** / **serves: 4 to 6**

Once I learned about adding enchilada sauce to my chili, I never looked back. Enchilada sauce is so delicious that you can skip adding other spices to get the flavor just right. This quick and easy chili saves well in the freezer, makes meal prep easy, and saves your sanity when you know you're going to have a busy week ahead. I've brought it to new parents who need a little extra help, and to friends going through tough times. It's a feel-good meal—and packed with veggies as a bonus.

1 tablespoon extra-virgin olive oil

2 garlic cloves, minced

1 small yellow onion, diced

1 pound ground turkey

1 teaspoon dried oregano

½ teaspoon salt, plus more as needed

Pepper

2 teaspoons chili powder (or more, if eaters can handle spice)

1 tablespoon ground cumin

2 cups cubed butternut squash (or sweet potato, and both can be frozen)

1 can (15 ounces) diced tomatoes

Heat the oil in a large skillet over medium-high heat. Once the oil is shimmering, add the garlic and onion and let cook for 5 minutes or until the onion is translucent. Push the vegetables to one side of the skillet and add in the turkey. Season the turkey with the oregano and salt and pepper. Crumble the turkey and cook until browned and no longer pink on the inside, about 7 minutes. Stir the vegetables and the meat to combine.

Transfer the meat mixture to the pot of a slow cooker. Add the chili powder, cumin, and the ½ teaspoon of salt and stir well to coat. Add the squash, tomatoes, vegetable broth, enchilada sauce, and black beans, and stir well to combine. Cover and cook on low for 7 to 8 hours or on high for about 4 hours. Taste and season with more salt, if needed.

Serve warm, with your desired toppings.

1 cup low-sodium vegetable broth (if you like a thicker chili, omit the broth entirely)

1 jar (15 ounces) enchilada sauce

1 can (15 ounces) black beans, drained and rinsed

Lime wedges, cheddar cheese, green onions, avocado, cilantro, or other desired toppings, for serving

INSPIRALIZED TIP

You can substitute sweet potatoes for the squash.

FEEDING LITTLES TIP

Chili is a versatile leftover: serve it on top of pasta or a baked potato, as a dip for a quesadilla, or with a topping bar to make it a little more interactive.

I CAN'T EVEN

Use frozen butternut squash to save time instead of chopping it yourself.

PREP AHEAD

This entire chili can be prepared ahead of time and saved in the refrigerator for 3 to 5 days and up to 3 months in the freezer.

salmon fish sticks with mustard sauce

time to prep: 20 minutes / time to cook: 10 minutes / makes: 8 salmon sticks

The first seafood recipe I ever learned to make from my mom was a Dijon mustard salmon. For years, I stuck with it. When I cooked these fish sticks for my family and was searching the pantry for a dip, I went straight for the Dijon mustard and mayo. The tangy sauce brightens up the crunchy salmon, bringing in a much-needed zest. You'll find that it takes the same amount of time to preheat the oven and toast store-bought frozen fish tenders as it would to make them from scratch.

2 large eggs, beaten

2 cups panko breadcrumbs

1 teaspoon garlic powder

1 teaspoon paprika

½ teaspoon salt

Pepper, to taste

1 pound boneless, skinless salmon, sliced crosswise into 8 "sticks"

Cooking spray, for the air fryer

½ cup whole-grain mustard

½ cup mayonnaise (vegan works, too)

Preheat an air fryer to 400°F. Meanwhile, set up the egg wash and breadcrumb mixture. In one shallow dish, place the eggs and whisk them together with 2 teaspoons of water. In another shallow dish, place the panko breadcrumbs, garlic powder, paprika, salt, and pepper. Mix the panko mixture together so the seasonings distribute evenly.

With one hand, roll a piece of salmon in the egg wash and then lay it in the panko mixture. With your other hand, roll the salmon in the panko. Set aside on a plate and repeat with the remaining salmon.

Spray the bottom of the air fryer tray with cooking spray. Lay out the breaded salmon, spray the tops with cooking spray, and cook for 10 minutes, flipping halfway through, until browned on the outside.

While the salmon cooks, in a small bowl, whisk together the mustard, mayonnaise, and pepper. Set aside.

Serve the salmon sticks with the mustard sauce.

INSPIRALIZED TIP

If salmon is too strong a flavor, you can use cod here, too.

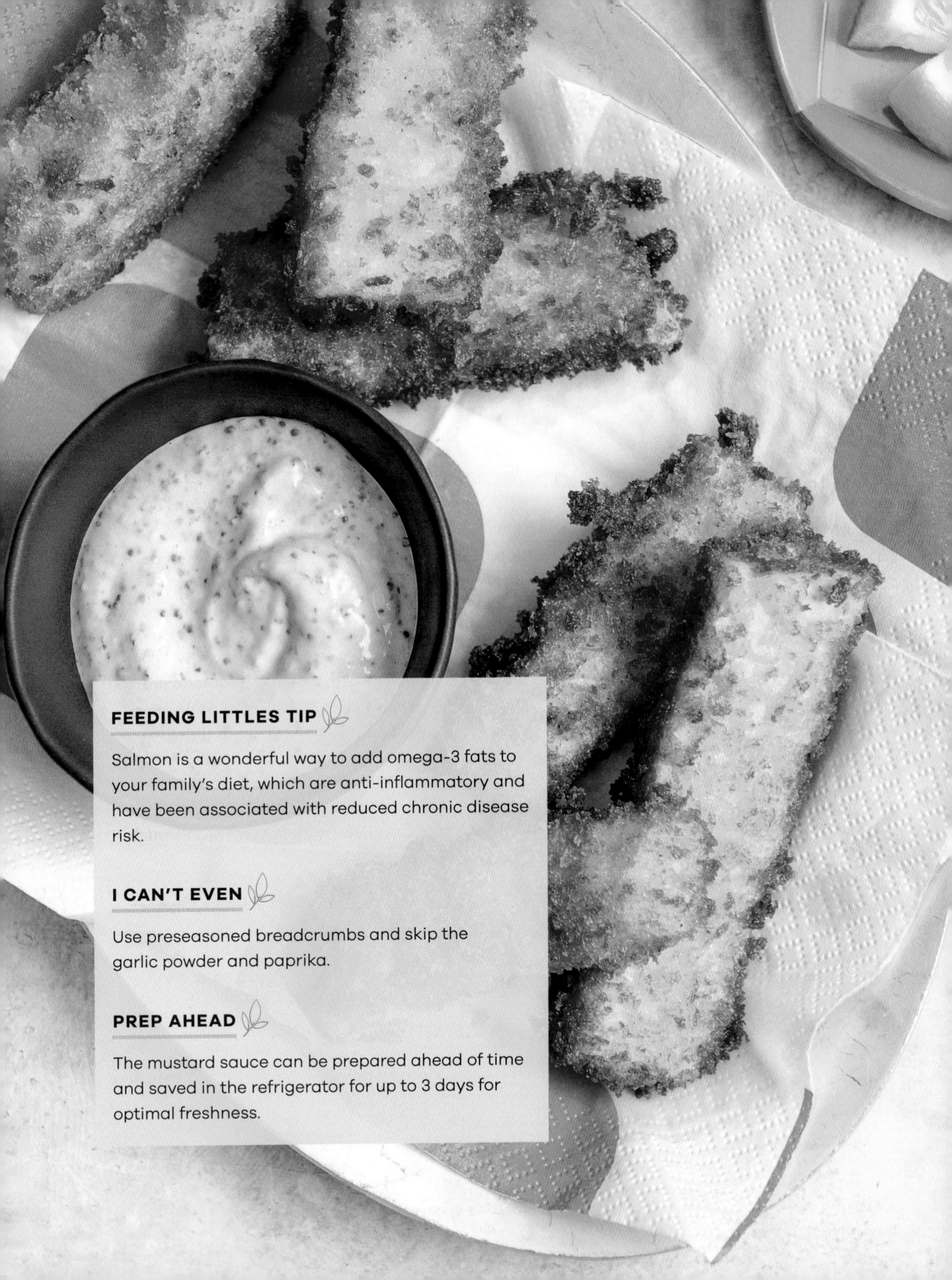

FEEDING LITTLES TIP

Salmon is a wonderful way to add omega-3 fats to your family's diet, which are anti-inflammatory and have been associated with reduced chronic disease risk.

I CAN'T EVEN

Use preseasoned breadcrumbs and skip the garlic powder and paprika.

PREP AHEAD

The mustard sauce can be prepared ahead of time and saved in the refrigerator for up to 3 days for optimal freshness.

slow cooker lentil taco soup

time to prep: 30 minutes / time to cook: 4 hours / serves: 8

This vegetarian chili swaps in lentils for ground meat and is bulked up with sweet potatoes and carrots for a nutritious, set-it-and-forget-it meal. Lentils are protein powerhouses, making this satisfying plant-based meal an easy way to add more protein to your diet. What makes this chili absolutely unbeatable is all the fixings, so load up on tortilla strips, avocados, cheese, and cilantro for extra flavor and a heartier texture. My family loves crushing tortilla chips up for a topping, but tortilla strips are an effortless way to get the same effect.

1 tablespoon extra-virgin olive oil

1 medium onion, diced

4 garlic cloves, minced

1 jalapeño, seeded and minced (you can use ¼ teaspoon cayenne pepper, instead)

1 cup dry green or brown lentils

2 cups peeled and diced carrots

2 cups peeled and diced sweet potatoes

4 cups low-sodium vegetable broth

1 tablespoon ground cumin

1 teaspoon salt, plus more as needed

2 teaspoons paprika

Heat the oil in a large skillet over medium-high heat. Once the oil is shimmering, add the onion, garlic, and jalapeño, and let cook for 1 minute or until fragrant. Transfer the mixture to a slow cooker and stir in the lentils, carrots, sweet potatoes, vegetable broth, cumin, the teaspoon of salt, the paprika, oregano, chili powder, and tomatoes, and season with pepper. Taste and add more salt if needed.

Cover and cook on high for 3 to 4 hours or until the lentils are tender. Let the corn sit out to thaw. Once the soup is ready, stir in the corn, cover, and let the corn warm through, about 5 minutes.

Uncover, divide the soup into bowls, and top with the avocados, tortilla strips, cilantro, and cheese. Serve with lime wedges.

1 teaspoon dried oregano

1 tablespoon chili powder

1 can (28 ounces) crushed tomatoes

Pepper, to taste

1 cup frozen corn

2 medium avocados, peeled, pitted, and diced

Tortilla strips, cilantro leaves, shredded cheddar cheese, and lime wedges, for serving

INSPIRALIZED TIP

To make this a thicker chili, use an immersion blender to blend half of the soup. If you don't have an immersion blender, pour half of the soup into a high-speed blender, blend until creamy, and pour back into the slow cooker and stir.

FEEDING LITTLES TIP

Tortilla chips or strips can be a choking hazard for kids younger than four. If you're using them, make sure to stir them into the chili so they're softened by the liquid.

I CAN'T EVEN

Instead of measuring out all the spices, just add 2 tablespoons of taco seasoning.

PREP AHEAD

This entire dish can be prepped ahead and saves well in the refrigerator for 3 to 5 days.

unstuffed turkey pepper skillet

time to prep: 15 minutes / time to cook: 25 to 30 minutes / serves: 4 to 6

Before we had children, stuffed peppers were on my weekly rotation; after kids, they went by the wayside because they were time consuming and not exactly functional for little eaters. At a certain point in parenthood, you reach the shortcut phase, and thus this "unstuffed" pepper casserole was born. Although it's made entirely in a pressure cooker, I like to serve it in a casserole. Old-school stuffed peppers will always have a place in my heart, but these have a special place in my mama heart.

- **1 tablespoon extra-virgin olive oil**
- **1 pound ground turkey**
- **1 teaspoon dried oregano**
- **Salt and pepper**
- **½ cup chopped red onion**
- **2 garlic cloves, minced**
- **3 bell peppers, seeded and diced**
- **1 teaspoon chili powder**
- **½ teaspoon ground paprika**
- **½ teaspoon ground cumin**
- **1 can (16 ounces) tomato sauce**
- **3 cups low-sodium vegetable or chicken broth**
- **2 cups dry brown short-grain rice**

Set the pressure cooker to the Sauté function and add the oil. Once the oil is shimmering, add the turkey and crumble. Season with the oregano and salt and pepper, and cook for about 7 minutes or until the meat is cooked through and no longer pink. Add the onion, garlic, and peppers to the pressure cooker and cook until lightly softened, about 5 minutes. Add the chili powder, paprika, cumin, tomato sauce, broth, and rice, and season with more salt. Stir well to combine. Press Cancel. Set the pressure cooker to High pressure and cook for 10 minutes. Quick release, uncover, stir, and fold in the cheese, stirring until melted. Transfer to a casserole-style dish for presentation, garnish with cilantro, and serve.

1½ cups shredded cheddar cheese

Chopped cilantro, for serving

INSPIRALIZED TIP

Top the pepper skillet with avocado and serve with chips (suitable for children older than four years old) for more texture, nutrition, and flavor.

FEEDING LITTLES TIP

This would be a great dish to serve in a ramekin, mug, or other small, novel container for a reluctant eater.

PREP AHEAD

This entire dish can be prepped ahead. It saves well up to 5 days in the refrigerator or 3 months in the freezer.

tuscan-style short ribs

time to prep: 10 minutes / time to cook: 20 minutes + 5 hours or more in the slow cooker / serves: 4

Every cook should have a standout meal when they have guests over, an intimate night in, or a celebration. This is also a superb option when you're craving something that tastes sophisticated without the big production. And like all great meals, it's made with love. Not only that, the slow cooker does all the work so that when you're ready to sit down and enjoy your meal, you're relaxed (or at least, as relaxed as you can be with little ones underfoot). The kids can join in on the special meal, too, thanks to the slow cooker that tenderizes the meat so it is soft enough for young mouths.

3 tablespoons extra-virgin olive oil

4 to 5 pounds beef short ribs (about 12 ribs)

Salt and pepper

3 garlic cloves, minced

6 carrots, peeled and sliced into 2-inch pieces

2 pounds small, round potatoes, halved (aka creamer potatoes)

1 tablespoon chopped fresh thyme

1 can (28 ounces) crushed tomatoes

2 tablespoons chopped fresh parsley, for garnish

Heat 1½ tablespoons of the oil in a large Dutch oven over medium-high heat. Once the oil is shimmering, season the short ribs generously with salt and pepper and add half of the short ribs to the pan. Brown the ribs on all sides, about 8 minutes. Transfer the short ribs to a slow cooker. Repeat with the remaining 1½ tablespoons of oil and short ribs. Place the browned short ribs in the slow cooker.

Place the garlic, carrots, and potatoes in the Dutch oven, and cook, stirring to scrape up any browned bits on the bottom of the pan, until the vegetables are browned, about 5 minutes. Stir in the thyme and transfer the vegetable mixture to the slow cooker along with any pan juices. Add the tomatoes to the slow cooker and season with salt and pepper. Cook on high for 5 hours or on low for 9 to 10 hours or until the meat is tender and falling off the bone. Uncover, stir well, and spoon the juices over the short ribs.

Using tongs, transfer the meat and vegetables to a serving dish, spooning half of the juices from the slow cooker pot over them.

Garnish with the parsley and serve.

INSPIRALIZED TIP

Baby new potatoes work well here, too.

FEEDING LITTLES TIP

Because the short ribs are tender, they are a suitable way to expose babies to beef while also offering an easy handle for them to hold.

PREP AHEAD

Cut the carrots ahead of time and store in a bag to save time.

the crispiest chicken nuggets

time to prep: 30 minutes / time to cook: 15 to 30 minutes / makes: about 24 nuggets

We debated not including a chicken nugget recipe in this cookbook because there are millions out there—but we want this book to be a one-stop shop, and what would a family cookbook be without a nugget recipe (especially one with our fresh spin)? To avoid the time-consuming and messy task of frying nuggets in a skillet, the air fryer is key. These can also be made into tenders if you skip slicing them into nugget-sized pieces. However these end up on your plate, they're just as crispy and tasty as the freezer aisle versions, but just elegant enough for adults' palates. Try serving them over a simple Caesar salad or rolled up in a wrap with crunchy veggies and ranch dressing.

Cooking spray, for the parchment paper

½ cup arrowroot powder (cornstarch or all-purpose flour also works)

2 large eggs

⅔ cup panko breadcrumbs

½ cup finely grated Parmesan cheese (if dairy-free, this can be omitted)

½ teaspoon garlic powder

1 teaspoon dried oregano

¼ teaspoon salt

Pepper, to taste

1 pound chicken tenders, chopped into nugget-sized pieces

Preheat an air fryer to 400°F. If using the oven, preheat the oven to 400°F. Line a baking sheet with parchment paper and spritz with cooking spray.

Prepare the nuggets. Place the arrowroot powder in a baking dish or on a plate. Whisk the eggs in a second baking dish or bowl. In a third baking dish or bowl, mix together the breadcrumbs, cheese, garlic powder, oregano, salt, and pepper. Arrange the dishes next to one another in this order: arrowroot, eggs, and breadcrumb mixture. Then, to the right, set the prepared baking sheet. Working left to right, take a chicken nugget, roll it in the arrowroot, dip it in the egg, then roll it in the breadcrumb mixture to coat. Set aside on the prepared baking sheet. Repeat this process until all the nuggets are coated.

If using an air fryer: spritz the basket with cooking spray and lay the nuggets in an even layer. Spritz the nuggets with cooking spray and cook for 12 to 15 minutes or until they are crispy and browned, flipping halfway through.

If using the oven: transfer the baking sheet with the nuggets to the oven and bake for 17 minutes or until the chicken is cooked through and opaque, flipping halfway through.

Serve.

INSPIRALIZED TIP

For a more basic nugget, omit the Parmesan and oregano and add ¼ teaspoon paprika. If you don't have an air fryer but want to make these nuggets, see the instructions for cooking them in the oven—they won't have the same crunch, but they'll still taste the same!

FEEDING LITTLES TIP

If your kiddo only likes nuggets, making them homemade is a first step in helping them to learn to like other types of meat. Serve them with a familiar dip like ketchup or barbecue sauce if your kiddo is still hesitant to try them.

PREP AHEAD

These nuggets can be completely prepped ahead of time.

crispy brussels sprouts dinner inspiration

time to prep: 1 minute / time to cook: 7 to 20 minutes / serves: 1

Brussels sprouts are no longer the feared vegetable of childhood. With the rise of Brussels sprouts as both a leading appetizer and side dish (think kung pao Brussels sprouts), we've seen this tiny cabbage transform before our eyes. Needless to say, lackluster steaming is out and novel preparations are in.

There are so many surprising ways to prepare Brussels sprouts that we thought we'd give them a dedicated section with our favorite way to serve them: crisped up in the air fryer. They're almost like chips, and they're so salty and savory that even the littlest of eaters will love them. These are some starting ideas using our base Crispy Brussels Sprouts, so that you can create your own restaurant-worthy version. There's also an oven recipe, but you may want to buy (or borrow) an air fryer to make them as crispy and delectable as can be.

We consider this reinvented vegetable to be the main event, so we've provided suggestions for protein pairings to inspire you to create your own meals around Brussels sprouts, too.

Crispy Brussels Sprouts: Base Recipe

Here's your base recipe, the one you can refer to when you're craving crispy sprouts, no bells or whistles needed. This recipe makes 1 serving, so adjust accordingly; everything can be evenly doubled, tripled, and so on.

1½ tablespoons extra-virgin olive oil

1½ cups thinly sliced or shredded Brussels sprouts

Salt and pepper

Cooking spray, for greasing the baking sheet (for oven method)

Air fryer method: Preheat an air fryer to 400°F. In a large bowl, toss the oil and sprouts together. Season generously with salt and pepper and toss again. Spread the Brussels sprouts out in the basket, trying to lay them out as evenly as possible. Cook for 7 minutes, shaking the basket halfway through and removing any sprouts that are burnt (you want a little burnt crispness, but not totally black). Remove those pieces and continue to cook the others until all are mostly crispy. Transfer to a bowl and serve.

Oven method: Preheat the oven to 425°F. Grease a baking sheet with cooking spray. Toss the oil and sprouts together in a large bowl. Season generously with salt and pepper and toss again. Spread the Brussels sprouts out evenly on the baking sheet, trying to lay them in one layer. Bake for 15 to 20 minutes, shaking the pan halfway through and removing any sprouts that start to burn (you want a little burnt crispness, but not totally black). Remove those pieces and continue to bake the others until all are mostly crispy. Transfer to a bowl and serve.

Crispy Balsamic Brussels Sprouts

These sprouts are superbly tart with a salt and vinegar flavor that's savory enough to pair with any protein—try them with the chicken from the Baked Bean Rice Bowls with Barbecue Chicken (page 212) or store-bought rotisserie chicken.

Base recipe

½ tablespoon balsamic vinegar

Generous pinch of garlic powder

To cook the sprouts, follow the base recipe, but add the vinegar and garlic powder when tossing the sprouts with the oil to prep before cooking.

Garlic Parmesan Brussels Sprouts

Nothing adds depth of flavor like finely grated Parmesan cheese. It's savory, nutty, and it takes these sprouts to the next level. The richness of the cheese complements a heavier protein, like a steak or burger, but the Brussels sprouts also go with roasted tofu with marinara sauce, too. Try serving these as a side dish with the Sweet Potato Spaghetti with Chicken Meatballs (page 150). You may need to reduce the air-fryer cook time by 2 minutes, as the cheese burns more quickly than the sprouts, so be sure to check as they cook.

Base recipe

Generous pinch of garlic powder

2 tablespoons finely grated Parmesan cheese, plus more for garnish

To cook the sprouts, follow the base recipe, but add the garlic powder and 2 tablespoons of Parmesan when tossing the sprouts with the oil before cooking. Once the sprouts are done cooking, immediately garnish with more Parmesan.

Soy Sesame Brussels Sprouts

Soy sauce is the ultimate umami, or savoriness, infuser. If you haven't tried adding soy sauce to your vegetables, you're about to experience its power. If you have a soy allergy in the family, coconut aminos are a good substitution. We love serving these salty sprouts with seafood—try serving them with the Teriyaki Salmon Bite Bowls (page 200).

1½ tablespoons sesame oil

1 tablespoon low-sodium soy sauce, plus more as needed

1½ cups thinly sliced or shredded Brussels sprouts

Pepper

Cooking spray, for greasing the baking sheet (for oven method)

Air fryer method: Preheat an air fryer to 400°F. Whisk together the oil and soy sauce in a large bowl. Add the Brussels sprouts and toss all the ingredients together. Season with pepper and toss again. Spread the Brussels sprouts out in the basket, trying to lay them out as evenly as possible. Cook for 15 minutes, shaking the basket halfway through and removing any sprouts that start to burn (you want a little burnt crispness, but not totally black). Remove those pieces and continue to cook the others until all are mostly crispy. Transfer to a bowl. Taste, and if the sprouts aren't flavorful enough, drizzle soy sauce on top.

Oven method: Preheat the oven to 425°F. Grease a baking sheet with cooking spray. Whisk together the oil and soy sauce in a large bowl. Add the Brussels sprouts and toss all the ingredients together. Season with pepper and toss again. Spread the Brussels sprouts out evenly on the greased baking sheet, trying to lay them out in one layer. Bake for 25 to 30 minutes, shaking the pan halfway through and removing any sprouts that start to burn (you want a little burnt crispness, but not totally black). Remove those pieces and continue to bake the others until all are mostly crispy. Transfer to a bowl. Taste, and if the sprouts aren't umami enough, drizzle soy sauce on top.

INSPIRALIZED TIP

Buy pre-shredded Brussels sprouts to save time.

FEEDING LITTLES TIP

Let your little one help you prep these sprouts. Even if they don't want to eat them just yet, they're more likely to try them in the future.

visual index

If you've been asking yourself, *"All of these recipes are great, but how do I plate them for my baby?!"* you've come to the right place.

This Visual Index shows images of how you can serve each recipe in the book to your baby, six months or older (see page 9 for more information on starting baby-led weaning). These suggestions are just that—suggestions. You do not have to serve your baby every component of the meal shown, and you also don't have to cut or serve the food in this way.

Keep in mind that these suggestions are for babies who don't yet have a pincer grasp and can't pick up small pieces of food (typically six to ten months of age). If your baby can pick up smaller pieces, feel free to cut the food up further.

We have omitted or modified any possible choking hazards. Furthermore, we are not including images from the Baked Bites section here (see page 57), as many of those foods are desserts that parents might not be comfortable serving to their babies just yet.

You may notice that since we are omitting parts of the recipe that aren't suitable for babies younger than one, some plates may appear light. You can use our Starter Fruit and Vegetable Guide, on page 20, to supplement any meal with fruits, veggies, grains, and more. For example, with the Everything Bagel Broccoli and Cheddar Egg Donuts, feel free to serve with fruit and toasted and buttered bread or full-fat yogurt.

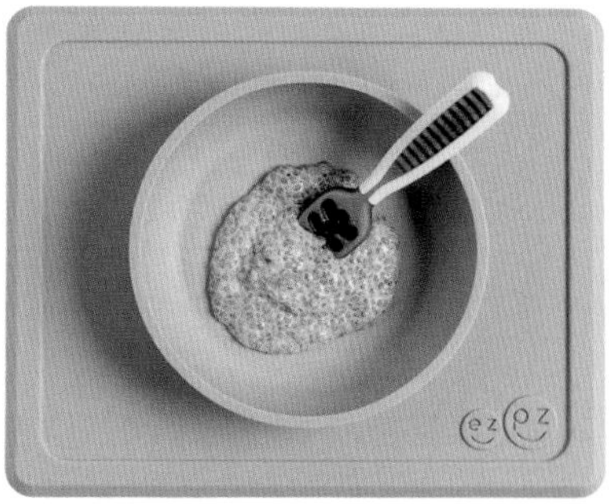

AB&J Chia Seed Pudding, page 45

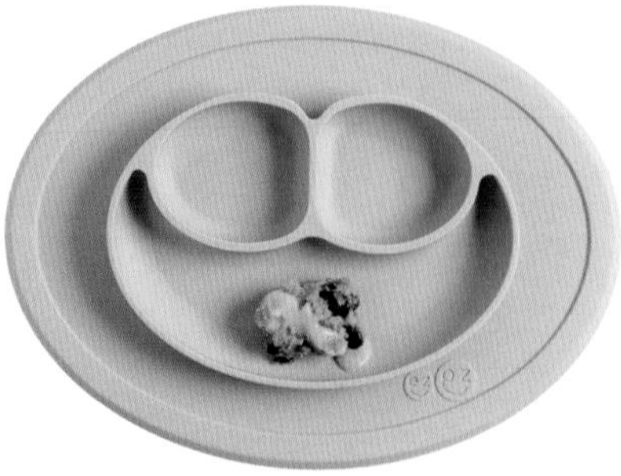

Air Fryer Sweet Potato and Black Bean Taquitos, page 253

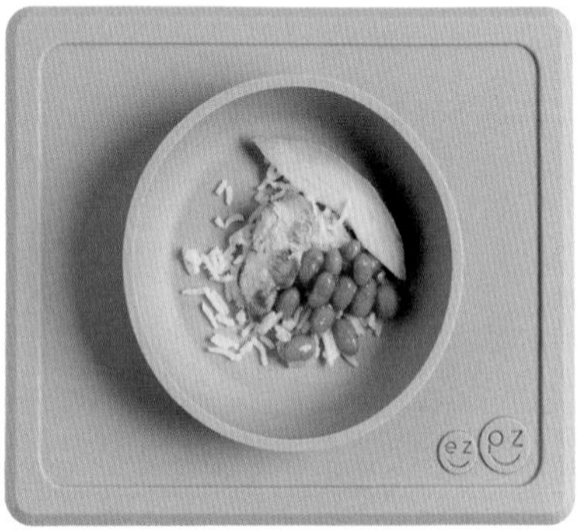

Baked Bean Rice Bowls with Barbecue Chicken, page 212

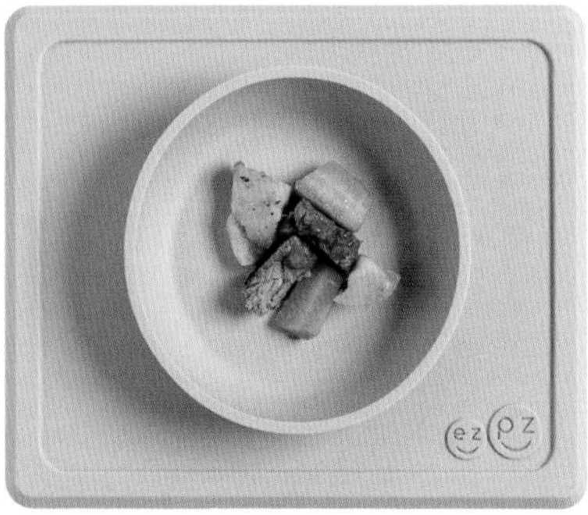

Baked Beef Stew with Parsnips, page 159

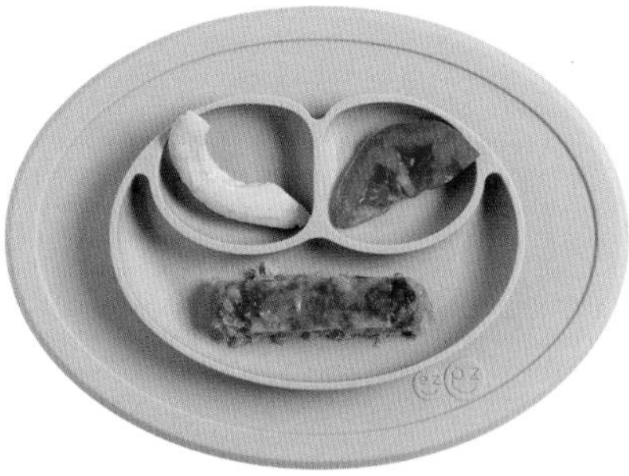

Barbecue White Bean Veggie Burgers, page 179

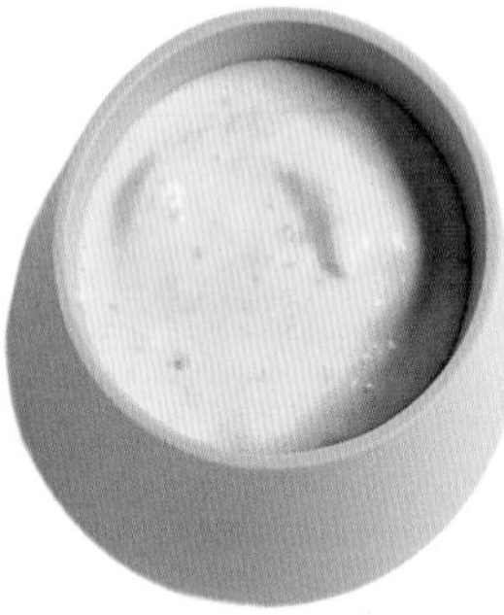

Beach Vacation Breakfast Smoothie, page 54

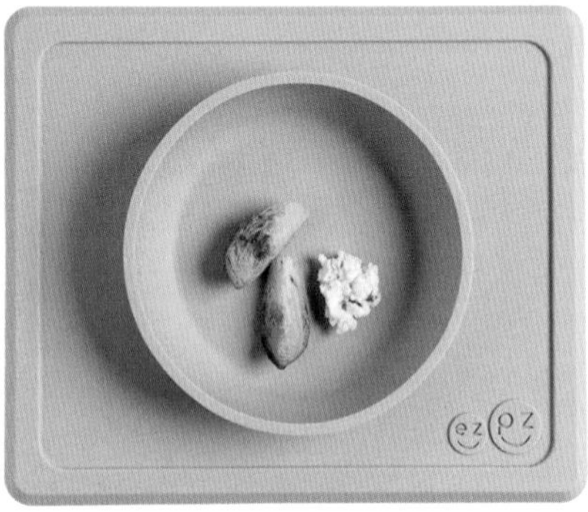

Brussels Sprouts and Bacon Harvest Kale Salad, page 234

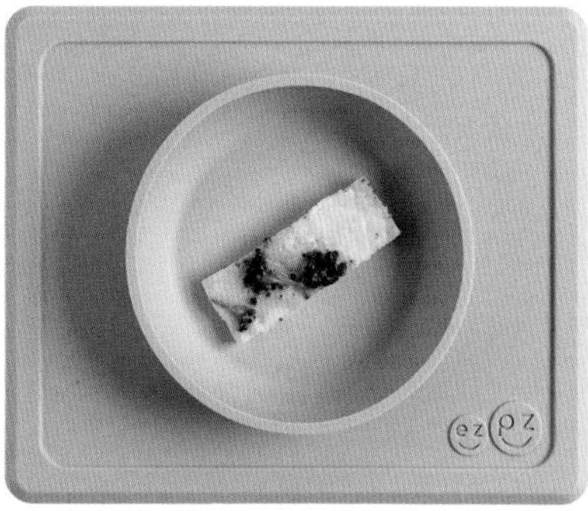

Build Your Own Sheet Pan Eggs, page 47

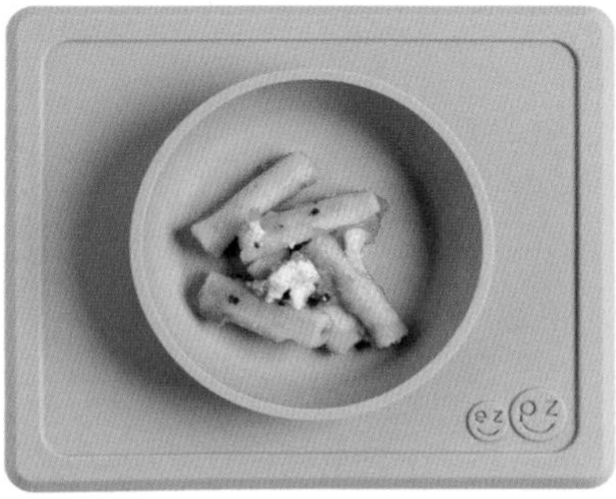

Butternut Squash Sage Baked Ziti, page 153

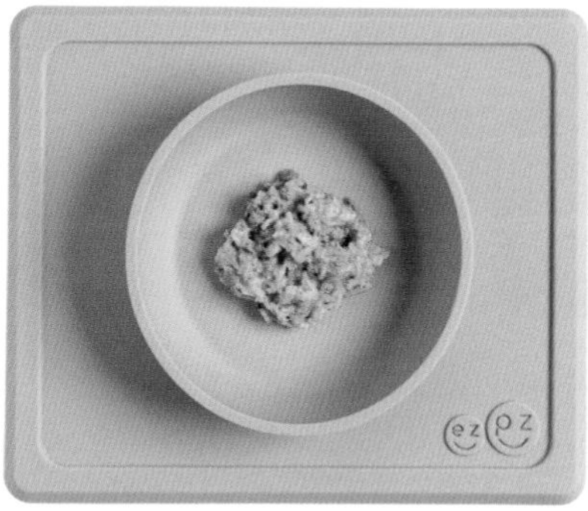

Carrot Cake Overnight Oats, page 44

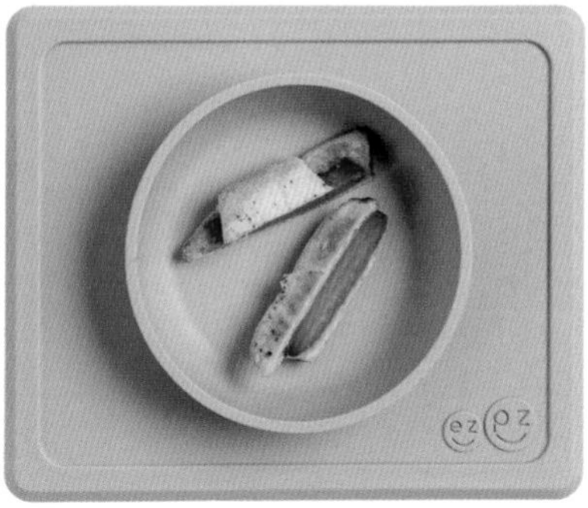

Carrot Crescent Roll Puffs, page 176

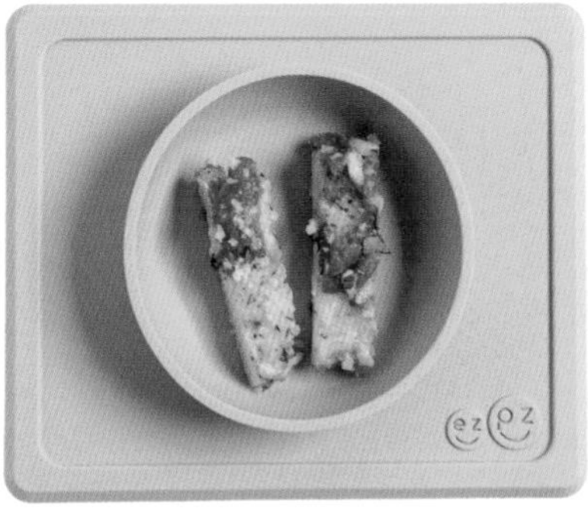

Cauliflower Parmesan Bake, page 143

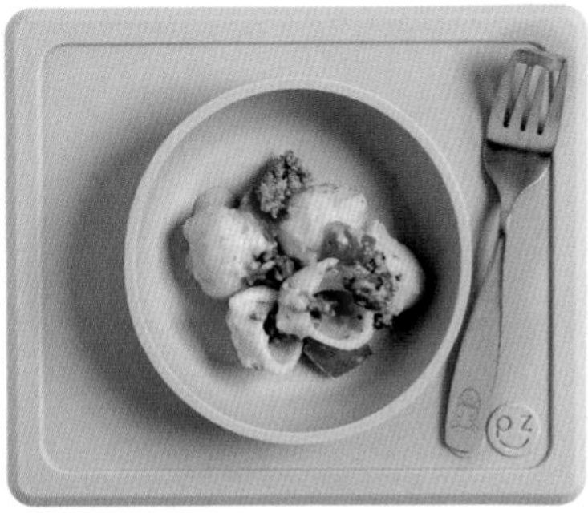

Cheesy Cheeseless Hamburger Pasta, page 79

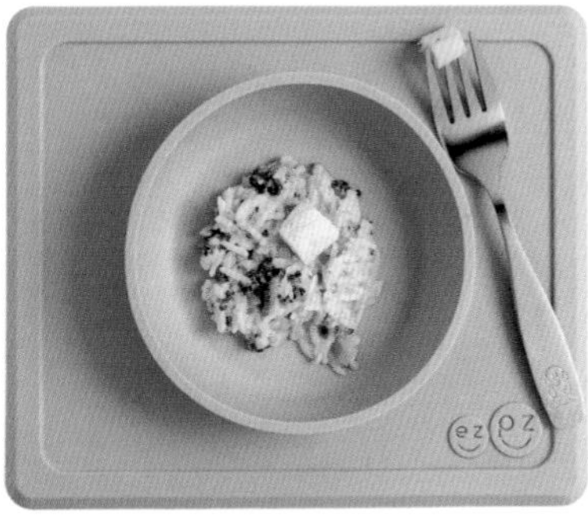

Chicken and Broccoli Rice Casserole, page 191

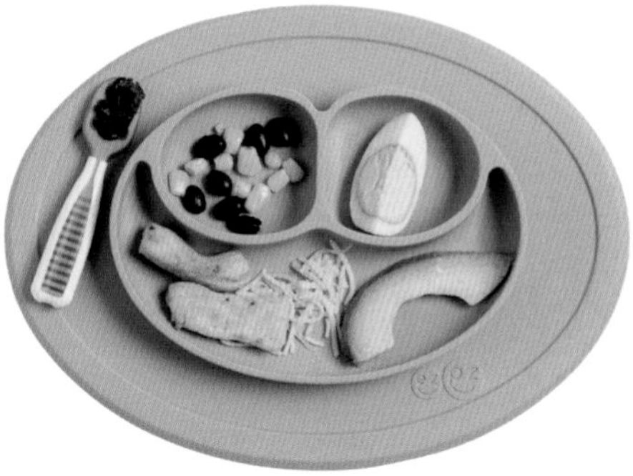

Chicken Cobb Salad with Cilantro-Lime Dressing, page 221

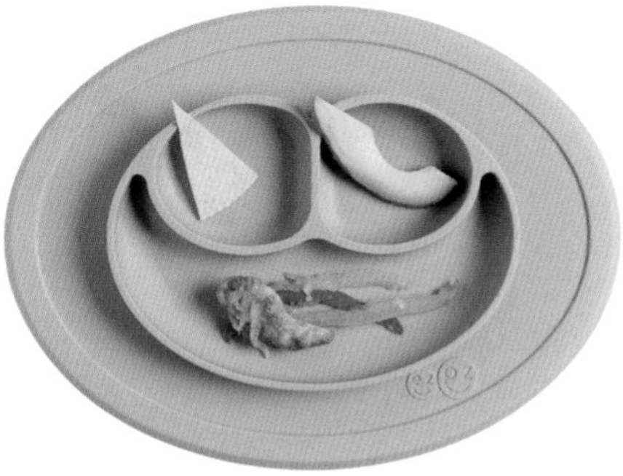

Chicken Fajita Casserole, page 156

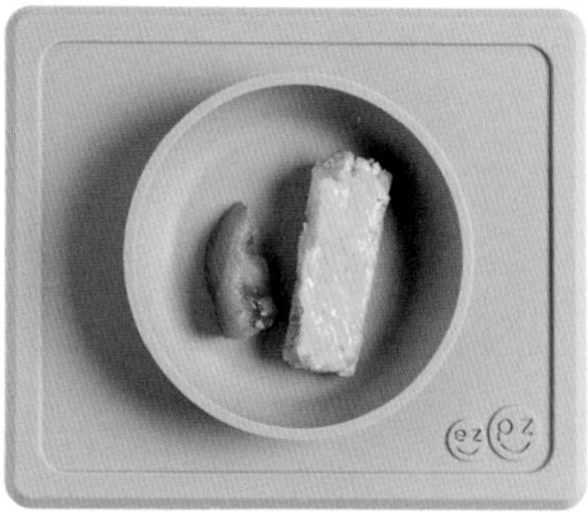

Chickpea "Tuna" Melts, page 90

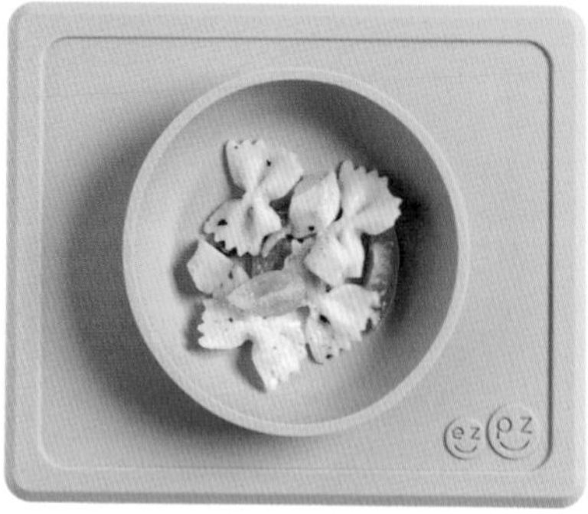

Creamy BLAT Pasta Salad with Bowties, page 83

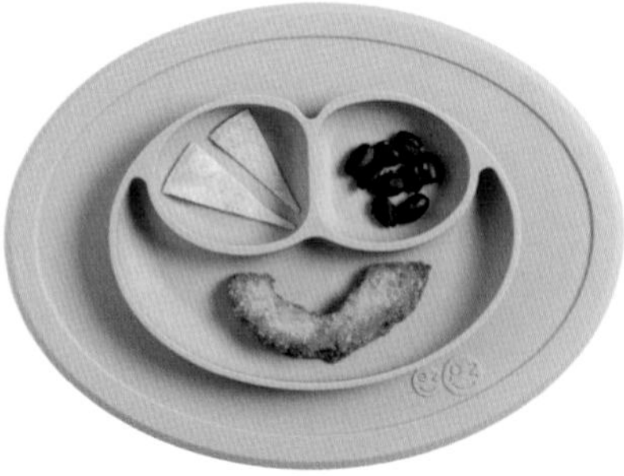

Crispy Avocado and Black Bean Tacos with Chipotle Crema, page 243

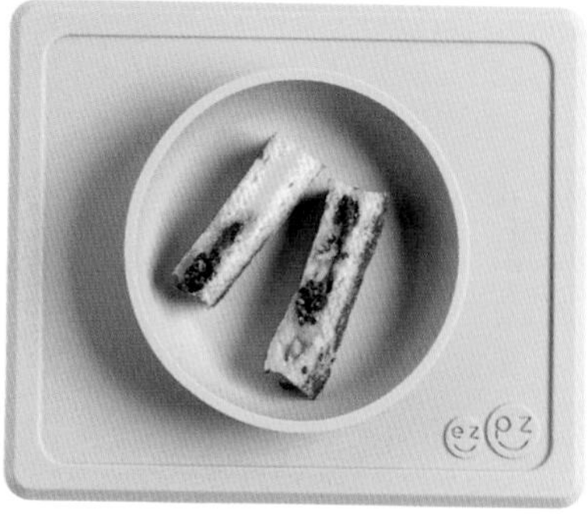

Crunchy Oven-Baked Grilled Cheese with Broccoli, page 125

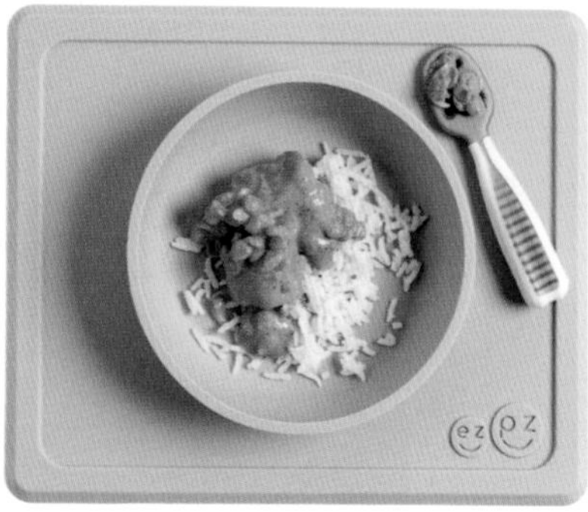

Curried Lentils and Carrots with Rice, page 256

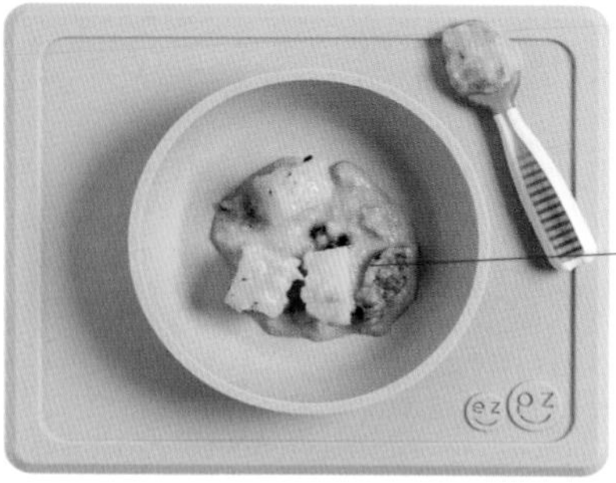

Dairy-Free Creamy Potato and Sausage Soup, page 108

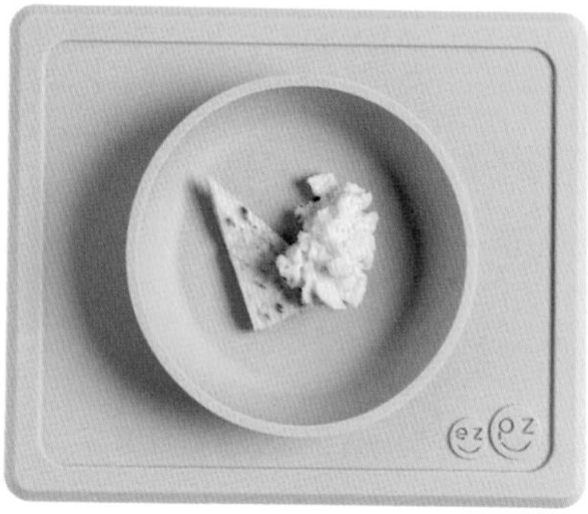

Egg Salad Pitas with Carrots, page 82

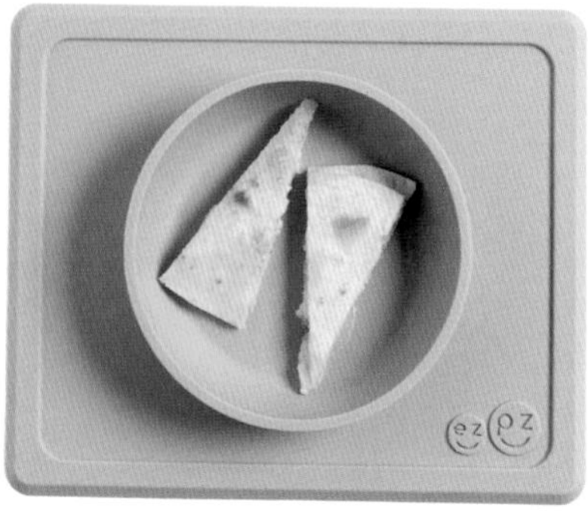

Egg-adilla with Pepper Confetti, page 42

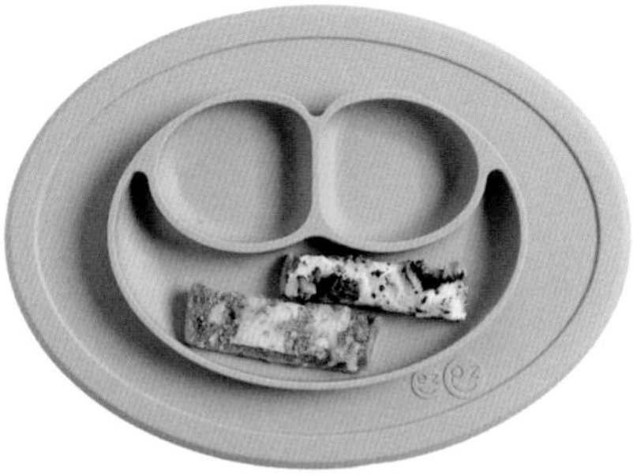

English Muffin Mini Pizzas, page 132

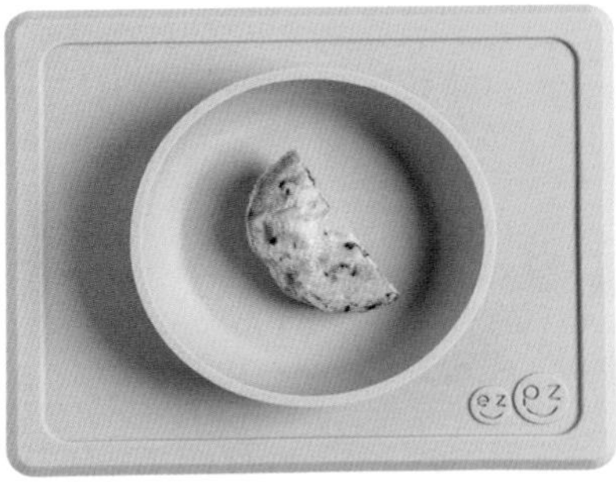

Everything Bagel Broccoli and Cheddar Egg Donuts, page 55

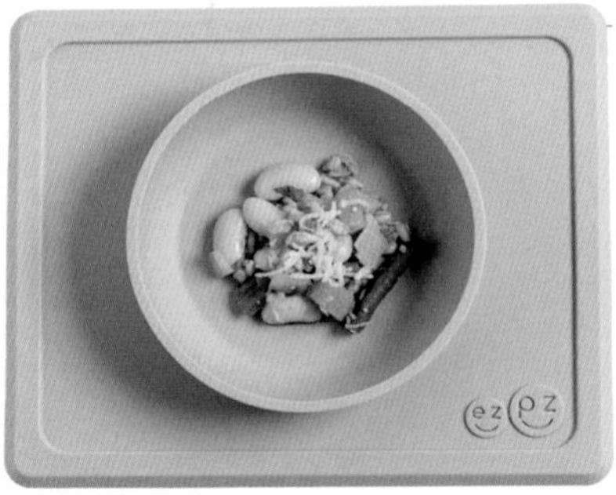

Farro Minestrone Soup, page 110

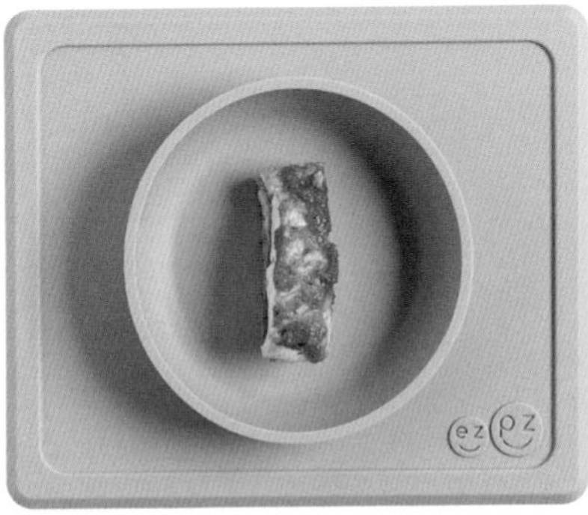

Felicia's Eggplant Parmesan in Stacks, page 101

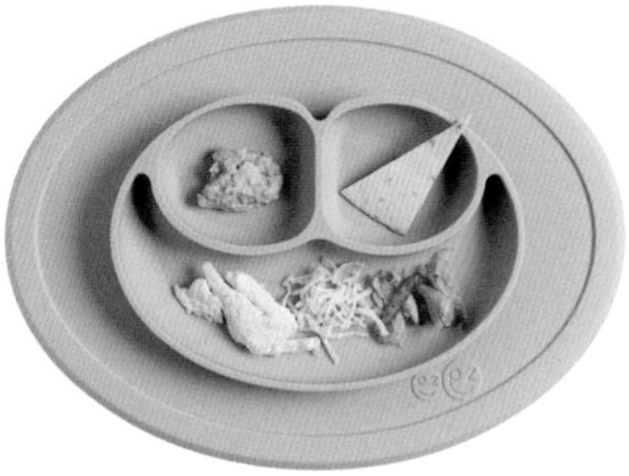

Freeze-Ahead Breakfast Burritos, page 198

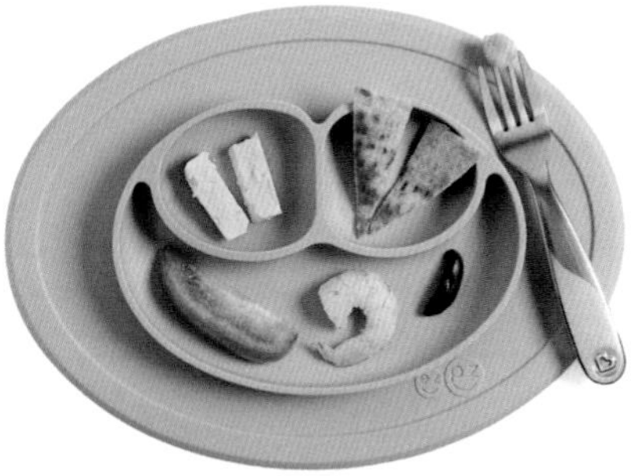

Greek-ish Salad with Lemony Shrimp and Pita, page 227

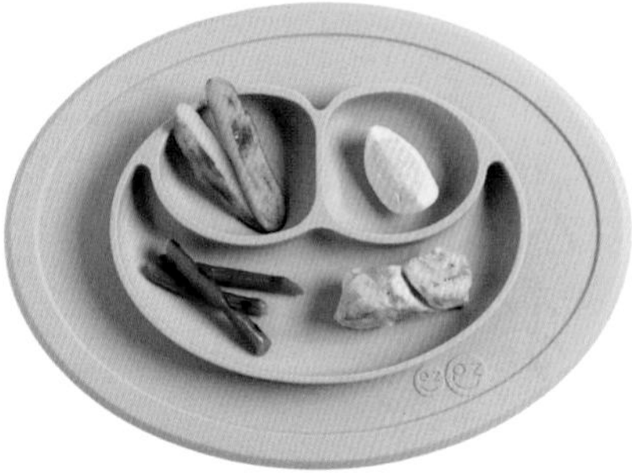

Grilled Salmon Niçoise Salad with Fingerlings, page 224

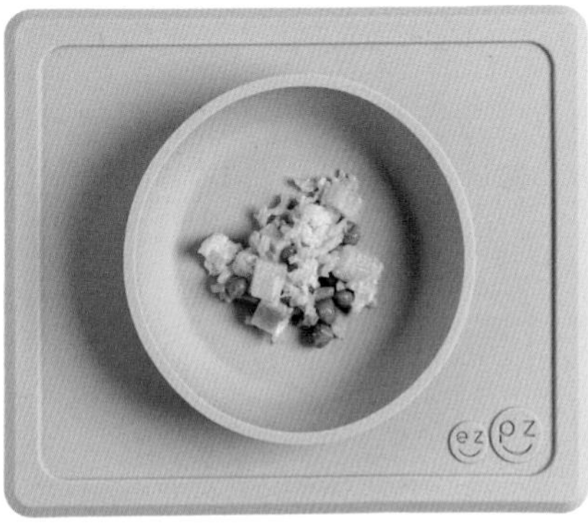

Hawaiian Fried Rice with Veggies, page 129

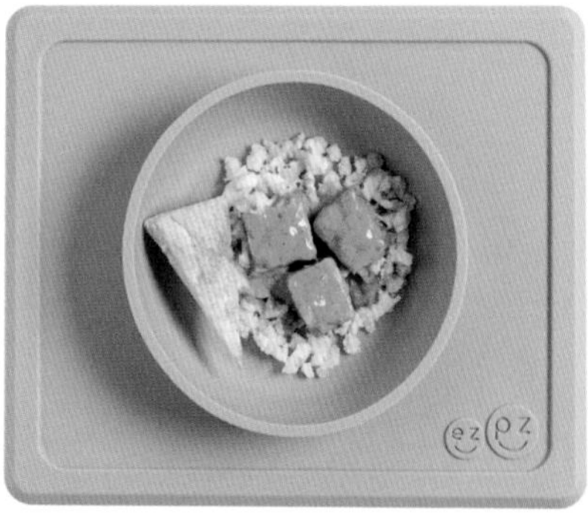

Indian Butter Tempeh with Cauliflower Rice, page 181

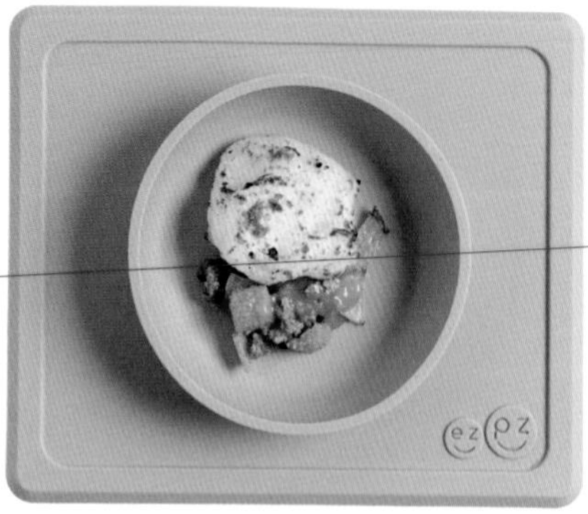

Judy's Shepherd's Pie, page 163

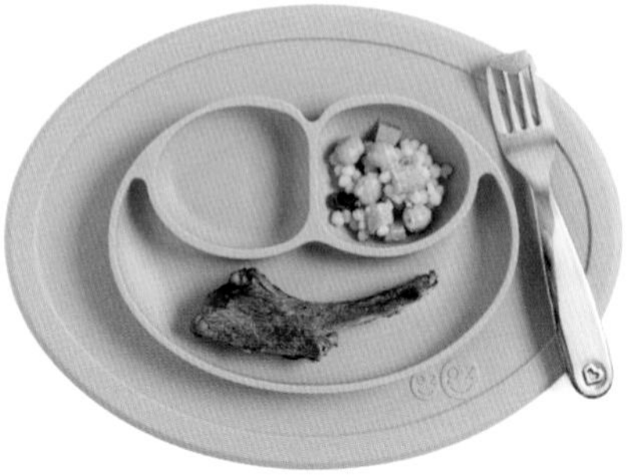

Lamb Chops with Curried Tahini Couscous and Chickpeas, page 88

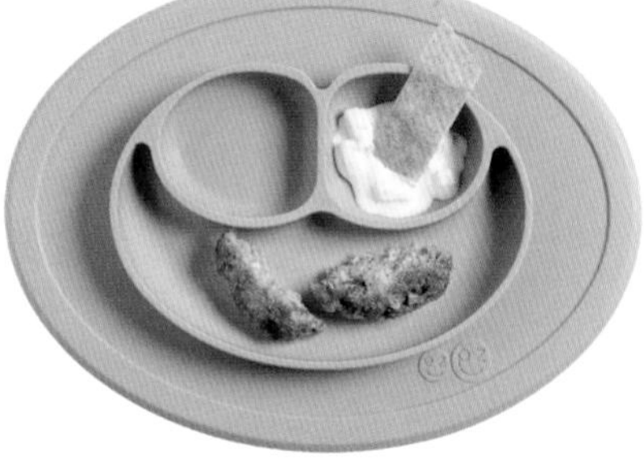

Lentil Gyro Wraps with Tzatziki and Avocado, page 215

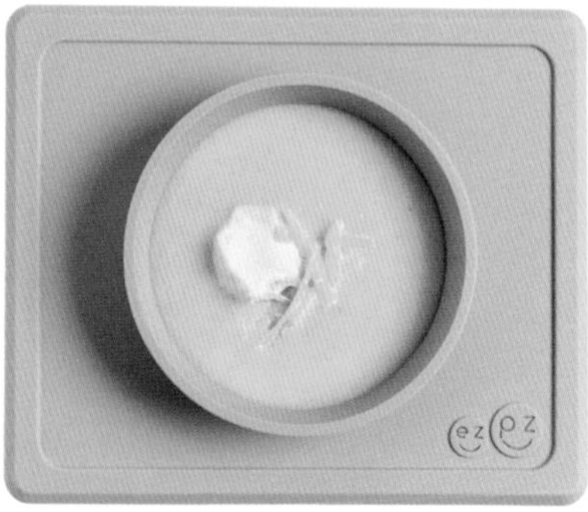

Loaded Baked Potato and Zucchini Soup, page 190

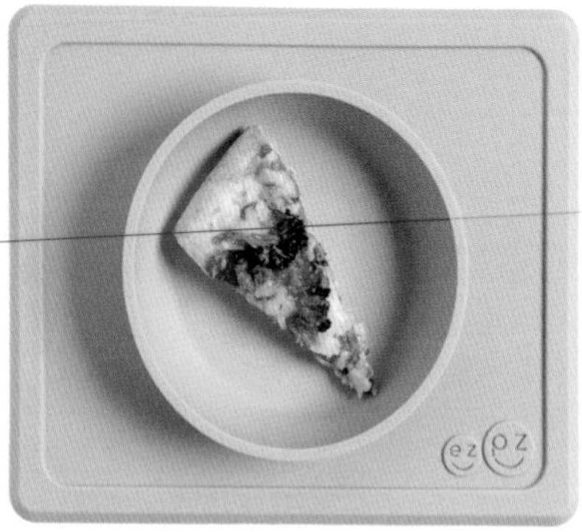

Mama's Trees and Sausage Pizza, page 209

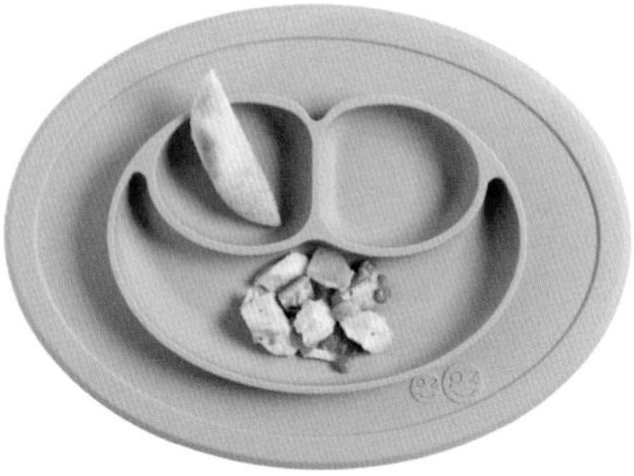

Mini Biscuit Turkey Potpies, page 203

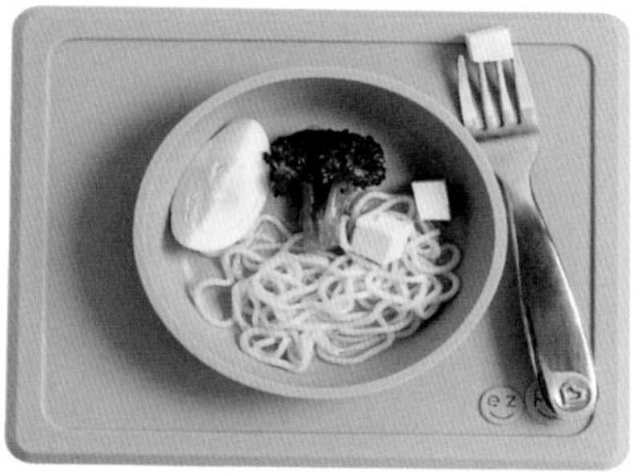

Miso Noodles with Tofu and Roasted Broccoli, page 105

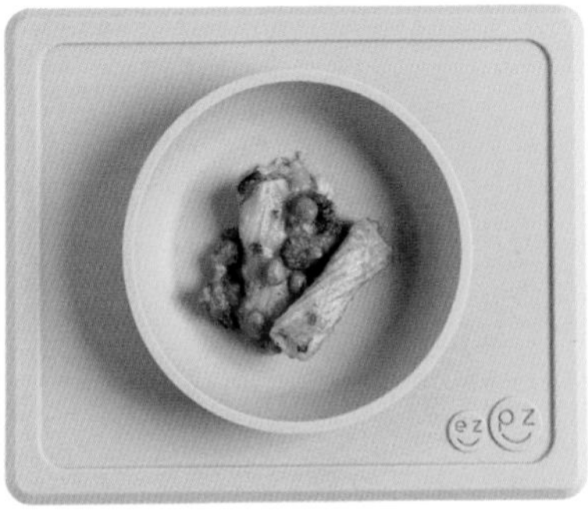

No-Boil Tomato, Pea, and Sausage Rigatoni, page 155

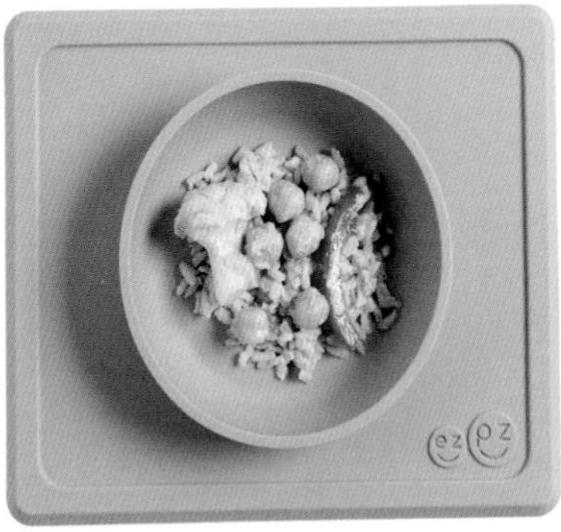

One Pot Cauliflower and Chickpea Coconut Curry, page 93

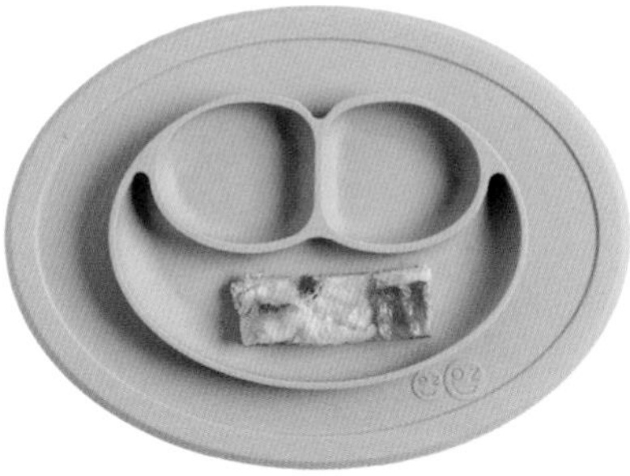

Overnight French Toast Casserole with Coconut Whipped Cream, page 52

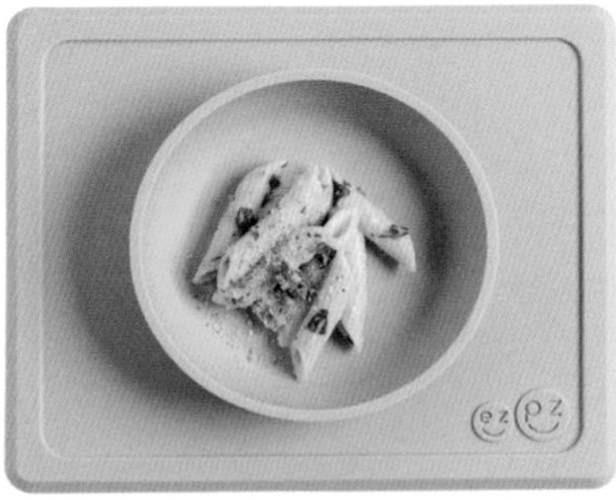

Penne with Chickpea Sauce and Spinach, page 131

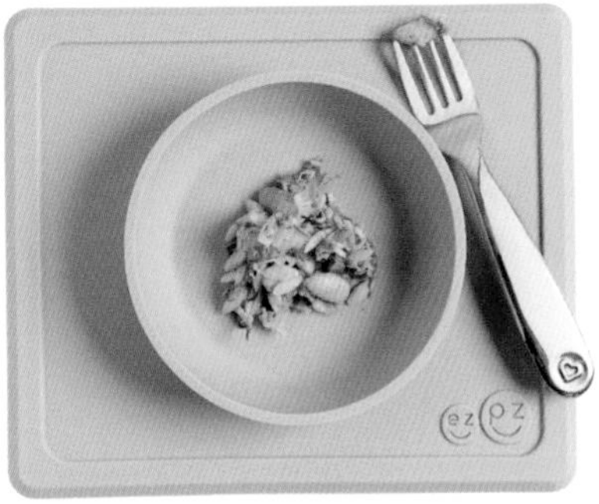

Pesto Orzo with Crispy Beans and Brussels Sprouts, page 80

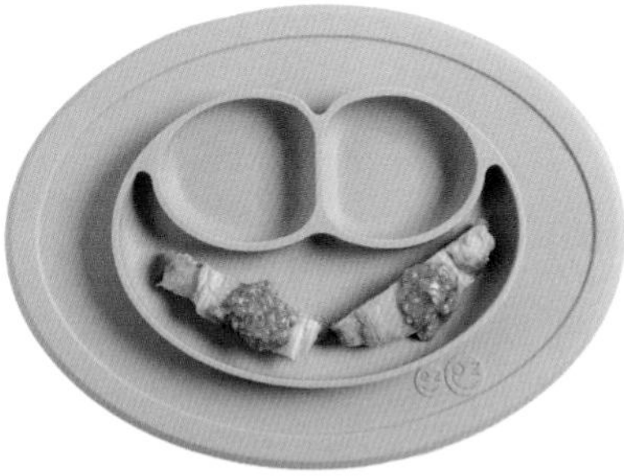

Pizza Rolls with Spinach, page 95

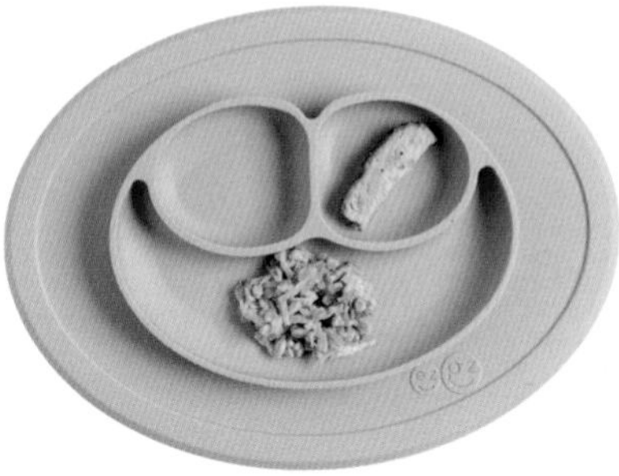

Pork Chops in Sun-Dried Tomato "Cream" Sauce, page 103

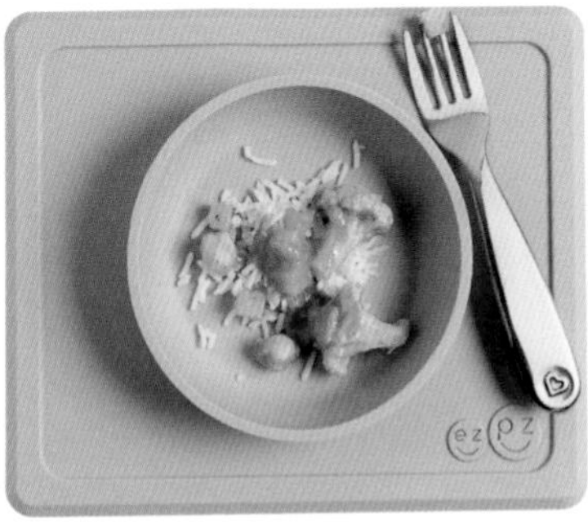

Pressure Cooker Aloo Gobi with Chickpeas, page 240

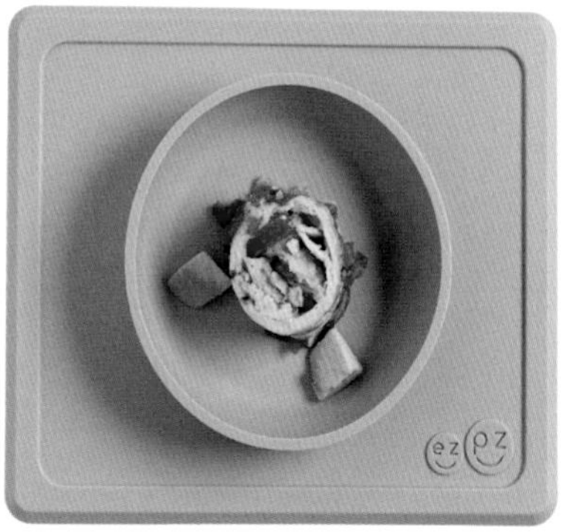

Pressure Cooker Chicken Salsa Kinda-chiladas, page 261

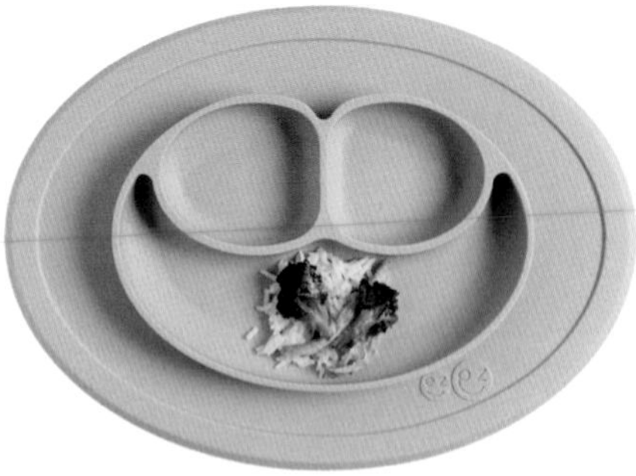

Pressure Cooker Chicken Teriyaki and Rice Bowls with Broccoli, page 245

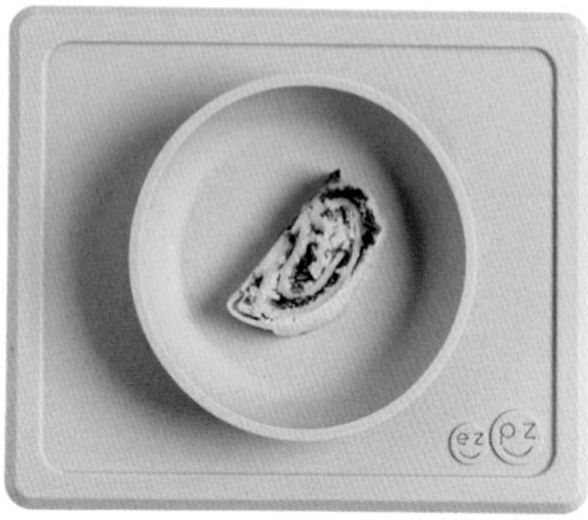

Pumpkin and Kale Lasagna Roll-Ups, page 165

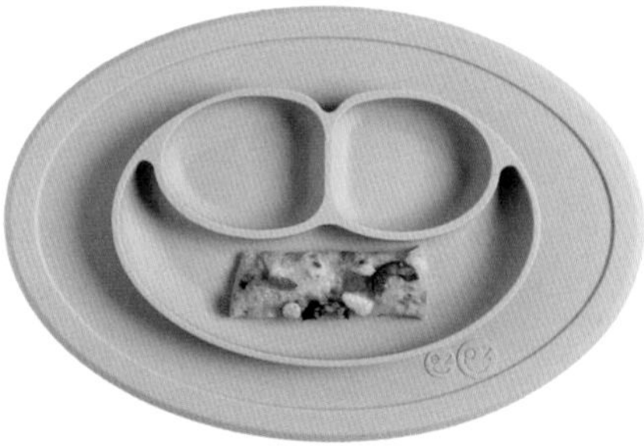

Refried Bean Flatbreads, page 214

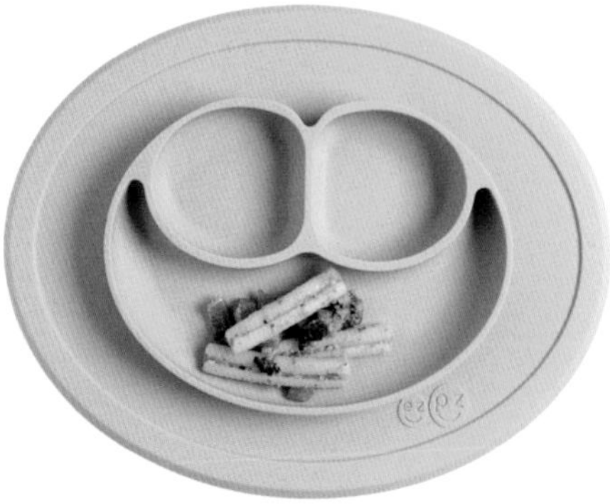

Roasted Vegetable Pasta with Pesto, page 98

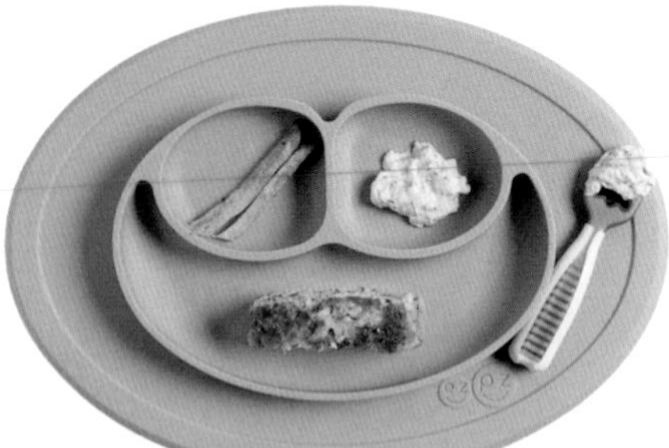

Salmon Cakes and Fries with Avocado Dill Aioli, page 193

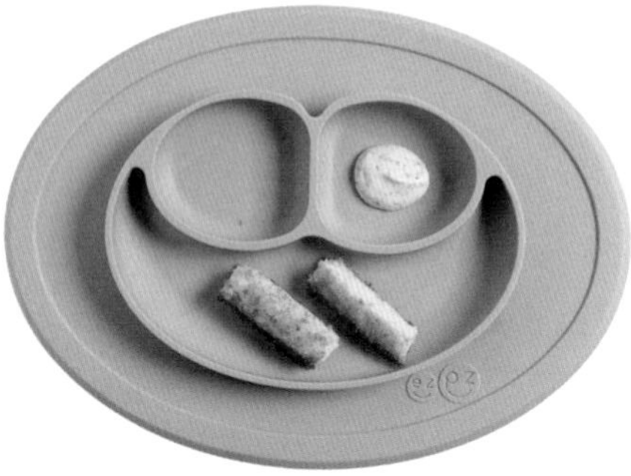

Salmon Fish Sticks with Mustard Sauce, page 266

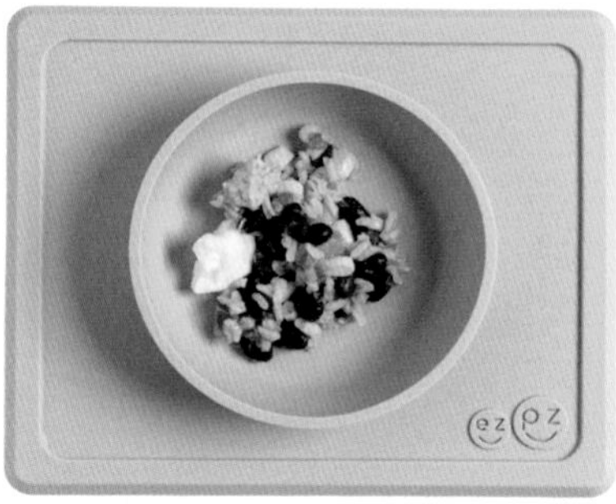

Secret Salsa Black Bean Burrito Bowls, page 130

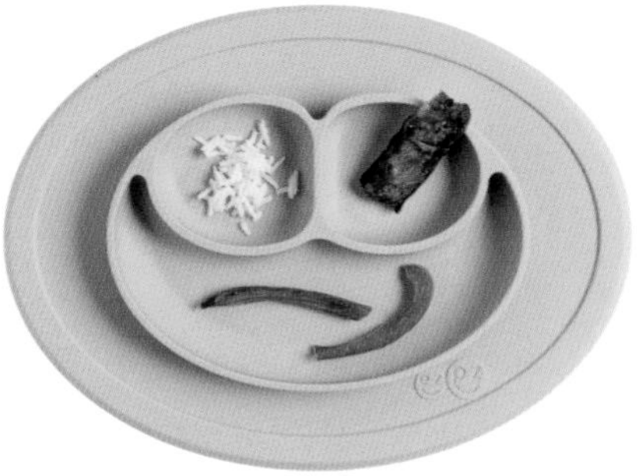

Sesame Ginger Steak, Pepper, and String Bean Stir-Fry, page 86

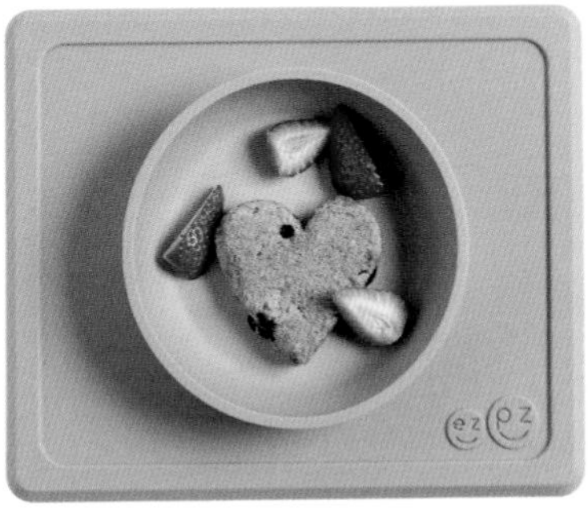

Sheet Pan Blueberry and Butternut Squash Pancakes, page 50

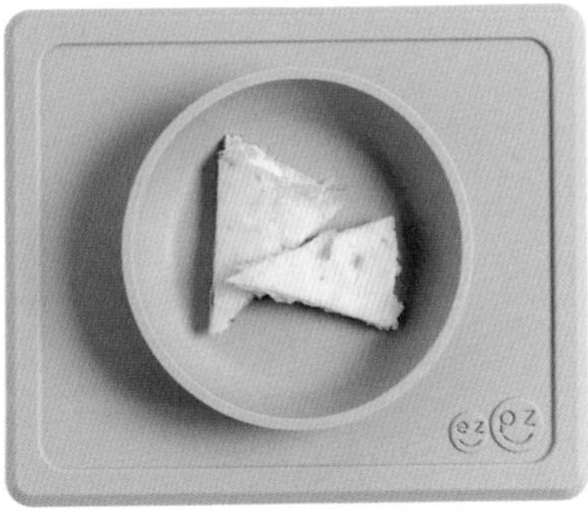

Sheet Pan Chicken and Veggie Quesadillas, page 146

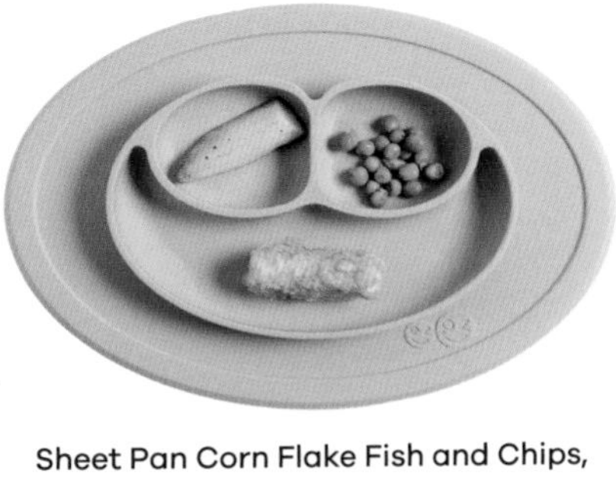

Sheet Pan Corn Flake Fish and Chips, page 141

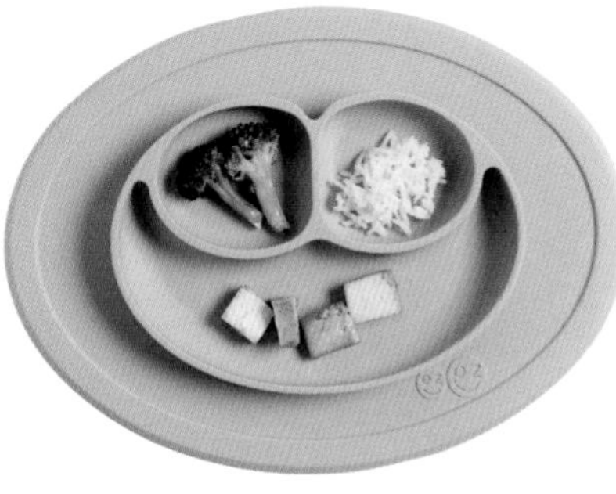

Sheet Pan Sesame Tofu and Broccoli Trees, page 167

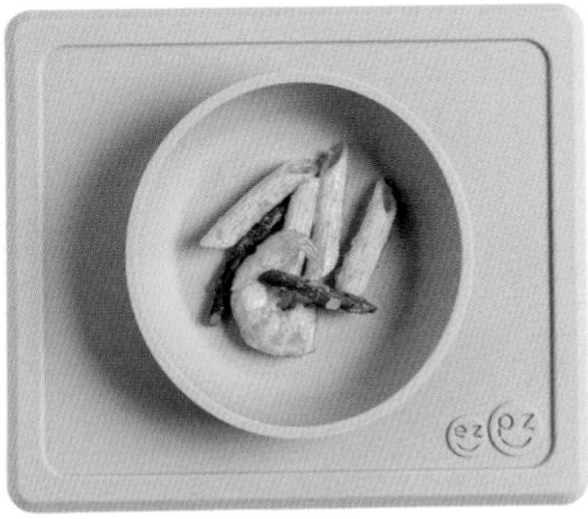

Shrimp and Asparagus in Red Pepper Sauce with Penne, page 172

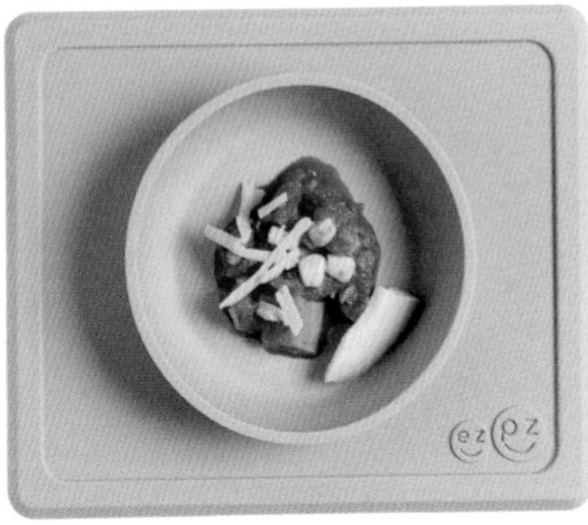

Slow Cooker Lentil Taco Soup, page 268

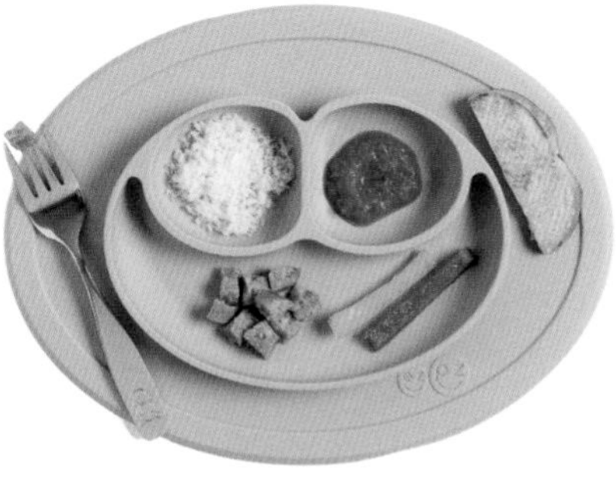

Slow Cooker Sausage and Pepper Hoagies, page 259

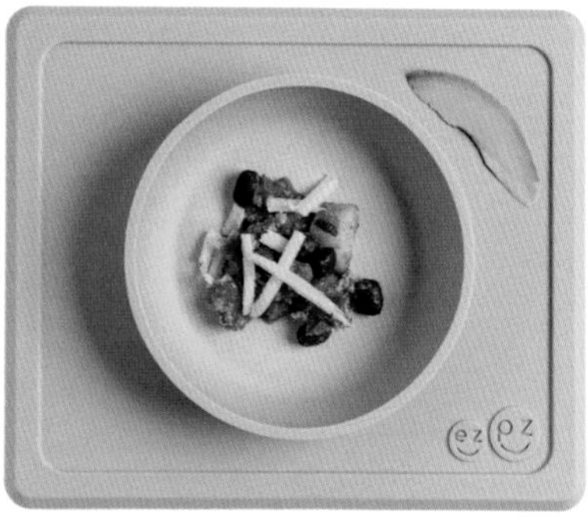

Slow Cooker Turkey and Butternut Squash Enchilada Chili, page 264

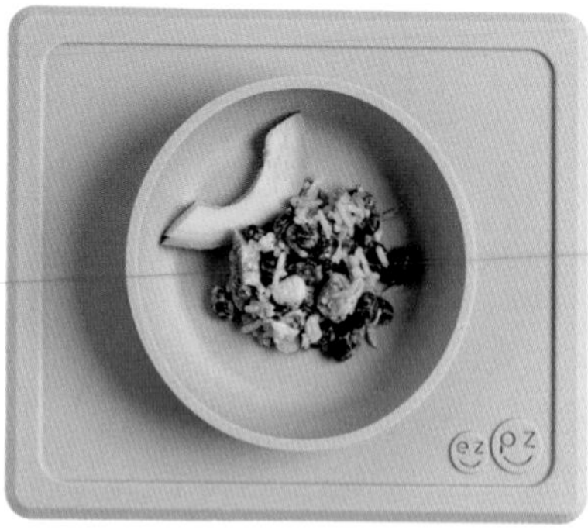

Southwestern Salsa Rice Bake with Chipotle Sauce, page 161

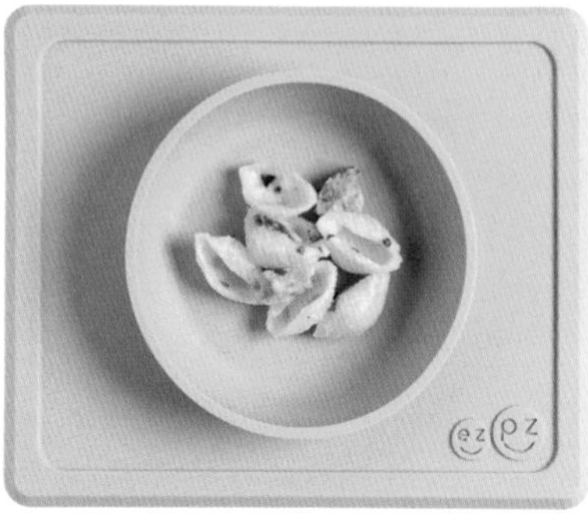

Spinach Alfredo Shells with Sausage, page 112

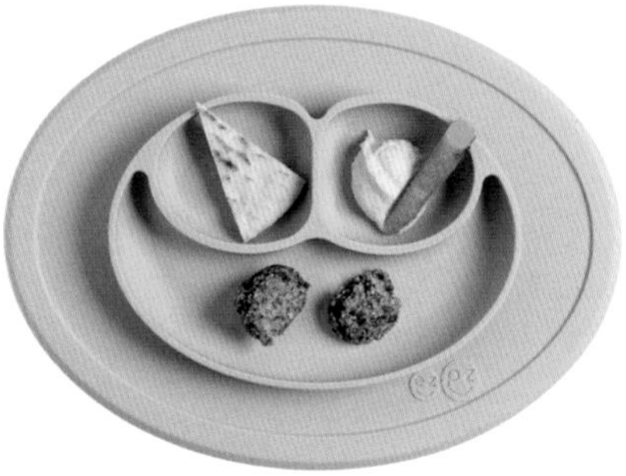

Spinach Falafel with Carrots and Hummus, page 186

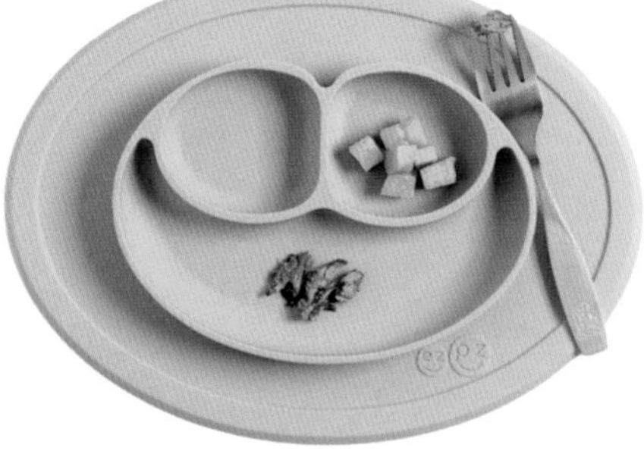

Steak Bites and Sweet Potatoes with Chimichurri, page 247

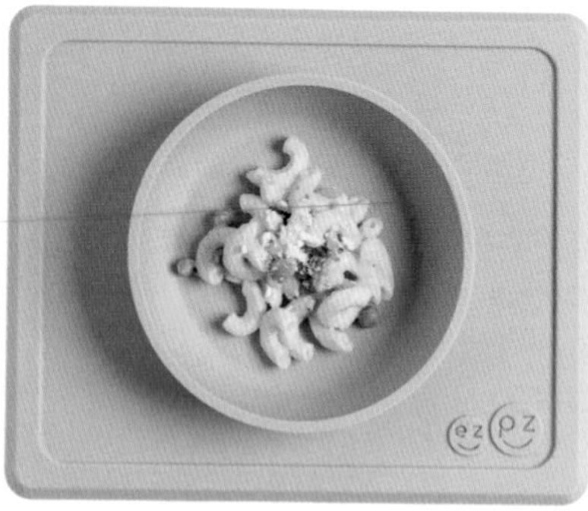

Stovetop Butternut Squash Mac and "Cheese," page 188

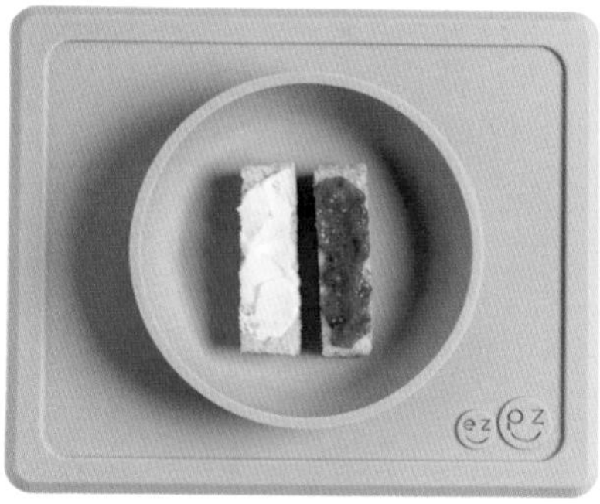

Strawberry Chia Jam and Cream Cheese Squares, page 128

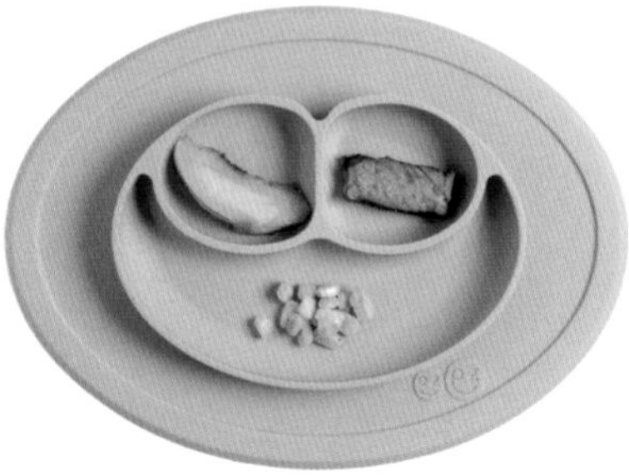

Summer Steak and Peach Salad with Greek Yogurt Balsamic, page 236

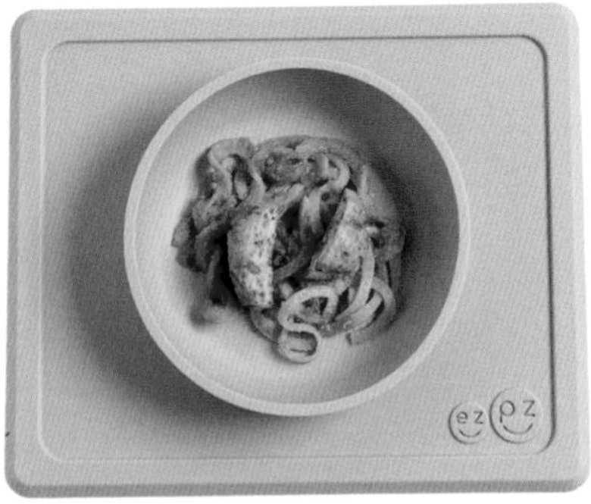

Sweet Potato Spaghetti with Chicken Meatballs, page 150

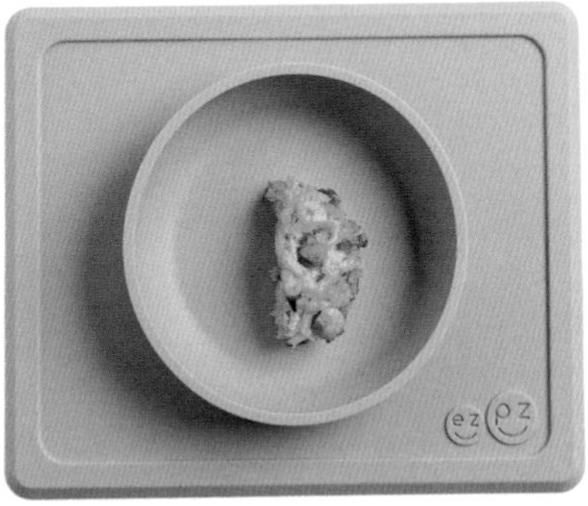

Sweet Potato, Ham, and Cheese Cups, page 126

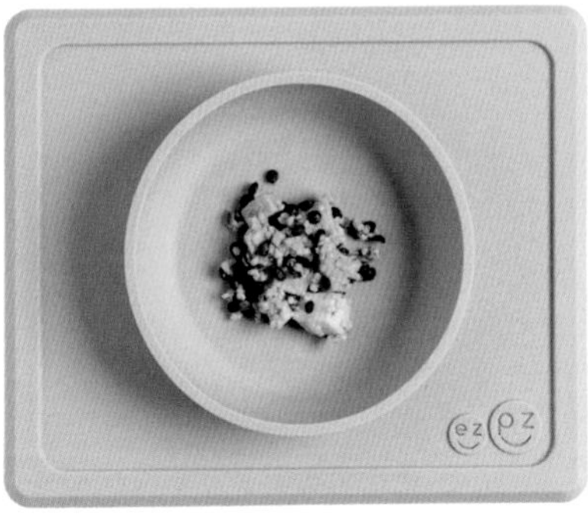

Sweet Potato, Quinoa, and Lentil Arugula Salad, page 232

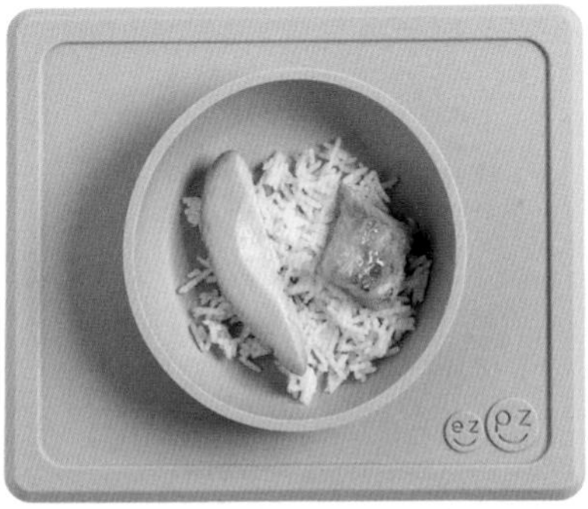

Teriyaki Salmon Bite Bowls, page 200

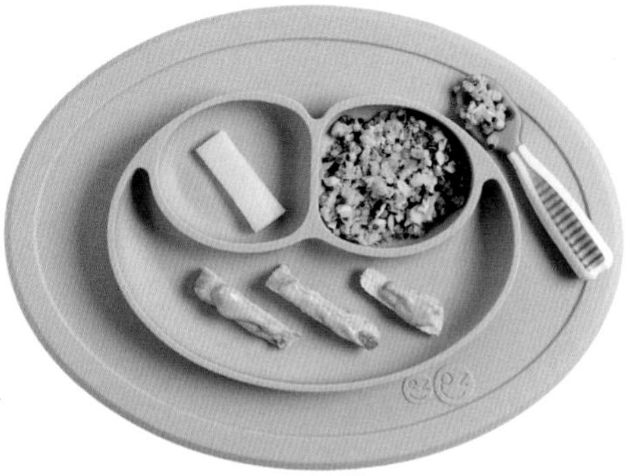

Thai Peanut Chicken Quinoa Bowls, page 250

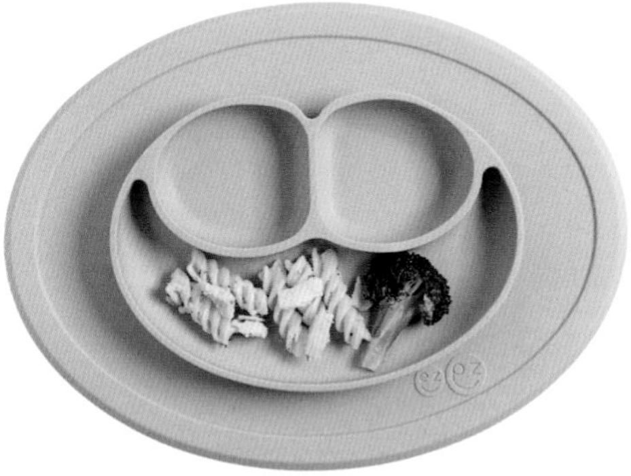

Tuna, Broccoli, and Kale Caesar Pasta Salad, page 230

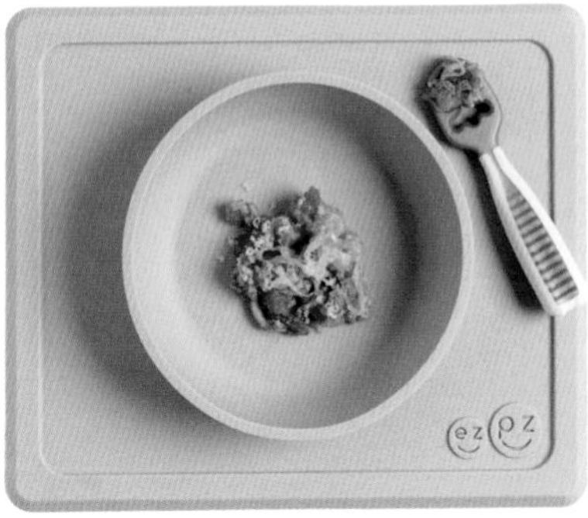

Turkey Bolognese with Spaghetti Squash, page 205

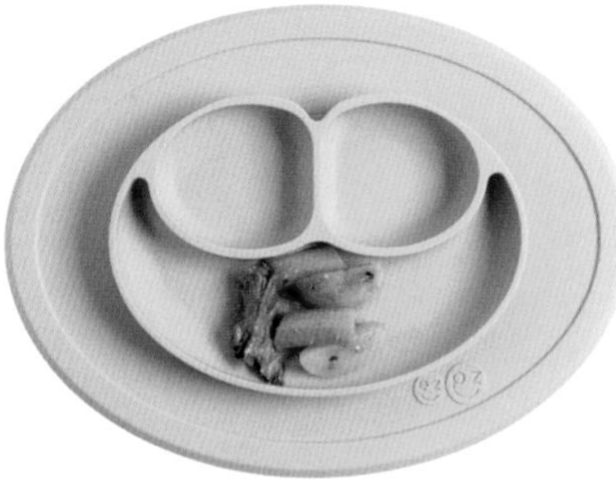

Tuscan-Style Short Ribs, page 272

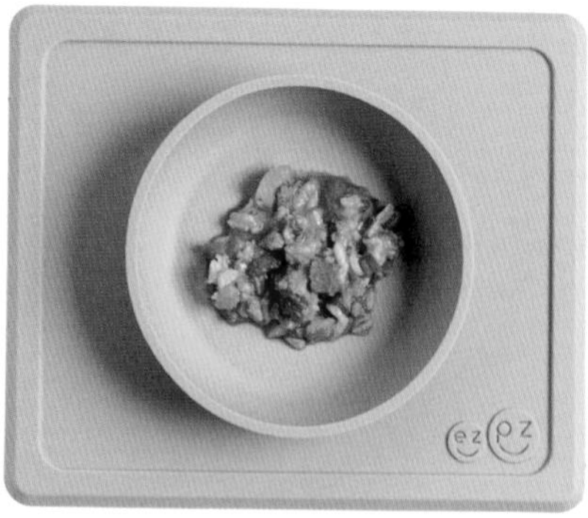

Unstuffed Turkey Pepper Skillet, page 270

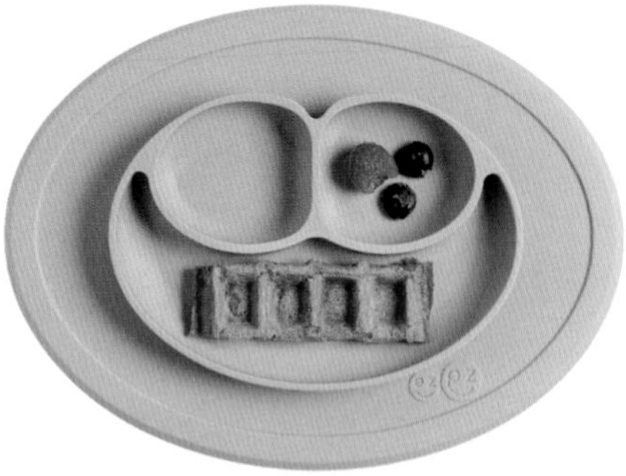

Vegan Pumpkin Waffles, page 49

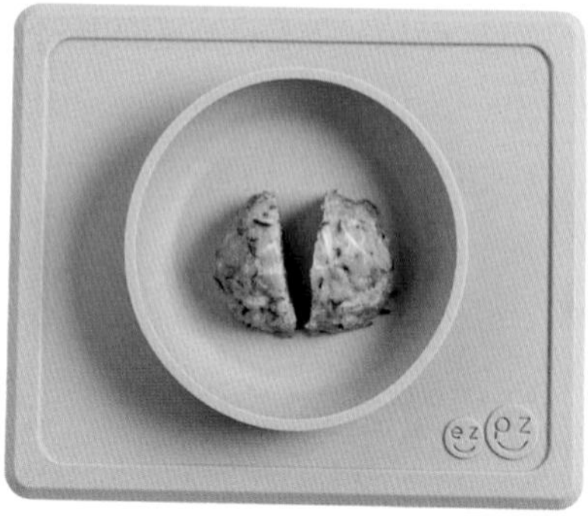

Veggie Bites Two Ways, page 123

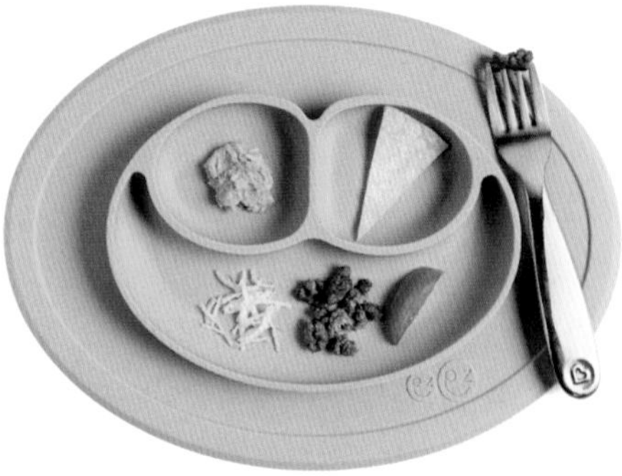

Weeknight Beef Tacos with Edamame Avocado Mash, page 184

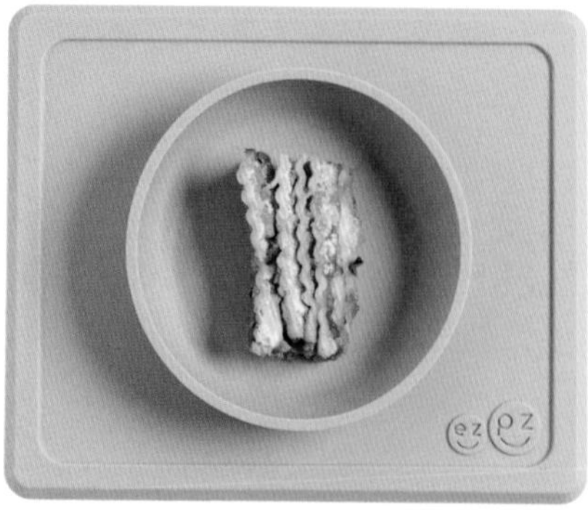

Zucchini and Quinoa Lasagna, page 149

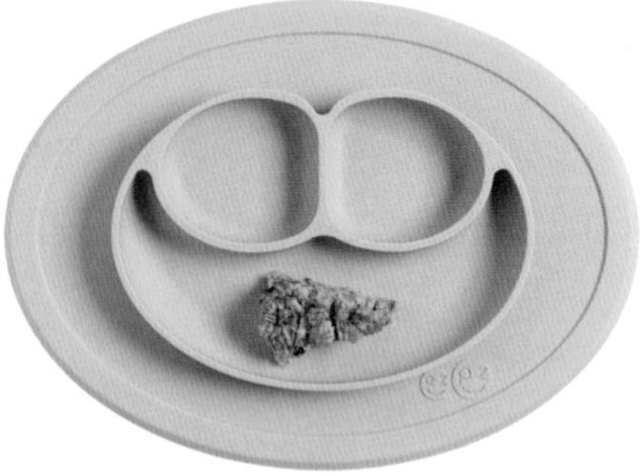

Zucchini Bread Oatmeal Bake, page 41

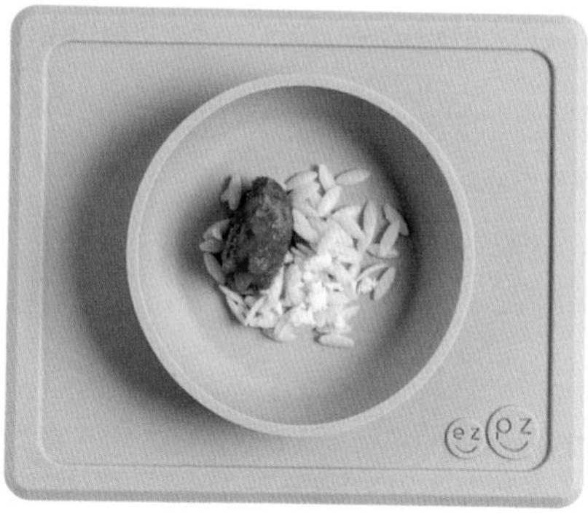

Zucchini Lamb Meatballs with Orzo and Feta, page 207

acknowledgments

While there is a very specific list of people who made this book happen logistically (which we gratefully appreciate below, as Megan, Judy, and Ali together), we also owe immense thanks to our families, who we'd like to take a moment to individually appreciate.

from ali

Needless to say, as I sit here and write my fourth cookbook, a lot of thanks need to be given. Without my Inspiralized community and team, my friends, my family, and everyone who supported or believed in Inspiralized along the way, this book you're holding wouldn't be possible. So let me start thanking, as I'm endlessly grateful and appreciative of everyone who has helped me do what I love: show people how to incorporate more vegetables into their meals in a tasty, creative way!

To Meaghan Prenda, we've been through a lot since 2015 when you started working with me for the launch of my first cookbook, and I'm so proud that we're coming out with our fourth. I say "we" because without you, I could never run Inspiralized and write these books. Thanks for running team Inspiralized, always.

Felicia, forever my "baby" sister, I am so grateful for all the time we got to spend together in 2020 and early 2021, a positive side effect of the COVID pandemic. We ate your eggplant Parmesan so much during that time, I had to memorialize it in this cookbook—thank you for the recipe, it'll always remind me of you! I'm so proud to be your sister and even prouder to be Brooks's aunt!

Mom and Dad, I love you, and thank you for letting me use your kitchen for two months to test over one hundred recipes—and for tasting the good and the bad (sorry for the bads, you're welcome for the goods!). Along with Lu, you'll always be my OG taste testers.

Speaking of, thank you to my husband, Lu, who keeps me laughing every day and inspired to create. I love you, and I'm so excited to cook through these recipes for you and our kids. May I always fill your plate—and cup!

And to my kids, Luca, Roma, Rio, and Sol—as I wrote in my third cookbook to Luca, "everything from this point on is for you," and that is now true for all four of you. The best gift in life has been you, and I'm so proud to be your mama. I can't wait for all of us to sit at the table and eat these recipes together!

from megan and judy

First and foremost, thank you to Ali for allowing us to coauthor a book! A *real* book! This has been a dream come true for us, and we could not have done it without your vision, flexibility, creativity, and amazing cooking skills. We are and have always been in awe of you.

Thank you to our mentors for inspiring us to go big, do more, think differently. Specifically, thanks to Elyse Resch and Evelyn Tribole, coauthors of *Intuitive Eating*, for changing our lives and how we think about food. We will be forever grateful for your work.

Behind our courses, content, and everything we create at Feeding Littles is an amazing group of women who work hard every day. To our team—we are so lucky to know you. Thank you for the support you give to parents across the world every day and for helping us do the work we love. We literally could not do this without you.

To Sarah and Chris, baby Jack's parents... losing your son was the most devastating experience of your lives. And yet, you have managed to turn it into something meaningful, something beautiful. Thank you for introducing us to one another many years ago. Because of you, millions of families worldwide can find more happiness, connection, and fun at the dinner table. Jack's influence will live on for generations. We are honored to be a part of his legacy.

from megan

I am blessed to have some really supportive friends, who have watched Feeding Littles grow from a singular Facebook group to the brand it is today. Thank you for being my sounding board and support system throughout this entire process. You know who you are... and you are greatly appreciated!

It takes most people a long time to find their passion, but I knew I wanted to be a dietitian in high school. Thank you to my parents and sister for always supporting my journey, no matter how challenging it was. You believed in me, even when I didn't always believe in myself. I can't wait to share these recipes with you!

To my husband and fellow entrepreneur, Greg, I have so much love and respect for you. You inspire me to be better every day. You lead by example, and our kids are blessed to have you as their dad.

Speaking of kids... to Hannah and Mia, you are why I do this work. My entire world changed when you were born, and I feel inspired to help other parents because I know how much they love and want to protect their kids. It's the same way I feel about you. I look forward to cooking and enjoying these recipes together, and perhaps one day you'll share your favorites with your families, too.

Lastly, to Judy. What a crazy ride this has been! Thank you for being the most perfect partner for me. You have allowed me to grow in ways I never thought possible. I am so lucky to call you my colleague and friend.

from judy

First, I want to thank the babies, toddlers, and kids over the last thirty-nine years who have taught me about feeding, allowed me to be a part of their lives, and showed me what it feels like to struggle with eating. To the parents, family members, caregivers, and teachers who have given me their trust and confidence along the road and know that we are in this together. I celebrate you every day!

To my OT mentors along the way, A. Jean Ayres, Audrey Yasukawa, Robin Glass, and Lynn S. Wolf, and to the babies and Grandmother Rocking Chair program that I started at Children's Haven on the South Side of Chicago back in the 1970s, where I knew I had found my niche in feeding.

My deepest appreciation and love to Louie, who has always believed in me! And our two children, Prescott and Elise, who taught me about feeding my own children with patience, joy, and laughter.

And to my business partner, Megan, holy guacamole! Who knew that our initial three-hour phone call could ever take us to this point! Thank you for your creativity, entrepreneurial spirit, and strong influence on my life. You are the best business partner I could have ever asked for and I am lucky to call you my friend.

from ali, megan, and judy

To the Avery publishing team, thank you for believing in the concept of this book and bringing it to life. Nina Shield, you have been kind and receptive throughout this entire process, and although you gave us creative freedoms, you also cleverly guided us when we needed it and helped us write the best cookbook for families ever written! To Lorie Pagnozzi and the designers who labored over the cover concepts with us, we appreciate your patience and commitment. We are so proud to be on the Avery author list!

To Alyssa Reuben, thank you for making it possible for all of us to seamlessly come together and write a cookbook that's much needed in the family space. With three Inspiralized cookbooks under your belt, we're humbled to add another one, this time with the Feeding Littles powerhouse—and hopefully many more to come!

To the photography team, we can't stop staring at this book; you so perfectly captured our recipes, you can practically smell them off the page. Along with prop extraordinaire Carla Gonzalez-Hart and food stylist phenom Hadas Smirnoff, photographer Evan Sung masterfully made family-friendly food look simultaneously approachable and elegant. Carla, we're still in awe of how you incorporated adult sophistication and whimsical childhood innocence into each photo. Hadas, we couldn't have cooked the food better ourselves—no, really, you made our food shine while keeping us company and laughing. And Evan, your skills can't be complimented enough, but your photos aren't all that sets you apart from the rest—it's your commitment to capturing our vision for each photo (a.k.a. reading our minds), your patience, and your kind demeanor and sensibility. You've captured all of the Inspiralized books, and now we're excited to keep the tradition going with the Feeding Littles brand now included.

To our recipe testers, you had the most important job: making sure these recipes worked! Without you, this cookbook wouldn't have the good bones it does (tried-and-true recipes fit for the whole family!). We hope you had some great meals while testing, and sorry for the ones that didn't work out—they've been fixed, we promise! Thanks Laura, Karen, Brooke, Jamie, Samantha, Hillary, and Meaghan.

To our baby models (Arin, Cora, Remi, and Evie) and their families, thank you for your willingness to participate in this project. Your babies' precious faces fill this book with so much more love and energy and are a reminder of why we do what we do: to be a part of your family's first food memories (what a privilege!).

To everyone who follows Feeding Littles and Inspiralized, it is because of you that we are able to help bring families together at the table. Without you sharing our brands with your dear friends and family, tagging us when you make our recipes or on your Messy Mondays, we wouldn't be where we are today. We wrote this cookbook for you and with you in mind; you've helped us feed so many families and get through so many seasons of life. Thank you for being there for us every step of the way, and we are so humbled for this cookbook to have a place on your shelves.

index

Note: Page numbers in *italics* refer to images in visual index or starter guide.

C

D

E

M

N

Q

R

S